W9-BWD-070

WITHDRAWN

Social and Behavioral Foundations of Public Health

For A.B. and Juanita Coreil, Jim Lindenberger, and Matthew, Kara, and Gabriela Henderson

Social and Behavioral Foundations of Public Health

Jeannine Coreil · Carol A. Bryant · J. Neil Henderson

With contributions from Melinda S. Forthofer and Gwendolyn P. Quinn

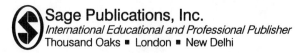

Sage Publications, Inc.
International Educational and Professional Publisher
Thousand Oaks ▪ London ▪ New Delhi

147949

Copyright © 2001 by Sage Publications, Inc.

All rights reserved. No part of this book may be reproduced or utilized in any form or by any means, electronic or mechanical, including photocopying, recording, or by any information storage and retrieval system, without permission in writing from the publisher.

For information:

Sage Publications, Inc.
2455 Teller Road
Thousand Oaks, California 91320
E-mail: order@sagepub.com

Sage Publications Ltd.
6 Bonhill Street
London EC2A 4PU
United Kingdom

Sage Publications India Pvt. Ltd.
M-32 Market
Greater Kailash I
New Delhi 110 048 India

Printed in the United States of America

Library of Congress Cataloging-in-Publication Data

Coreil, Jeannine.
  Social and behavioral foundations of public health / by Jeannine
Coreil, Carol A. Bryant, J. Neil Henderson; with contributions from
Melinda S. Forthofer and Gwendolyn P. Quinn.
      p. cm.
  Includes bibliographical references and index.
    ISBN 0-7619-1744-6 (cloth: alk. paper)
    1. Public health—Social aspects. 2. Public health—Psychological
aspects. 3. Social medicine. I. Bryant, Carol A. II. Henderson, J.
Neil. III. Forthofer, Melinda S. IV. Quinn, Gwendolyn P. V. Title.
    RA418 .C673 2000
    362.1—dc21   00-0095190

01   02   03   04   05   8   7   6   5   4   3   2   1

Acquiring Editor:	Rolf Janke
Editorial Assistant:	Heidi Van Middlesworth
Production Editor:	Diana E. Axelsen
Editorial Assistant:	Candice Crosetti
Typesetter/Designer:	Barbara Burkholder
Indexer:	Jeanne Busemeyer
Cover Designer:	Ravi Balasuriya

Contents

Preface

This book is a collaborative effort of a group of professors who have shared responsibility for teaching social and behavioral sciences to public health students for the past 13 years. Increasingly dissatisfied with the lack of an introductory text that applies social science to *public health* as opposed to medicine, nursing, or general health sciences, we felt the need to fill this gap with a primer that encompasses the broad range of topics and issues in this multidisciplinary field. More narrowly focused volumes have been published that cover the interface of psychology, sociology, or anthropology with public health, but, with the exception of Angrosino's (1987) *A Health Practitioner's Guide to the Social and Behavioral Sciences*, no integrated volumes have been available. We hope this text fills this niche in a dynamic and growing field of research and practice in public health.

There are three main audiences intended for the book. The first is graduate students and upper-level undergraduate students enrolled in public health courses or other health science courses that share a focus on the behavioral, societal, and cultural bases of health. Some medical anthropology, medical sociology, and health psychology courses would fit in this category. The second audience is made up of sociobehavioral researchers, whose scholarly work relates to community health broadly defined. For them, the book can serve as a useful reference volume. Third, a wide range of practicing health professionals will find the book a valuable guide in applying behavioral science concepts and perspectives to real-world problems. The examples and case studies that illustrate various approaches throughout the volume were specifically selected to provide useful information that practitioners can readily apply in their work.

Although the field of social factors in public health is a relatively new domain compared to the more developed areas of epidemiology, environmental health, and health policy, its roots extend far back into history. If one considers public health in the broadest sense of knowledge about the health of populations and organized efforts to protect community health, then social aspects of public health have existed for a very long time. Concerns for the regulation of behavior and care for vulnerable populations were present in the earliest human settlements. The rituals and taboos of even the most "primitive" human societies incorporate social and behavioral factors in health. Prohibitions on immoral behavior, dietary restrictions, ceremonial resolution of social conflict, appeasement of willful spirits, isolation of the sick, and other organized actions reflect the efforts of ancient societies to protect the well-being of their members. The early Hebrew civilization placed strong emphasis on public health and sanitation, as codified in practices described in the Pentateuch and Talmud. Between the 15th and 12th centuries B.C., the Greeks followed the preventive philosophy of the goddess Hygeia, whose legends taught the importance of protecting the health of the human mind and body. Hippocratic writings from the fifth century B.C. stressed the importance of environmental forces in disease causation, including climate, diet, and occupation. Roman medicine also had important public health components, including systems of sanitation, sewage, and water supply, and social welfare elements were reflected in the assignment of physicians to tend the poor, hospitalized persons, and the armed forces. Between the fall of Rome in the fifth century A.D. and the Renaissance in the 15th century, Islamic medicine flourished, including the establishment of social services for the poor, women, and children.

During the Middle Ages, efforts to fight infectious diseases, particularly the bubonic plague and other epidemics, shaped the development of formal public health activities. In response to epidemics, the practice of quarantine was established as a way of protecting the health of citizens. Among the various theories that surfaced to explain the plague, such as miasmas, vapors, and punishment for sin, scapegoating of social groups occurred, including accusations that Jews had poisoned wells and that nobles, cripples, and physicians helped spread the malady. During the 16th through 18th centuries, new sociopolitical and economic beliefs arose that justified and supported the power of nation-states. An ideology of promoting the health of the populace to supply labor in support of state wealth gained acceptance. New methods of enumeration and surveillance advanced the quantitative study of social conditions as a fundamental public health practice.

The 19th century witnessed the rapid development of organized public health activities, as the focus shifted to the problems associated with industrialization and urbanization. Recognition of the role of poor working and living conditions gave birth to the sanitary movement, led by reformers in Britain, France, Germany, and the United States. The first public health departments were established in the latter part of the century. Efforts were directed at improving diet, housing, sanitation, factory conditions, and other lifestyle factors. A strong sense of humanitarianism characterized the emerging field of public health. The rise of bacteriology and the germ theory of disease in the early part of the 20th century led to new methods of disease prevention, including mass immunization programs and the application of technology to infection control.

The scope of public health knowledge and practice broadened immensely during the 20th century, as diverse disciplines were integrated into the fold. Programs for special populations such as mothers, infants, and schoolchildren were established. Since 1950, enormous growth has occurred in the application of social and behavioral sciences within public health. Subfields such as public mental health, health promotion, social epidemiology, community health education, and public health social work represent but a few of the many areas within public health that emphasize the influence of social factors in health. The range of topics subsumed in this area is now quite broad, as reflected in the chapters of this volume. Recognition of the importance of social and behavioral factors is reflected in current standards for training public health students. Accredited schools of public health are required to offer programs in social and behavioral sciences.

Like public health generally, the social and behavioral sciences subfield covers a disparate array of disciplines, problems, issues, and approaches. Professionals from very different backgrounds contribute to the literature, infusing their work with distinctive perspectives, worldviews, and occupational cultures. Consequently, no consensus exists regarding the use of concepts, theoretical frameworks, or methodologic approaches or the application of research findings to real-life problems. Different researchers often use the same concepts to mean quite different things. This poses a challenge to writers such as ourselves who attempt to describe the field in a coherent and unifying manner for the sake of readers.

Although presenting the subject matter through a common lens runs the risk of oversimplifying the content and misrepresenting reality, too little reframing tends to give the impression of a hodge-podge of disconnected topics. Our aim is a middle ground here, where we attempt to weave common themes throughout the chapters yet note important contrasts in approaches and terminology. In Chapters 1 and 3, we introduce unifying conceptual frameworks that are integrated into discussions of particular topics in later chapters. Three overarching frameworks serve this purpose: the Social Ecology of Health Model, the Health Impact Model (Chapter 1), and the Causality Continuum (Chapter 3). These frameworks reflect the central themes of the book, which are the analysis of public health problems within a systems perspective; the importance of understanding sociocultural context; and the complex, multifactorial genesis of health problems.

Although a contextualized, ecological systems approach to public health is hardly new (Last, 1998), ours attempts to go beyond the "risk factor" approach to social and behavioral analysis that has dominated the field in recent decades.

Studies that identify significant predictor variables for health outcomes clearly make valuable contributions to public health knowledge and practice. However, our social ecological approach builds on this type of analysis by seeking an in-depth understanding of sociocultural context, one that amplifies multiple contextual domains through the development and linking of social science concepts. Comparable to the "ecosocial" approach outlined by Krieger (1994), our perspective is based on the assumption that it is as important to study the social conditions and processes underlying the health of populations as it is to isolate determinants of individual health. In this view, *context* is considered an important focus of inquiry in and of itself and not simply as a background or contributing factor to some bottom-line health outcome. Consequently, we give ample attention to systemic analysis, such as our descriptions of the organization of health cultures (including the culture of public health), societal response to deviance, demographic processes underlying health transitions, and the multilayered components of the social environment.

By introducing the organizing frameworks in Part I, we inadvertently may contribute to the problem of "model overload" that characterizes the field of social and behavioral sciences in health. Readers unfamiliar with the literature of this field especially may find the reference to so many different models confusing and frustrating. This is particularly the case in Chapter 4, "Health and Illness Behavior," an area in which dozens of distinct models have been advanced to guide research. For this reason, we have been somewhat selective in which models are covered in the book, and some readers may take issue with the omission of one or more of their favored models.

Some readers also may note the uneven attention to industrial and developing countries across chapters. This stems from the fact that for some health problems and issues, developing countries have figured importantly, whereas for others the focus has been mostly industrial countries. For example, lifestyle change, aging, and chronic disease prevention have received a great deal more emphasis in industrialized nations, whereas infectious disease control and population problems have been addressed more intensively in Third World settings. For this reason, we felt it made sense to include a chapter on international health that highlights those issues particularly germane to less developed countries.

The book is organized into four parts: Introduction and Overview, Conceptual Foundations, Sociocultural Response to Illness, and Special Topics. In the first part, three chapters set the stage for the book and introduce key concepts and frameworks that organize the content of subsequent chapters. Chapter 1 makes the case for the importance of understanding the social and behavioral dimensions of public health problems. It briefly reviews the history of social and behavioral science research on health and the particular significance this field has for public health theory and practice. Examples are given to highlight the value of sociobehavioral approaches to health problems and their utility in diverse public health settings. The scope of the book is outlined by overviewing the core social science disciplines and noting the chapters that draw more heavily from different disciplines.

Chapter 2 takes perspectives from history, demography, and anthropology to examine long-term changes in disease patterns, social organization, and subsistence modes of human groups. Basic concepts of population dynamics, culture change, adaptation, and ecosystemic processes are presented. The specific processes of demographic, epidemiologic, and health transitions are included as underpinnings of the shift from infectious to chronic disease problems in public health. A historical perspective is developed through an examination of the five stages of disease history: foraging groups, settled village, preindustrial cities, industrial cities, and the present. Linkages between population processes, environmental factors, nutritional status, and disease are illustrated. The new field of evolutionary medicine is described and the implications for public health discussed. Case examples presented to illustrate relevant concepts include sickle cell anemia in Africa, early public health movements, an evolutionary perspective on allergies, and motor vehicle injuries in industrial societies.

If epidemiology is the core discipline of public health, as many would argue, then social epidemiology provides the foundation for the study of social and behavioral aspects of public health. Chapter 3, "Social Epidemiology," covers basic definitions, concepts, indicators, and goals of social epidemiologic research, highlighting important research on chronic disease etiology. Particular emphasis is accorded the link between poverty and health, including the concept of excess mortality and the problems with confounding the relation between socioeconomic status, race, and health. The case examples of low birth weight among African American infants, the paradox of Hispanic health, breast cancer in the United States, and the risk factor approach to cardiovascular disease are used to illustrate these issues.

The second part of the book contains three chapters that emphasize theoretical perspectives from the social and behavioral sciences that have relevance for public health research and practice. Chapter 4 organizes the discussion of health-related behavior into three general categories: health behavior (primary prevention), illness behavior (help-seeking), and sick-role behavior (response to medical advice). Each category is reviewed, first, by presenting the concepts and models that have guided relevant research, then by summarizing the current state of knowledge in the area, and ending with illustrative case studies. The health behavior section highlights research using the Health Belief Model, the Theory of Reasoned Action, Social Cognitive Theory, and the Transtheoretical

Model. Contemporary applications to research on smoking, exercise, diet, stress, injury prevention, and other public health issues are addressed. Research on illness behavior is reviewed from two perspectives—studies that focus on help-seeking processes within the illness episode and those that seek to predict health care utilization. Concepts and models for looking at illness behavior from psychology, sociology, and anthropology are discussed. Sick-role behavior is discussed from the standpoint of changes over time in the conceptualization of patient behavior and an awareness of the power relations inherent in the notion of compliance. Critical perspectives on sick-role behavior are illustrated through a focus on tuberculosis control ideology and practice in the 20th century.

The main objective of Chapter 5, "The Social Environment and Health," is to show how people's wider social relationships (e.g., family, work, community, society) can affect their health status and their response to illness. The discussion is organized into sections on gender and health, stress, social support and health, health-related support groups, and family systems. Within these areas, topical highlights include men's health issues and the impact of maternal employment on child health. Rather than present a single theoretical perspective on the social environment, multiple approaches are illustrated through reviews of the topical areas, including feminist theory, social support theory, role theory, household production theory, and family systems theory.

Chapter 6, "Social Differentiation, Cultural Diversity, and Community Health," addresses public health issues in relation to community and individual sociocultural complexities. Basic components of communities are identified, including biologically defined racial distinctions; nonrandom habitation patterns; and social differentiation, such as ethnic, occupational, and class distinctions. The effects of the foregoing on the health of individuals and communities are discussed in terms of epidemiologic patterns, response to illness, and the organizational culture of intervention programs. The chapter also focuses on strategies for studying sociocultural dimensions of health problems by analyzing cases of social differentiation and cultural diversity affecting health issues, including the challenge of detecting subtle cultural issues within one's own behavior and thinking. A recurrent theme of the chapter is the notion that communities are complex, multidimensional entities requiring interventions that take into account, in a deliberate and nonsuperficial way, the intrasocietal differences to optimize program impact.

As stated previously, an organizing framework for the book is the notion that social and behavioral factors affect health both as antecedents and as responses to the occurrence of health problems. In keeping with this view, the content of Part II can be viewed as covering the conceptual antecedents of illness, and Part III addresses the different ways in which society responds to illness. The first two chapters in Part III discuss naturally occurring social responses to illness, and the remaining two focus on directed change strategies to improve health.

Chapter 7, "Deviance and Social Control," begins with a general discussion of why deviance is considered a threat to society and the common means by which groups impose limits on human behavior—through formal (regulation, legislation, policy) and informal (ostracism, stigma, discrimination) means. The tendency for public health to be concerned with the welfare of socially marginal and stigmatized groups is addressed, and the tendency for sickness to be attributed moral significance is noted. The discussion then turns to the conceptualization of illness as deviance and the social control mechanisms put in place to minimize its disruptive effects on the group. Drawing on role theory and labeling theory, the chapter overviews the concepts of the sick role; the "at risk" role; normative, situational, and secondary deviance; compliance; and medicalization. The special case of collective behavior in response to epidemics is examined in historical perspective, drawing comparisons and contrasts among the Black Death of the Middle Ages, cholera epidemics of the 19th century, and the modern-day AIDS epidemic. The social construction perspective and metaphorical analysis are used to explain irrational societal reactions to epidemics based on fear, moral judgment, and scapegoating. A discussion of social and behavioral issues in political violence, community violence, and family violence concludes the chapter.

Chapter 8, "Comparative Health Cultures," begins with the premise that all contemporary health care systems are pluralistic in that multiple healing traditions coexist and interface in variable ways. Taking a historical and cross-cultural perspective, the chapter overviews aspects of health culture from the standpoint of universal components found at all levels of cultural development. A closer look is taken at Western medicine as an ethnomedical system, highlighting the basic assumptions and core values that underlie its theories and practices. Focusing even more narrowly, the culture of public health in the United States is described and critically examined for its impact on programs and policies. Case studies of the cultures of medicine and public health are presented involving the instrumental ethos of medical practice and the sometimes contradictory nature of "scientific" versus "folk" beliefs in disease control programs.

Chapters 9 and 10 examine two approaches to planned health interventions at the population level, "Community-Based Approaches to Health Promotion" and "Social Marketing." Both draw heavily on social and behavioral science concepts and methods. Chapter 9 begins by defining what we mean by *community* and then discusses the major features and types of community-based approaches to intervention. Principles of participatory research are highlighted as integral to this approach. An in-depth discussion is presented of a widely used model for participatory intervention, the Planned Approach to Community Health (PATCH), illustrated with a case study from a school-based program. The chapter concludes with an overview of the advantages and challenges of implementing successful community-based interventions. Although a relatively new approach to planned change, social marketing is one of the fastest-growing strategies in public health. Chapter 10 examines the conceptual and methodologic bases of social marketing as an organized effort to achieve health goals. It outlines the steps for planning a social marketing intervention and illustrates the process with a case study involving the marketing of the Texas Special Supplemental Nutrition Program for Women, Infants & Children.

The special topics that make up the final part of the book were selected as representative of topical areas within public health that have integrated social and behavioral science perspectives in fundamental ways and that therefore provide arenas for illustrating practical application. The four topical areas include international health, gerontological health, nutrition, and mental health. Other areas that also could have been given separate treatment are maternal and child health, environmental health, and health policy. The latter topics have been covered more selectively in other chapters of the book.

The reprinted chapter "Health Behavior in Developing Countries" begins by outlining the defining characteristics of developing countries; comparisons then are made between industrial and less-developed countries on basic health indicators. The contrast between health conditions and public health priorities in the two areas is emphasized, referring back to the concepts of demographic, epidemiologic, and health transitions introduced previously. The implications of these differences for research on health behavior are discussed. The chapter overviews health behavior across the life span in developing countries, including infancy and childhood, the reproductive years, and adult and older years. Issues in primary health care, child survival, reproductive health, safe motherhood, tropical diseases, and AIDS control are discussed. The chapter concludes with an overview of current and future trends in health research in developing countries, examining issues such as the role of maternal education in family health, increasing attention to adult and men's health, and health issues of elderly people.

In Chapter 12, "Food and Society," the social context of diet and nutrition is examined. Following a review of the biological and psychological determinants of food practices, the chapter discusses the influence of culture on people's definitions of what is edible, how groups get and prepare their food, and the ways that food is distributed. Food is shown to fulfill important economic, social, aesthetic, and religious functions other than nourishment. People's relationships to food are discussed in terms of various forms of social organization. Dietary habits are linked to gender, age, social class, and ethnicity. Finally, the relations between food practices and worldview, religion, and health beliefs are examined.

"Public Mental Health" begins by reviewing the history of the public mental health movement and the public health significance of mental health problems today, including attention to the interface between mental and physical health. Major conceptual perspectives on mental health and illness are discussed. Two sections highlight the applicability of the Social Ecology, Health Impact, and Causality Continuum models to public mental health through an exploration of the contribution of social and behavioral factors as determinants and/or consequences of mental health. The importance of social and behavioral science theory for development and evaluation of mental health intervention programs is illustrated through case examples. The Epidemiologic Catchment Area Survey and the National Comorbidity Survey are used to show how basic research informs theory development. Interventions aimed at reducing the negative consequences of mental illness for families illustrate the translation of mental health theory into practice. The chapter concludes with an analysis of emerging strategies aimed at the primary prevention of mental illnesses.

The final chapter, "Public Health and Aging: The New Imperative," overviews the rapidly growing field of gerontological health. It begins with a discussion of the reasons why health issues of elderly people have emerged as an important arena of public health research and policy. Current demographic trends make the aged population a major concern of industrial nations. The health effects of aging as well the geriatric patient profile are described. Attention is given to the importance of prevention programs for improving the long-term health prospects of elderly people. The chapter concludes with a discussion of future needs in the evolving field of gerontological health.

Although we have attempted to cover the full range of theoretical and substantive issues that make up our collective view of the social and behavioral foundations of public health, by necessity we had to make choices about the attention devoted to different topics. Some readers undoubtedly will feel we have neglected some important aspects and overemphasized others. Such is the nature of any field. We hope the quibbles of omission and emphasis are minor and that readers come away with a greater appreciation of the value of social and behavioral science perspectives for public health research and practice.

Acknowledgments

This book has been a truly collaborative effort in many ways. Not only did it bring together five instructors with a common goal; many other faculty, staff, students, colleagues, and practitioners contributed in various ways along the way. We thank other faculty who have taught the core course in Social and Behavioral Sciences Applied to Health at University of South Florida over the years, whose knowledge and insights indirectly found their way into the book: Martie Coulter, Stan Graven, and Mike Angrosino. In addition, the many guest lecturers, too numerous to list, planted nuggets of ideas we digested and incorporated in some form or another. Special thanks go to our department chair, Robert McDermott, for encouraging and supporting this project throughout, and to all the students who helped us figure out what material was important and how to present it. For critical feedback on earlier drafts of the manuscript, we are indebted to many people. The students who took the course in Spring 1999 generously provided their evaluations of draft chapters and made extremely helpful suggestions for making the text "user-friendly." A number of colleagues reviewed drafts of chapters or steered us toward better presentation and content: Ann McElroy, Kokos Markides, David Himmelgreen, Howard Jacobson, Charlie Mahan, Jim Lindenberger, Karen Liller, and Larry Green. Suggestions from five anonymous reviewers were most welcome and appreciated. Andre Holmes, Rajeeb Das, and Graham Coreil-Allen provided creative assistance with graphic design. Hanna Osman generously organized our many references, and other research and bibliographic assistance was provided by Chitra Krishnaswamy, S. K. Kabir, Irene Pintado, Roberta Rossell, Moya Alfonso, Ivette Lopez, Hamisu Salihu, Monica Tucci, Adebayo Akintobi, and Ravish Behal. Joyce Harper patiently helped with manuscript preparation. Finally, we thank the many colleagues, friends, and family members who cheered us along and put up with us during the writing process.

I.

Introduction and Overview

The three chapters that comprise this part introduce the overarching frameworks for the book and provide the historical background for understanding relationships between human populations and disease. Drawing on perspectives from all the social and behavioral sciences and integrating these with epidemiologic perspectives from public health, the organizing frameworks locate health problems in the context of multilayered social systems and temporal processes of change.

The central framework of the book, presented in the Social Ecology of Health Model, can be viewed as a three-dimensional representation of social processes that influence health at the level of individuals and groups. It is a composite of social and cultural determinants that shape behavior through complex interaction. The Health Impact Model depicts the same phenomena from a temporal perspective, locating the problem at variable points in the illness process, that is, before or after the occurrence of a focal problem. From yet a different perspective, the Causality Continuum orders the multiple determinants of health according to relative directness of impact, with some kinds of factors having more proximate effects than others. Throughout the book, we elaborate on specific components of these models.

The historical perspective presented in Chapter 2 sets the stage for understanding the evolving nature of public health problems as human populations adapt to changing conditions within their social and physical environments. An understanding of the past provides timeless lessons for contemporary challenges, and we refocus the evolutionary lens on several current public health problems in subsequent chapters.

1

Why Study Social and Behavioral Factors in Public Health?

PUBLIC HEALTH THEN AND NOW

Imagine you are living in the mid-18th century. Smallpox, cholera, typhus, tuberculosis, and other infectious diseases are rampant. Both experts and common folk believe these afflictions are caused by moral and spiritual depravity. Public health measures to impede contagion are limited primarily to quarantine and isolation. Now, envision yourself in the 19th century. The same infectious diseases are still widespread, but officials now attribute their spread to foul air emitted from decomposing waste in crowded cities, in addition to immoral behavior of the poor. The Sanitary Reform Movement has introduced systems of sewage and other waste disposal as basic public health services. Next, move to the turn of the 20th century. Science has revealed that infectious diseases are caused by germs, leading to new preventive strategies such as water purification and immunization. Public health is a growing enterprise concerned with infection control, community sanitation, occupational health, and the well-being of children and families. Now, you are once again in the present, looking back over the past century, in which not only the kinds of diseases prevalent changed dramatically and understanding of etiology continually evolved, but organized actions to protect the public's health expanded enormously in scope and complexity.

In the 20th century, the field of public health underwent tremendous change and diversification. In the early part of the century, infectious diseases posed the greatest challenge to the health of the people, whether they lived in industrialized countries or developing nations. Control of communicable diseases was the focus of public health practice, through organized efforts such as provision of safe water and sanitation, immunization services, and monitoring and surveillance of disease outbreaks. After 1930, antibiotic therapy became an essential component of infection control, and it remains an important aspect of public health programs that deal with sexually transmitted diseases and other communicable illnesses. In the second half of the century, however, with the emergence of chronic diseases, injury, substance abuse, and other health problems as the focal public health challenges, the dominant paradigm has shifted toward social and behavioral approaches to disease prevention and health promotion. Although the more traditional activities of infection control and environmental protection remain important in today's world, much attention and effort is now focused on changing the social conditions underlying health as well as the behavioral patterns that put people at risk for illness and injury.

Sometimes referred to as the *new public health*, this emergent paradigm in public health parallels the reconceptualization of individual health within the field of medicine along similar lines (Frenk, 1993). Whereas in the past, the germ theory of disease dominated medical research and practice, we now view individual health as shaped by complex interacting systems of biological, social, and environmental factors. Although tremendous advances in biomedical technology have improved our ability to treat illness and prolong life dramatically through use of sophisticated diagnostic testing, powerful drugs, and advanced surgery, medicine increasingly has recognized the importance of cultural context, social organization, and lifestyle choices for individual health. Variously labeled *social medicine, behavioral medicine,* and *medical ecology,* the new medical model shares with public health a broadened framework for analyzing health problems in terms of complex biosocial systems.

A number of developments contributed to the rise of the social ecology paradigm in medicine and public health (Krieger, 1994). One was the shift in epidemiologic patterns from infectious to chronic diseases noted previously. This shift was part of a broader postindustrial transformation of society involving changing demographic trends and patterns of morbidity and mortality. People now live longer and healthier lives, and the health problems they do face involve conditions that cannot be "cured" in the traditional sense. The major illnesses affecting industrial populations today, such as heart disease, cancer, and diabetes, can be controlled only through primary prevention or "managed" over the long term to improve quality of life. Prevention and treatment of chronic diseases depend heavily on behavioral practices such as diet, exercise, substance use, and stress reduction. Likewise, behavior and social conditions are central components of preventive approaches for other leading public health problems such as unintended pregnancy, substance abuse, motor vehicle accidents, and violence. Even with the new and emergent (or resurgent) infectious diseases such as HIV/AIDS, tuberculosis, and sexually transmitted diseases, sociobehavioral factors are widely recognized as critical for their control.

Another important contribution to the social ecology model of public health has been the wealth of scientific discoveries linking biology, behavior, and culture. Nearly all diseases and health conditions are now known to have multifactorial etiologies involving complex interactions of processes located inside and outside people's bodies. We know, for example, that stress is an underlying component of all illness, including both acute infections and chronic disorders, and that physical and psychological stress can affect one's ability to fight disease and restore health. In fact, illness is increasingly viewed as a breakdown in the body's natural defense system, which is highly sensitive to internal emotions and external stressors in the social environment (see Chapter 5, this volume). The negative impact of social discord, whether from family relationships, the work setting, or school pressure, can be as important in whether someone gets a cold or flu as exposure to specific pathogens. Indeed, some argue that psychosocially mediated immunity is the primary factor in most people's susceptibility to infection (Kaplan, 1991). It is worth noting that only 25 years ago, researchers were just beginning to investigate the relation between stress and illness; today, the role of stress in health is well documented, and research has spawned a dynamic field of study called *psychoneuroimmunology.*

Research on stress and health is closely linked to studies of social support—the way in which our connections to other people have a protective effect on well-being. It has been shown, for instance, that people who interact with a large network of friends and family members get sick less often and recover from illness faster than do those who do not. Similarly, people who live alone have higher rates of death and suicide than do those who live with others (Syme, 1986). These trends illustrate one kind of mechanism through which the social environment can affect health status. The social environment also can influence health through social structural arrangements, which position people at different places in society and mediate access to resources such as education, income, medical services, status, and prestige (Link & Phelan, 1995). Because people occupy different positions in the socioeconomic structure, disease and mortality are not evenly distributed within a population. The field of study that addresses such variation in health risks is known as *social epidemiology*. Many advances in understanding social risk factors have occurred in recent decades, leading to redefinitions of health as "socially produced" and increased attention to interventions focused on organizational change (Goodman, Steckler, & Kegler, 1997).

We also have learned a great deal about how cultural factors influence health, such as the ways that people think about and behave regarding food, the relative value they place on work and leisure, how health and illness are perceived and managed, and the role of ethnic identity in shaping disease patterns. Approaches to studying cultural influence have broadened to encompass notions of gender culture, family culture, organizational culture, and corporate culture, all having important lessons for public health research and practice. In Chapter 2, we take a closer look at disease history in relation to long-term cultural evolution, highlighting the relation between human subsistence strategies and patterns of disease and injury.

Another development that has enlarged the scope of public health is the expansion into new arenas of social welfare, including primary care services, reproductive health, child and family protection, injury prevention, and the health consequences of war and political violence, to name but a few. Contemporary public health encompasses an enormous diversity of specialized fields, which in turn draw on the knowledge and perspectives of many disciplines. The social and behavioral sciences have become increasingly relevant in this robust endeavor, contributing new conceptual, methodologic, and policy perspectives to the field. Nowadays, it is just as likely to find public health professionals talking about consumer satisfaction, political advocacy, and community empowerment as it is the more traditional issues such as disease surveillance and government regulation. Although the "new public health" has been widely endorsed by diverse disciplines and constituencies within the health arena, it is not without critics (Bunton, Nettleton, & Burrows, 1995; Petersen & Lupton, 1996). The latter apply poststructuralist perspectives to highlight the ever-expanding control public health institutions tend to exert on everyday life, through social constructions; the creation of expert knowledge; and moral discourse on behavior, interpersonal relations, and other health "risks."

To illustrate the holistic approach outlined previously, the following section presents two case studies analyzing the impact of social and behavioral factors on two very different public health problems. The first case involves the repercussions of the 1989 oil spill in Prince William Sound, Alaska, and subsequent efforts to clean up the area. The second case uses the example of the AIDS epidemic to show the importance of sociocultural and psychological concepts for a comprehensive understanding of public health issues.

CASE STUDIES: SOCIAL AND BEHAVIORAL DIMENSIONS OF PUBLIC HEALTH PROBLEMS

The *Exxon Valdez* Oil Spill

The grounding of the *Exxon Valdez* oil tanker released 11 million gallons of crude oil into a once-pristine environment where Native Alaskans depended heavily on marine resources for their livelihood. The damage from the oil spill, along with ensuing efforts to clean up the area, set off a chain of events with profound social, cultural, and psychological impacts on affected communities. A year after the accident, anthropologist Lawrence Palinkas, with Downs, Petterson, and Russel (1993), conducted a population-based survey of nearly 600 households in 13 localities. The researchers measured demographic variables, levels of exposure to the spill, impact on social relations within families and the community, changes in traditional subsistence activities, and indicators of mental and physical health. By comparing respondents with high exposure scores to those with less exposure to effects of the spill and clean-up, a dose-response relation could be established for different consequences.

Exposure status was significantly associated with degree of reported decline in social relations, including conflicts among family members, neighbors, friends and coworkers. Not only did the spill dominate daily conversation in the year following the accident, but a large proportion of residents were involved directly in the intensive clean-up efforts, which required a large labor force over several months. The high wages offered to attract workers made it difficult for local communities to retain unskilled employees, and many families were disrupted when one or both parents worked long hours away from home. Only the able-bodied could handle the work, so not everyone benefited from the clean-up operation, causing some resentment among those excluded. Conflicts with outsiders who came for the lucrative work were commonplace. In some villages, more than 40% of respondents reported friendships ending over clean-up disputes, often related to whether one worked on the clean-up or not. Those who worked in the clean-up reported spending less time with friends, less participation in religious activities and festivals, and less time in volunteer activities compared to those less exposed to the spill.

Economic disputes were also rampant, over issues such as equitable distribution of monetary compensation among permit holders and crewmen for lost fishing. Furthermore, involvement in the spill and its aftermath had a dramatic effect on subsistence activities for this population. Hunting, fishing, and harvesting of certain traditional foods had long played an important symbolic role in maintaining native identify, culture, and family solidarity. These activities were curtailed drastically because of environmental pollution from the spill and because so many people were working long hours in the clean-up. Issues of cultural survival in relation to the disaster were discussed seriously.

Finally, in the health arena, high-exposed individuals scored significantly higher than low-exposed persons on measures of psychiatric disorders and physical health status, and they reported higher perceived increases in community levels of substance abuse and domestic violence. Exposure status was associated with generalized anxiety disorder, posttraumatic stress disorder, and depression. It also was linked to higher numbers of physician-verified illness conditions occurring after the spill as well as self-assessed decline in health status. These data were corroborated by documented increases in visits to community clinics for primary care and mental health services throughout the region.

The *Exxon Valdez* oil spill illustrates the extensive ways in which environmental disasters can produce direct and indirect social and psychological effects in affected communities. At a more general level, it illustrates the harmful impact of rapid sociocultural change in a case example that is likely to recur in other areas of the world. It allows the examination of the association of processes of sociocultural change and subsequent health and well-being.

The AIDS Epidemic

In the early 1980s, the AIDS epidemic burst on the international stage with alarming threat and sobering challenges. Here was a highly lethal infection with unclear etiology and transmission, spreading rapidly among disparate social groups, and with no effective treatment in sight. In North America and Europe, the disease primarily affected gay men, hemophiliacs, and intravenous drug users. In time, the microbial agent Human Immunodeficiency Virus (HIV) was identified, along with transmission routes involving sexual practices and contaminated blood. Screening of blood supplies eliminated the risk of infection from transfusions, but altering sexual and drug use practices proved to be a much bigger public health challenge. It soon became clear that, more than any other major health problem addressed to date, AIDS was a disease in which social and behavioral factors played a dominant role in etiology and control. Primary prevention was the only effective intervention available. Moreover, efforts to curb the epidemic through behavior change (i.e., safer sexual practices) encountered overwhelming obstacles at both the individual and societal level. Of particular interest were the ways in which social responses to the disease revealed disturbing patterns of moral condemnation, stigmatization of marginal groups, and questionable ethics in research and medical care.

Before long, the heterosexual transmission pattern dominant in developing countries emerged as a serious problem in the North as well. However, as noted previously, not everyone in the population was equally at risk, and, not surprisingly, it was those groups living in poverty at the margins of society who were most affected—ethnic and racial minorities, sex workers, and people living in high-crime urban neighborhoods. The social epidemiology of AIDS mirrored the health situation of the world's cities.

The epidemic served as a lightning rod for a host of psychosocial issues (Rushing, 1995). Everything related to the illness was charged with intense emotion: the fear of diagnosis for its victims, who could anticipate immediate rejection and discrimination and a horrifying deterioration ending in certain death; the anxiety among health workers, whose job put them at risk of infection; and the collective moral outrage of society at large, which tended to scapegoat "undesirable" groups who deviated from the norms of the privileged majority. A striking example of the latter unfortunate response was the labeling of Haitians in general as a "risk group" for several years, clearly a reflection of racially based fears of social contamination from foreigners. Most telling was the stark exposure of deep-seated homophobia triggered by the crisis. Incredibly, scientific thinking was suspended as the dogma of "punishment for sin" was espoused from pulpit to podium, and government officials blocked efforts to increase public funding for AIDS research and to educate the public about safe sex. The social control functions of illness labeling were clearly operating in many domains of the epidemic. Cultural taboos about sex silenced open discussion of the problem for a long time. The pernicious effects of gender stratification also were evident in the epidemiology of and failure to control the spread of HIV, particularly in poor countries where women's economic dependence on sexual relations with men placed them at risk for infection.

The social impact of the epidemic on families, communities, and health care systems was profound. Many people with AIDS were abandoned by their families out of fear, shame, and economic hardship. The devastating effects included family disintegration, orphaned children, and infants infected through their mothers. In some areas, the magnitude of adults affected seriously diminished the productive workforce. To its credit, the gay community responded positively by organizing for political advocacy and spearheading local educational campaigns. Because the disease involved expensive medical care for multiple conditions over an extended time period, issues of access to care surfaced quickly, highlighting ongoing ethical dilemmas about who should bear the burden of health care costs and how to allocate limited therapeutic resources. Even with the advent of effective drug treatment that has reduced health care costs, issues of equitable distribution remain unresolved. Likewise, ethical controversies continue in the realm of research, involving participants from poor countries who cannot afford the costly new medicines.

CONCEPTUAL FRAMEWORKS

The foregoing case studies highlight a variety of social and behavioral factors that are relevant to a holistic analysis of public health problems. These dimensions were presented without reference to a particular organizing framework; however, in the remainder of this volume, we use several conceptual models to systematize the discussion and provide coherence to the material covered. In this section, we present two general organizing frameworks for the book, the Social Ecology and Health Impact models, and in Chapter 3 we present the Causality Continuum. More focused conceptual models are integrated into subsequent chapters. The Social Ecology of Health Model is an overarching view that integrates the physical and social environment with individual, group, and societal spheres of influence. The Health Impact Model conceptualizes social and behavioral factors as both antecedents and responses to illness. Finally, the Causality Continuum groups factors into distal, intermediate, and proximate determinants of disease.

The Social Ecology of Health Model

Public health research and practice always has had a strong ecological orientation because of its focus on populations and disease transmission within and across groups (Last, 1998). The traditional model of host-agent-environment framed thinking around the notion of infectious organisms (agents) surviving within human hosts, who lived and interacted within a larger environment, which may include disease vectors, reservoirs for pathogens, and other biotic and physical features affecting disease ecology. In the expanded view of public health described previously, a more complex social ecology model has evolved that incorporates social environmental variables into the picture. As depicted in Figure 1.1, the Social Ecology of Health Model is a general ecosystemic model of human relations to disease and health within a social and physical environmental context. The relations can be ordered into different levels of organization from the individual through linkages to larger social networks, such as the family, community, social institutions, the state, and global systems. Like other ecological models, the Social Ecology Model derives from general systems theory, which views phenomena as open systems—systems composed of mutually interacting components (Catalano, 1979).

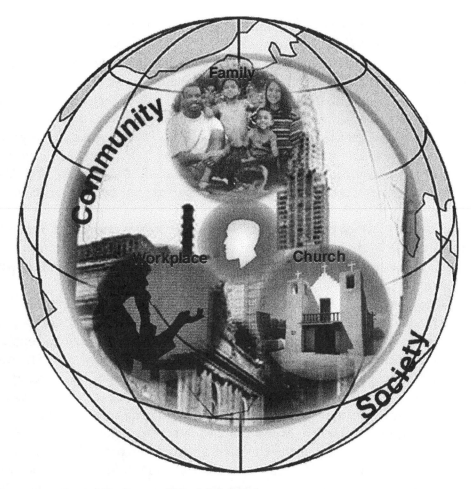

Figure 1.1. Social Ecology of Health Model

Key elements of systems models are integration, change, and adaptation. In the Social Ecology of Health Model, different parts of the system are integrated through social relationships among individuals and groups. For example, a mother has a relationship to her child and the family unit, she likely interacts with work and other community groups, and she belongs to social class and ethnic groups within the larger society. How she responds when her child gets sick is influenced by factors at different levels of the system. She may evaluate certain symptoms, such as a runny nose or cough, as minor and not needing medical attention, based on norms shared with her reference group. A fever, however, she may view as warranting professional attention, yet her ability to seek care likely is constrained by her work situation. Depending on the type of job she has, she may or may not be able to take time off for a doctor visit.

Although systems strive toward equilibrium, perfect balance is never achieved because systems are open to internal and external changes and thus constantly require adjustment or adaptation. Because of integration, change at any level of the system may require adjustment at other levels. The process of adaptation in response to change is one way of conceptualizing stress, and, again, it can occur at different levels, including psychological distress, family dysfunction, community disruption, rapid culture change, and environmental degradation. Sociocultural or environmental change can have repercussions that eventually affect communities, families, and individuals (Ell & Northen, 1991). For example, an economic recession often leads to high unemployment rates; within families, a provider may lose his or her job, leading to loss of medical benefits and reduced income, which affect access to health care. Social support can buffer the negative effects of stress at different levels of the system, such as through close friendships, strong families, community resources, and one's integration with (or alienation from) the larger society.

Although we have emphasized social environmental factors, because of the subject matter of this book, the Social Ecology of Health Model also incorporates aspects of the physical environment. At the household level, we can consider housing conditions and hazards in the home; at the community level, we must take into account physical aspects such as water quality, air pollution, precipitation, toxic waste, noise, crowding, and other features; at the societal level, examples of physical environmental concerns might include atmospheric change (e.g., ozone depletion), changes in flora and fauna (e.g., deforestation, vector habitat), climatic stress (e.g., heat waves, cold spells), and natural disasters (e.g., floods, tornadoes, hurricanes). The impacts of these biophysical phenomena are always mediated through social system arrangements, which shape how humans respond and manage environmental events.

In public health, we are concerned with changes emanating from the larger social system, including government legislation, regulation, and budgetary matters that affect health issues directly. The health of the economy almost always has social welfare repercussions. We are also concerned with more local-level institutions, such as state politics, community health services, the school system, and law enforcement. The Social Ecology of Health Model provides a framework that allows one to locate these disparate public health issues within a coherent organization.

The Health Impact Model

It is useful to consider health and sickness as an evolving process with an underlying time dimension, which allows one to examine influences "before" and

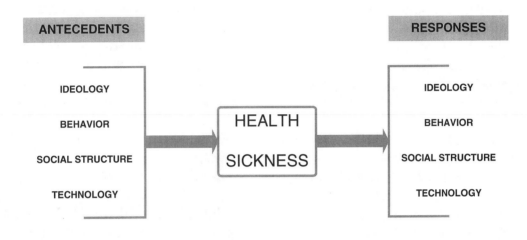

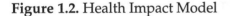

Figure 1.2. Health Impact Model

"after" the event in question. This process is illustrated in the Health Impact Model (see Figure 1.2). *Antecedents* are factors that affect the etiology of a health problem, and *responses* include the intentional and unintentional consequences of the event. The scope of potential antecedents and responses is quite large, so we focus on four areas for illustrative purposes, using the same categories on both sides of the model. *Ideology* encompasses the system of beliefs, attitudes, and values that shape how people think and act in the world and how they respond to events in their lives. *Behavior* includes the actions and activities of individuals and groups; it is patterned by the social and cultural context in which they function. *Social structure* derives from people's relationships to groups that make up the social system. Finally, *technology* is based on the manner in which tasks are accomplished using knowledge and technical methods.

Ideological antecedents to ill health might include perceptions of risk that lead people to take precautions or disregard them, such as beliefs about the need for prenatal care or regular check-ups. In response to illness, belief systems determine what signs and symptoms are recognized as indications of illness and what steps should be taken to deal with the problem. In the behavioral realm, commonly noted antecedents to illness include day-to-day lifestyle activities, such as eating, sleeping, exercising, and tobacco use, whereas behavioral responses might include taking time off from work or following a therapeutic regimen. Social structural antecedents can range from the macro level of the socioeconomic system, which can deprive people of the means to live healthy lives, down to the micro level of family dynamics, in which gender roles create different health risks for men and women. Technological advances have transformed our lives immeasurably, and, in the process, they have affected health in many ways. Examples of antecedent effects include our dependence on automobiles for local transportation, which makes motor vehicle accidents a major cause of death in developed nations. Yet, our sophisticated technology also provides life-saving emergency medical transportation and trauma care.

The public health enterprise is concerned with understanding both antecedents and consequences of health problems. In recent years, greater emphasis has been given to primary prevention, that is, reducing the incidence of disease, which in most cases is the most cost-effective approach to intervention. At the same time, improving secondary prevention through early detection and treatment remains an important strategy for control. The deleterious consequences of health conditions are addressed through tertiary prevention, such as rehabilitation and support services that aim to improve the quality of life of people affected by health problems. Social and behavioral factors affect all three levels of prevention.

THE SOCIAL AND BEHAVIORAL SCIENCES

Like the health sciences, the social and behavioral sciences have undergone considerable development and specialization in the past 50 years. The various disciplines include sociology, anthropology, psychology, demography, economics, geography, history, political science, communication, and gerontology. All these disciplines have made important contributions to understanding health and illness, and each has developed specialized fields of inquiry related to medicine and public health, such as medical anthropology, medical sociology, health psychology, health communication, and gerontological health. Medical sociology focuses on the health effects of people's relationships to groups through various forms of social organization, such as role behavior, family relationships, and social stratification. Chapter 5, "The Social Environment and Health," and Chapter 7, "Deviance and Social Control," draw heavily on sociological theory and research. Medical anthropology examines health and illness in the context of biocultural systems, including the evolutionary history of disease in human populations and the cultural construction of illness. Chapter 2, "Historical Perspectives on Population and Disease," and Chapter 8, "Comparative Health Cultures," are informed primarily by anthropological perspectives. Individual determinants of health-related behavior are the main subject matter of health psychology, which has contributed importantly to health education theory and practice. Chapter 4, "Health and Illness Behavior," and Chapter 13, "Public Mental Health," incorporate some of the key concepts in this area.

Chapter 3, "Social Epidemiology," applies principles and concepts from demography and other social science disciplines. Likewise, the Special Topics chapters incorporate multidisciplinary perspectives in addressing specific topics such as international health, diet and nutrition, aging, and mental health.

Much cross-fertilization has taken place among the sociomedical sciences so that today most research on public health topics integrates a variety of concepts and methods from different social science traditions. It is truly an interdisciplinary field, very dynamic and evolving, offering an exciting agenda for research in the 21st century.

2

Historical Perspectives on Population and Disease

In the introductory passage of this book, we asked the reader to imagine being alive during different historical periods and to envision the kinds of public health problems confronting society at various points in time. In this chapter, we delve even further back into human prehistory to examine the scope of health changes that have affected human populations since ancient times. Our discussion reveals how aspects of human population demography and cultural organization interact to produce distinctive sets of disease challenges. In particular, the discussion focuses on the interrelation between settlement patterns and subsistence technology—the organized system for procuring food, shelter, and other necessities of life. To lay the groundwork for this discussion, we begin by overviewing basic principles and processes of population dynamics.

POPULATION DYNAMICS

Demography is the branch of science that investigates the vital statistics of a population, such as births, deaths, marriages, and divorces. It is an important area of research for public health because epidemiologic patterns are linked closely with population parameters and because public health practice is organized around defined populations and their unique health profiles. Needs assessment and program planning in public health rely heavily on standardized demographic indicators. Thus, it is important for public health students and professionals to understand and evaluate the significance of these various measures.

The demographic indicators most commonly used in public health work relate to fertility, mortality, and population growth. *Fertility* concerns the rate of childbearing in a population and is measured in several ways. *Total fertility* refers to the mean number of children born per woman in a particular population. On average, this figure ranges between 1 and 10. For example, in 1998, the total fertility in the United States was 2.0, and in Niger it was 7.1. The *crude birth rate,* on the other hand, is based on the number of children born in a given year per 1,000 population. This indicator may range from 10 to 50. The indicator often seen in the literature is the *age-adjusted fertility rate,* determined by the number of live births per 1,000 women who are 15- to 44-years-old or some other defined age group. The fertility of certain subgroups of society often receives special attention, such as adolescent childbearing, because of social concerns related to health risks, morality, and human welfare (see the following section). Also, fertility patterns of different ethnic groups sometimes generate discussion because of the implications for changing demographics and majority-minority group relations.

Mortality rates usually are computed for specific age groups and phases of life. The *crude death rate,* however, refers to the number of deaths in a year per 1,000 population. *Infant mortality rate* (IMR) is one of the most widely used demographic measures in public health because it has come to be recognized as the most sensitive indicator for overall health and quality of life of a population. The IMR is determined by the total number of deaths among infants in the first year of life, per 1,000 live births. Over the course of human history, infant mortality has varied considerably, from as high as 500—analogous to a 50% death rate in the Middle Ages—to less than 10 today in most industrialized countries. Because deaths among adults occur less frequently than among infants and children, the *adult mortality rate* is calculated using a larger denominator than infant mortality; it is the number of deaths over a year per 100,000 population. In Chapter 3, we discuss how adult mortality is often used to determine excess mortality among socially disadvantaged subgroups in a population. *Maternal mortality* is a specialized indicator based on reproductive deaths, broadly defined to include those attributable to contraception and abortion, as well as pregnancy and childbirth. Like infant mortality, it is calculated in relation to the number of live births to control for fertility (i.e., exposure to maternal mortality risk), and like adult mortality it uses the 100,000 denominator because of the lower frequency of the event. The indicator is called the *maternal mortality ratio* and is based on the number of deaths among women related to reproductive causes, per 100,000 live births. Great disparities exist in maternal mortality between developed and developing countries, where the ratios vary from as low as 5 in Scandinavian countries to over 500 in sub-Saharan Africa.

The third demographic process of concern to public health is the *population growth rate,* the speed at which groups increase or decrease in size. Overall population growth is a function of the two processes just defined, fertility and mortality; in addition, *migration* must be taken into consideration, as seen in the basic formula for determining population growth.

$$P_1 + B - D \pm M = P_2 \text{ where}$$

P_1 = population size at Time 1,

B = births,

D = deaths,

M = net migration ("in" – "out"), and

P_2 = population size at Time 2.

The magnitude of the difference between P_1 and P_2 indicates the absolute increase or decline in a population. If converted to a percentage of P_1, this statistic represents the population growth rate, which typically ranges between 0 and 4.0.

The pace of population growth is often described as "slow," "moderate," "rapid," or "explosive." Table 2.1 depicts the population growth rates associated with these labels, along with the corresponding "doubling time" (the number of years it takes for the population to double itself) and examples of countries currently experiencing different rates. Population problems arise when human welfare (any value held by the people concerned) suffers because of the number, composition, distribution, or growth rate of a population. Overpopulation occurs when there are too many people to meet their basic needs, but having too few people—underpopulation—also can pose problems, such as inadequate numbers to sustain communities. *Composition* refers to the sociodemographic profile of the group, such as ethnic breakdown and gender ratios. A markedly skewed gender ratio, for example, can affect fertility patterns. Maldistribution of the population can take a variety of forms, including geographic and social dimensions. For example, regional and urban/rural concentrations can create problems for city planning, water resource management, and health service organization. On the social side, age structure is important for broad human welfare concerns, such as the challenges posed by the increasing elderly population in industrial countries. When we think of population problems, however, it is rapid population growth rates that come to mind first, particularly in poorer countries that still have agrarian economic systems and that value large families.

TABLE 2.1   Population Growth Rates, Doubling Time, and Representative
Countries

Growth Rate[a]	Doubling Time	Descriptive Label	Representative Countries
0.0-0.4	140 years	Slow	Japan, United Kingdom
0.5	130	Moderate	Sweden, Cuba
1.0	70	Moderate	U.S.A., China
2.0	35	Rapid	Haiti, Malaysia
3.0	23	Explosive	Nigeria, Congo
4.0	18	Explosive	Yemen, Jordan

a. Average growth rate 1990-1997 (UNICEF, 1999).

Overpopulation leads to malnutrition, high infant and child mortality, environmental degradation, political tension, and severe strain on social services. It has been linked to famine, disease, and war. Maldistribution of food resources within countries exacerbates precarious food security situations. In addition, one of the saddest casualties of war is the widespread starvation that often ravages the most vulnerable segments of the embattled populations. Refugee camps fill with displaced families, women, children, and elderly people uprooted from their homes, who are weakened by disease and food deprivation. The international community and relief agencies mobilize food and medical aid, but too often such goods become weapons of war themselves, used by military groups to perpetuate the destructive conflicts (Maren, 1997).

But there is another side to population pressure, and that is overconsumption and waste, the misuse of resources to the detriment of well-being (Crocker & Linden, 1998). The picture of this malady is widespread obesity, overflowing landfills, and toxic chemicals in breast milk. They are the spoils of postindustrial societies whose populations produce waste and control global resources vastly out of proportion to their numbers. Ecologists use the term *net primary productivity* (NPP) to refer to the amount of energy captured from sunlight by green plants and transformed into living tissue. It is the base of all food chains and provides the energy that powers all of nature. A single species among millions, human beings consume about 40% of land-based NPP. Such "overgrazing" has been linked to global warming, ozone depletion, topsoil degradation, species extinction, and loss of tropical rainforest. Consuming such a huge proportion of the earth's resources, some argue, leaves too little for the natural world to maintain conditions for the long-term well-being of the ecosystem. Furthermore, the 40% of NPP is disproportionately consumed by the wealthiest segments of the richest countries; 20% of the world's people consume 82% of global resources, leaving the vast majority of people with far too little (Weston, 1997). For example, a person living in the United States consumes, on average, more than 500 times the energy used by someone who lives in a poor country such as Ethiopia.

Worldwide population growth reached an all time peak of 2.0 in 1960, sparking vocal alarm and debate among demographers regarding the maximum number of people the earth can support in a healthy state without degrading the environment (i.e., *carrying capacity*). Some doomsday scenarios predicted dire consequences before the end of the 20th century, although more moderate perspectives are tempered by the anticipation of natural and socially engineered population controls. By 1970, global population growth had slowed considerably, quelling fears of imminent catastrophe, but recent increases have renewed concerns about overpopulation. Experts identify the optimal world population growth rate to be 0.5%, yet the current global population is increasing at a rate of 1.5% per year.

What is particularly noteworthy about the demographic history of the human species is the rapid acceleration of population growth rates in recent centuries. As shown in Table 2.2, for thousands of years human numbers across the globe were quite low and population size increased very slowly. A significant increase occurred about 10,000 years ago with the Neolithic Revolution, the development of agriculture. Another swell began in the 18th century with the Industrial Revolution and its concomitant urbanization and mass production of goods and services. Now, we have entered the postindustrial era characterized by slower rates of population growth, although many parts of the world have only recently begun the process of industrialization. Demographers predict that

TABLE 2.2   Human Population Growth Rates Through Time

Year	Rate (%)
100,000 B.P.	0.002
10,000 B.P.	0.05
1800 C.E.	0.4
1900 C.E.	0.7
1960 C.E.	2.2
1970 C.E.	2.0
1980 C.E.	1.7
1990 C.E.	1.5
2000 C.E.	1.3
2050 C.E.	0.4

NOTE: B.P. = Before Present (the number of years prior to current day); C.E. = Common Era (replaces the traditional "*anno Domini* (A.D.)").

sometime near the middle of the 21st century, the world population will reach a plateau and then slowly decline. Futurists differ considerably, though, in their visions of how desperate the human welfare situation will become before that point is reached.

Current Challenges and Approaches to Population Problems

Since 1600, the human population has increased from about half a billion to nearly 6 billion. The increase in the last decade of the 20th century exceeds the total population in 1600. Compared to human history prior to World War II, the world's population growth rate is unprecedented. Within the lifetime of some people now alive, the world's population has tripled. If global total fertility drops to the highest projection—2.5 in the 21st century—by 2050, there will be 12 billion people on earth, and this number will continue to rise. If it falls to 1.7, the lowest prediction, global population will peak at 7.8 billion in 2050 and then begin to decline. Even the latter scenario might give cause for concern, because estimates of the earth's carrying capacity range from fewer than 1 billion to more than 1 trillion people, with most estimates falling between 4 and 16 billion.

Proposals for solutions to the world's population problems confront formidable intellectual and ideological minefields. The various approaches can be grouped into three categories or "schools of thought" (Cohen, 1995). First, the *Bigger Pie School* subscribes to the liberal philosophy that more resources can be produced through improved technology, such as the agricultural "green revolution" based on genetically engineered crops and advanced chemical fertilizers. Second, the *Fewer Forks School* seeks to reduce the number of people and/or the expectations of people served, such as through family planning programs and by encouraging people to eat lower on the food chain and reduce waste. Third, the *Better Manners School* advocates changing the terms under which people interact both politically and economically and includes solutions based on freer markets, socialism, wealth redistribution, and less corruption.

The biggest source of population growth is what is called *population momentum*, the very high fraction of young people in developing countries who begin having children at an early age themselves. Approaches to counteract population momentum include raising the average age at childbearing, inducing women to have fewer children, and making contraceptive services more available to adolescents.

The second-largest source of increased population is unwanted fertility. In developing countries, one birth in four is estimated to be unwanted. In many places, families still desire large numbers of children. Surveys in the late 1980s of 27 countries in Africa, Asia, and Latin America found that desired family sizes everywhere exceeded two children. In sub-Saharan Africa, people wanted nearly six children. Approaches to reducing fertility, including wanted and unwanted, generally encompass some form of investment in human development, such as improved access to education, enhancing the status of women, and improving the health and survival of children.

In October 1993, representatives of 58 scientific academies from around the world signed a report titled *Population Summit of the World's Scientific Academies* (1994). The document urged that all reproductive health services be implemented as part of a broader strategy to raise the quality of human life. Specific proposals included far-reaching reforms, such as reducing inequalities between men and women in sexual, social, and economic life; provision of convenient reproductive health services regardless of ability to pay; elimination of unsafe and coercive practices (e.g., abortion in some areas); and more attention to safe water, sanitation, primary health care, and power for poor people, particularly women.

It is interesting to note a minority dissent report submitted by the African Academy of Sciences (1994):

> For Africa, population remains an important resource for development, without which the continent's natural resources will remain latent and unexplored. Human resource development must form part of the population/resource issue. Many of the so-called impediments to family planning have a rationality which require careful assessment. Whether or not the earth is finite will depend on the extent to which science and technology are able to transform the resources available for humanity. The potential for transforming the earth is not necessarily finite. (Quoted in Cohen, 1995, p. 376)

Indeed, some heavily populated African nations have adopted pronatalist positions encouraging high fertility. These views show that population control is not uniformly considered a desirable goal everywhere in the world.

Case Study: Adolescent Pregnancy

Although levels of sexual activity among U.S. adolescents have increased significantly in recent decades, the rate of unintended pregnancy among sexually active teenagers has steadily declined (about 19%). Still, each year, about 1 million, or 1 in 9 women, aged 15 to 19 in the United States become pregnant. Over three quarters of these pregnancies are unplanned. About 51% have the baby, 35% have abortions, and 14% miscarry. Rarely do teens put their babies up for adoption (Guttmacher Institute, 1999). Despite significant declines in U.S. ad-

TABLE 2.3   Cross-National Trends in Adolescent Fertility

Selected Countries	Year	Age 15-19 Fertility Rate
Cuba	1991	70.0
United States	1994	60.0
United Kingdom	1996	30.0
Hungary	1996	29.5
Canada	1993	24.7
Denmark	1995	8.3
Italy	1994	7.3
France	1994	7.2
China	1994	5.2

SOURCE: U.N. Development Program (1999).

olescent childbearing, when put in cross-national perspective, the U.S. teen fertility rate is extremely high (see Table 2.3).

Adolescent pregnancy gained recognition as a serious public problem during the 1970s, when rates of childbearing among young teenage girls (14- to 15-year-olds) reached the highest levels of the 20th century. However, births to older teens aged 16 to 19 years continued to decline during the 1970s from their high during the postwar baby boom (National Center for Health Statistics [NCHS], 1999). Public concern about adolescent fertility has not always corresponded with the magnitude of the problem. For example, despite declining rates of teenage pregnancy in the past few decades, there continues to be considerable discussion of the issue as a social problem of substantial proportions. There are serious risks to mother and infant associated with adolescent childbearing, particularly among very young girls. The leading problems in this population include premature births and low birth weight in infants and nutritional and physiological stress on the growing mother.

In addition to health issues, the source of public concern about adolescents having children is more closely related to the fact that the majority of young girls who have babies are not married. In 1997, 78% of girls aged 15 to 19 years who had children were unmarried (Ventura, Martin, Curtin, & Mathews, 1997). Although nonmarital fertility has increased for all ages of the population, it is most elevated among adolescents. Whereas in earlier periods, pregnant teenage girls were expected to marry before the baby was born, today it is quite common for the girl to remain living in her parents' home as a single mother.

During earlier periods of human society, the concept of adolescent pregnancy and childbearing held little significance. Puberty occurred late in adolescence, was followed by a period of sterility lasting 1 to 4 years, and girls entered marriage at a much earlier age than today. In prehistoric populations, for example, menarche (onset of menses) occurred between 15 and 17 years of age, and a woman did not bear her first child until she reached 18 to 22 years (Hassan, 1980; Lee, 1980). In preindustrial agrarian societies, age of menarche occurred sooner than in foraging groups, but young girls also were paired off with husbands at a very early age (Davis & Blake, 1956). There was no waiting to complete an education or to get settled in a stable job, or postponing starting a family until the time was right. Thus, the concept of adolescent pregnancy did not yet exist. In fact, the notion of "childhood" as a separate period in the life course did not emerge until the 19th century, and the concept of "adolescence" is a product of the 20th century. In contemporary industrial societies, average age at marriage has become increasingly higher at the same time that menarche has occurred at younger and younger ages (12-13 years). These trends have created a lengthy period of adolescence and young adulthood in which people are sexually mature but are not expected to form families and have children. "Out of wedlock" childbearing has been increasing for all ages, not just teenagers. More than 32% of all births in the United States are to unmarried women. Between 1980 and 1994, nonmarital fertility in the United States increased from 29.4 per 1,000 to 45.2 per 1,000, a 54% rise (U.S. Department of Health and Human Services [DHHS], 1995b).

In her book *Dangerous Passage,* Constance Nathanson (1991) argues that it is not teenage childbearing per se or nonmarital pregnancy per se that gives the problem of adolescent childbearing its symbolic weight. What really upsets society is nonmarital sexuality. In the United States, socially acceptable sexuality is confined to legally sanctioned marital relationships. For this reason, the idea of teenagers practicing contraception and, by inference, sexual behavior raises all sorts of moral and social issues. The root issue, according to Nathanson, is society's need to control female sexuality, particularly young women's sexual behavior.

As noted previously, since 1920 the fertility rate among 15- to 19-year-olds has decreased and among 14- to 16-year-olds has increased only slightly. In 1920, the birth rate for teenage girls was 65.0. Following the general fertility patterns in the United States, adolescent fertility peaked around 1960 near 100 per 1,000 and has declined steadily since. Also, since 1982, birth rates have continued to fall in all teenage categories. Most recently, between 1991 and 1997, teenage birth rates fell in all U.S. states, with declines ranging from 6% to 30% (DHHS, 1997). In 1997, the birth rate was 52.3 per 1,000 among women aged 15 to 19 years, compared to 62.1 in 1991. Yet, a press release from the NCHS issued in September 1997 stated that "Despite the recent decline in teen birth rate, teen pregnancy remains a significant problem in this country" (NCHS, 1997).

The press release went on to note that the reason adolescent childbearing remains a problem is that most teen pregnancies are "unintended" (i.e., not planned for within a marital relationship):

> They are also far more likely to be poor. About 80 percent of the children born to unmarried teenagers who dropped out of high school are poor. In contrast, just 8 percent of children born to married high school graduates aged 20 years are poor. (NCHS, 1997, p. 1)

What this points to is another source of the concern surrounding the problem, and that is the poverty issue. Children of poor, unmarried teenage mothers must be cared for by society. Their basic needs must be met, and their health care costs are high. Infants born to teenage mothers have a higher mortality rate than do babies of older women, and they have a higher tendency to be born prematurely, with low birth weight and subsequent health problems. Adolescent mothers also suffer health and nutritional costs from early childbearing.

The United States has one of the highest rates of both unintended pregnancy and teenage pregnancy among Western nations. Lack of access to contraceptive services is usually cited as the main cause of this disparity. For almost 50% of the 6 million women in the United States who become pregnant annually, pregnancy was an accident. Eight in 10 teenage pregnancies are not intended.

In January 1997, President Bill Clinton announced a comprehensive federal initiative to prevent teenage pregnancy. The program called for a national strategy to prevent out-of-wedlock teen pregnancies and a directive, under the new welfare law, to assure that at least 25% of communities in the United States have a teenage pregnancy prevention program. The strategy aimed to encourage adolescents to remain abstinent and "sends the strongest possible message to all teens that postponing sexual activity, staying in school, and preparing to work are the right things to do" (NCHS, 1997).

The forgoing overview of adolescent fertility in the United States reflects three competing perspectives on adolescent pregnancy (Nathanson, 1991, p. 149). First, there is the public health perspective, which highlights the health risks for early childbearing (prematurity, infant mortality). Second, the moral perspective repudiates the behavior as socially unacceptable ("Children having children!"). Third, the economic perspective emphasizes the burden to society involved in supporting the offspring of young, unmarried individuals (high proportion born in poverty, families need public assistance). Within the broad scope of this book, all three perspectives can be viewed as bearing on the public health issues surrounding adolescent pregnancy. We noted in Chapter 1 that all illness has a moral dimension; this is probably true of all public health problems as well. Also, al-

most invariably, big public health issues have important economic considerations involving the use of public funds. Viewed from these perspectives, perhaps it is not at all surprising that adolescent childbearing continues to draw
attention.

DEVELOPMENTAL TRANSITIONS

Demographic and health researchers have described a number of large-scale
population changes—*transitions*—that accompany developmental change in human societies. Originally proposed to explain changes that occur as countries undergo industrialization, much of the focus of these discussions has focused on
contemporary developing countries, with extrapolation to earlier historical periods. Developing societies are undergoing complex transitions in the areas of population trends, disease patterns, and health behavior. These processes have been
described, respectively, as the *demographic, epidemiologic,* and *health transitions.*
Each of these is briefly discussed in turn, with further elaboration in Chapter 11
on the health consequences for transitional societies.

Demographic Transition

History has shown that as societies undergo the shift from rural agricultural
economies to urban industrialized ones, population processes follow a predictable course of change, referred to as the demographic transition (Notestein,
1983). The pretransition period is characterized by high rates of fertility and mortality, particularly infant and child mortality, producing moderate rates of population growth. During the period of transition, death rates first begin to decrease
in response to improvements in living conditions and health care, but there is a
lag time during which fertility remains high because the factors favoring large
family sizes, such as expectations for high mortality among children, are slow to
change. This results in elevated population growth rates, which is the situation
characteristic of many developing countries at the turn of the 21st century and
the reason that population growth is sometimes used to define underdevelop-
ment. Over time, fertility decreases in response to falling mortality, producing
the low growth rates characteristic of industrialized nations.

Epidemiologic Transition

Along with the demographic changes just described, corresponding changes
occur in the pattern of diseases that dominate the health profile of a society. The

pretransition situation is characterized by high rates of infectious disease, including diarrheal diseases, respiratory infections, and parasitic diseases, which, coupled with poor nutritional status, leads to excess deaths in the younger age groups. As infectious diseases decline, more children survive to adulthood, life expectancy increases, and chronic diseases affecting the older population become the major health problems of a society, as currently seen in industrialized countries. These processes are referred to as the epidemiologic transition (Omran, 1983), and most developing countries are currently in the early stages of this transformation. Table 2.4 illustrates common health problems experienced by young and older age groups before and after the transition. However, it has become apparent in recent years that population subgroups within a single country may experience very different rates of disease change, creating an *epidemiologic polarization* between the disadvantaged and wealthier classes. It is also important to consider variation across ethnic groups, time periods, and geographic zones (Phillips, 1991).

Health Transition

The concept of the health transition is a more recently defined area of study that seeks to understand the cultural, social, and behavioral determinants of health that underlie the epidemiologic transition (Caldwell, 1993). Health transition research looks beyond changes in material standard of living and medical services to understand the behavioral and sociocultural factors that influence health conditions in all societies, with most work concentrated in poor countries. Some of the important findings to emerge from this work include the far-reaching effects of maternal education on a variety of health activities and the impact of household organization on health-related behavior. The accumulating body of research on health behavior in developing countries would fall within the health transition rubric, although many such studies are not explicitly identified as health transition research.

Shifts in demography and disease patterns do not occur in isolation fromother sociocultural changes. The ecosocial approach followed in this volume directs our attention to contextual conditions that both enable and limit the kinds of health problems encountered in a population. In the following section, we take a historical look at the various "stages" and transitions that have characterized human disease history, including what some anthropologists call the "first" demographic transition (Handwerker, 1983), which accompanied the Neolithic Revolution. We examine disease from the perspective of cultural evolution.

TABLE 2.4   Illustrative Health Problems of Children and Adults, Pre- and Postepidemiological Transition

	Pretransition	*Posttransition*
Children		
	Diarrhea	Congenital defects
	Acute respiratory infections	Growth failure
	Polio, tetanus	Micronutrient deficiency
	Undernutrition	Mental Development Problems
	Malaria	Injury
	Intestinal helminths	
Adults and Elderly People		
	Tuberculosis	Mental disorders
	Malaria	Circulatory disease
	AIDS/STDs	AIDS/STDs
	Parasitic diseases	Cancers
	Injury	Injury
	Maternity problems	Chronic pulmonary disease

SOURCE: Reproduced, with permission, from the Annual Review of Public Health, Volume 11, 1990, by Annual Reviews Inc. (see Mosley, Jamison, & Henderson, 1990).

DISEASE AND CULTURAL EVOLUTION

Key Concepts

One of the most important concepts in this discussion is human *culture,* the patterned ways of thought and behavior that characterize a social group, which are learned through socialization processes and persist through time. However, like all aspects of dynamic systems, culture is never static. It is constantly changing and evolving, at variable rates over time. *Culture change* can be described as long-term or short-term, depending on the time depth involved. *Long-term culture change* takes place over several generations, centuries or millennia, such as the shift from one form of subsistence to another. For example, the move from a hunting-and-gathering livelihood to food-producing subsistence is an example of long-term culture change. *Short-term culture change,* on the other hand, occurs within a single generation or a few years. Examples of short-term culture change include the introduction of automobiles, mass communication, Western medicine, and computer technology within a society. *Cultural evolution* refers to the process of long-term culture change that is slow and developmental, often described in terms of stages, in which one form builds on the previously existing phase.

Following Polgar (1964) and Armelagos and Dewey (1978), we organize the following discussion along five constellations of subsistence mode and settlement pattern: foraging groups, settled villages, preindustrial cities, industrial cities, and the present. The discussion draws on several sources related to historical trends in fertility, health, and nutrition in human populations (e.g., Cohen, 1989; Cohen, Malpass, & Klein, 1980; Fabrega, 1997; Stuart-Macadam & Dettwyler, 1995). Note that two abbreviations are used to denote time periods. "Before Present (B.P.)" indicates the number of years prior to current day, and "Common Era (C.E.)" replaces the traditional "*anno Domini* (A.D.)" designation.

1. Foraging Groups (3 million B.P.)

If the time depth of culture history were depicted as a continuous line across a wide surface, it would appear that almost the entire trajectory were taken up with the original human subsistence mode, the foraging group, with only a tiny segment at the end representing all the subsequent phases. The vast preponderance of human history was spent in the hunting-and-gathering stage, and some would argue that we are "hard-wired" to be most adapted socially, biologically, and emotionally to this form of life (see subsequent focus on Evolutionary Medicine).

Foraging, or hunting and gathering, is a subsistence technology that relies almost totally on human energy and simple tools to collect wild plants and kill free-roaming animals. All prehuman and human groups foraged for food until about 10,000 to 15,000 years ago. Today, fewer than 1% of human groups rely primarily (over 75%) on food gathering, hunting, and fishing. The few groups who remain are found in marginal lands not suitable for agriculture in the desert fringes of Australia, Southern Africa, and North America; in the forests of Asia, South America, and Central Africa; and in the frozen wastelands of Siberia and the Arctic. Even these groups have contact with technologically more complex groups, from whom they obtain food and other supplies. Competition for land and other resources with more complex societies places the technologically simpler foragers at a disadvantage, often with deleterious effects on their way of life and health status.

Foragers live in small groups that move frequently in their search for food—they are nomadic. Although there is a good deal of variation in the size of foraging groups, population density rarely exceeds one person per square mile. The exact size of a group and its density is constrained by the resources available and the nomadic lifestyle.

With the exception of a few groups living in extremely harsh regions, such as the Arctic, foraging tribes have enjoyed generally good nutritional status and leisurely work schedules. The !Kung Bushmen, studied in great detail by Richard Lee (1968), offer a good example. Typically, the !Kung woman collects enough food in 2 days to feed her entire family for a week or an average of 240 calories of plant food per hour. The rest of her time is spent cooking, fetching wood, embroidering, dancing, storytelling, resting, and visiting with friends. This steady mixture between work and leisure varies little throughout the year. The man's schedule is more uneven. Hunting may occupy an entire week followed by several leisurely weeks. As with the woman, 2 or 3 days of hunting produce enough food for the entire week. Even the most avid hunter in the tribe studied by Lee worked only 32 hours per week.

Most foragers' diets are high in complex carbohydrates and low in fat, especially saturated fats. The roots, leaves, berries, plant shoots, and the highly nutritious mongongo nut are among a surprising variety of the plant foods the !Kung gather from their desert environment. Meat is consumed less regularly than plant food, contributing 20% to 30% of the diet's calories. Groups living in the Arctic are an exception: They rely almost exclusively on hunting, with animal products contributing as much as 90% of the calories to their diet. Although this diet contains more than enough protein, the entire animal (entrails, organs, stomach contents, etc.) must be consumed to obtain the vitamins and minerals needed to sustain life.

Foragers tend to be lean, robust, and tall and suffer from few nutritional deficiencies. Nutritional surveys of contemporary hunters and gatherers show them to be generally free from severe protein-calorie malnutrition, scurvy, rickets, or vitamin B deficiency diseases. Although malnutrition and starvation are rare, loss of subcutaneous fat during leaner times of the year has been noted, suggesting that the amount of energy available at those times is not optimal. The chronic diseases we see in more modern societies are also rare in these simple societies. The active lifestyle and low fat content of many foragers' diets help protect them from cardiovascular disease. Also, fewer people reach the ages at which these illnesses occur.

In foraging groups, fertility remained low because women breastfed their infants for extended periods, often until a child reached 4 years of age. Frequent nipple stimulation from infant suckling inhibits ovulation in the lactating mother, leading to births spaced several years apart. In some cases, infanticide was practiced when a second child was born too soon after an older sibling. Child spacing was essential in these nomadic groups in which young children had to be carried from one camp to another. Population density remained low, so epidemic infectious diseases were not a serious problem. There was not a sufficient concentration of people living in close proximity to one another to maintain a reservoir of new hosts for disease organisms to flourish.

However, life expectancy was low in early human populations because of the hardships of life and the primitive state of medical care. Parasitic diseases were prevalent, and people were exposed to the risks of injury and trauma, animal predation (including insects and snakes), sepsis from wounds, and interpersonal violence (homicide and war). Maternal mortality was very high because prehistoric obstetrical care offered limited help for complications of childbirth. Feeble, handicapped, and sickly members of the group had lower survival chances with the vigorous demands of everyday life.

Focus: Evolutionary medicine. An interdisciplinary field of study emerged in the 1990s that draws heavily on what we know about human biocultural adaptation during the foraging phase of history. Evolutionary medicine examines current-day medical problems from the perspective of how ancient patterns of life continue to influence health and illness (Neese & Williams, 1996; Trevathan, Smith, & James, 1999). Also known as *Darwinian Medicine,* the specialty draws on the disciplines of human ecology, physical anthropology, archaeology, genetics, developmental psychology, and the clinical sciences. Evidence is pieced together from ethnographic studies of extant foraging groups, the fossil record, archaeological data, and primate research. The basic principles center on the tenet that culture evolves faster than biology, so physiologically humans are still primarily adapted to a foraging lifestyle. Consequently, certain modern cultural practices conflict with our biological makeup, leading to a variety of health problems.

Among the diverse areas of study, maternal and child health problems have received particular attention. For example, various malignancies including breast, endometrial, and ovarian cancers have been linked with the changes in fertility patterns noted previously. It is argued that Stone Age women ovulated and menstruated much less regularly than modern women, so today's women have much greater exposure to estrogen and other reproductive hormones than did their ancient sisters. Also, exposure to environmental toxins that mimic estrogen contributes to the estrogen load of women in industrial countries. Childbirth and infant feeding patterns are also drastically changed today compared with earlier times, with, some argue, significant health consequences. For example, current technological birth practices and loss of childbirth social support are cited as contributing to certain labor complications and increased Caesarean section rates. Finally, researchers have implicated the replacement of breast feeding with artificial feeding for the rise in childhood allergies and other disorders (Trevathan & McKenna, 1994).

In addition to changes in infant feeding practices, environmental modifications have been linked to the increased prevalence of allergic disease, including asthma, in developed country settings. In particular, modern domestic architecture creates tightly closed spaces that accumulate substances (e.g., dust mites, animal dander, insect pests, mold) that trigger allergic reactions in some people. The allergic response to inhaled substances may include bronchial constriction (wheezing), coughing, sneezing, and mucous secretion; food allergies may cause vomiting or diarrhea. Such reactions are mediated by the immunoglobulin IgE, which triggers the bodily reactions when it comes into contact with allergens to which the host is sensitive. Evolutionary researchers suggest that the allergic response serves (or did serve in the past) to protect people from various toxins they encounter in the environment. Some theorists propose that the IgE system evolved as a back-up mechanism to rid the body of harmful substances quickly when other defenses fail (Profet, 1991). Others propose that the IgE-mediated allergic response may be linked to a protective mechanism from our evolutionary past, as a defense against the highly prevalent helminthic (parasitic worm) infections in prehistoric populations (Barnes, Armelagos, & Morreale, 1999; Hurtado, Hurtado, Sapien, & Hill, 1999). The role of IgE antibodies in controlling damage from parasitic disease has been demonstrated. Furthermore, contemporary populations that carry a heavy parasitic load have very low rates of allergy, whereas those with low helminthic infestation have experienced a marked increase in allergic disease in recent decades. Proponents of the second theory argue that as changes in living conditions and disease patterns reduce the risk of parasites, the IgE system has been redirected to respond to other environmental toxins.

An example of evolutionary medicine that focuses on behavior—in particular, parental child care practices—involves the perplexing disorder Sudden Infant Death Syndrome (SIDS). Research on infant sleeping patterns suggests that there may be a link between the risk of SIDS and solitary sleep, and, conversely, infants sleeping with their mothers or parents (cosleeping) may be protective. In laboratory experiments, infants cosleeping with their mothers exhibited more regular breathing patterns that were synchronized with that of their mothers. They also had more arousals during the night and spent less time in deep sleep. Among breastfed infants, those sleeping near their mothers nursed more often and longer. In contrast, infants sleeping alone had more erratic breathing, deeper sleep, and less frequent breast-feeding, all factors that have been implicated in the etiology of SIDS (McKenna, Mosko, & Richard, 1999; Mosko, Richard, McKenna, & Drummond, 1996). Historically and cross-culturally, the cultural norm is for infants to sleep next to their parents, and, in fact, they spend much of their waking time carried by their mothers as well. This near universal pattern contrasts sharply with the modern Western practice of solitary infant sleep, often with the infant placed in a separate room.

Another area of investigation within evolutionary medicine relates to the effects of sedentariness and malnutrition of affluence (see Chapter 12, this volume). The abundance of food in industrialized societies contributes to obesity. Designed to enable people to survive in environments with fluctuating food supplies, the human body is equipped with efficient mechanisms for accumulating body fat and excellent defenses against the depletion of these energy stores. These biological mechanisms place people with access to an abundant food supply at risk for gaining excessive amounts of weight (Hill & Peters, 1998).

2. Settled Village (15,000 B.P.)

Roughly 10,000 to 15,000 years ago, a very different form of cultural adaptation evolved within the human species. In response to population pressure, people began to settle down in small villages to grow staple crops and raise livestock for consumption and production of raw materials. The shift to a sedentary population concentrated in a permanent community created a whole new set of ecological interactions with significant health consequences. With increased population density came problems of waste accumulation and the breeding of disease pathogens. Domestic animals living in close proximity to humans became a new reservoir for zoonotic diseases. Modifications to the natural environment for agricultural and settlement purposes altered ecological relationships among local plant and animal species, sometimes creating health hazards. Most important, the increased population density allowed the continuous transmission of communicable diseases in the population, marking the beginning of a long-term public health problem still with us today.

The first, and least complex, system of agriculture is called *horticulture.* Horticulture is a nonmechanized system that relies solely on human labor to cultivate plants in small garden plots. It is characterized by its reliance on human energy and a limited inventory of simple tools. Digging sticks and hoes are used rather than plows; neither irrigation nor terracing is employed. In traditional horticultural groups, food production is intended for home consumption rather than commercial sale. Each farmer controls his or her own production, and there is little interdependence between groups. Horticulture is still practiced by a large number of people throughout the world.

Today, many people relying on horticulture produce crops for sale and for home consumption are no longer independent. These farmers, sometimes called peasants, participate in a national and international marketplace. Peasants use the cash they obtain from these sales to pay tax or rent and buy necessities and luxury items produced outside their communities. Typically, the elite or wealthy members of the society rely on trade with peasants to enhance their own standard of living. This link between peasants and the elite is a key factor distinguishing peasants from more autonomous agriculturists. Most farmers in developing countries fit this pattern of the peasant economy.

As peasant societies shift from subsistence food crops to cash crops, their diets change radically, usually with deleterious effects. Typically, the most fertile land is used for the cash crop (e.g., coffee, peanuts, cotton, cocoa), thus lowering the production capacity of the land under food cultivation. The shift to a cash economy also means that a large part, if not the majority, of food is purchased instead of produced. The high cost of purchased protein-rich foods often makes them prohibitive, thereby forcing people into an affordable high-carbohydrate diet deficient in many vitamins and minerals as well as protein.

In contrast to the varied food consumption of foraging society, fewer types of foods made up the agrarian diet, and high-carbohydrate grains and root crops are the main staples. Because horticulturalists rely primarily on one or two crops, typically high in carbohydrates and low in protein, they are more vulnerable to episodic famines and nutritional deficiencies than are hunters and gatherers. A high-carbohydrate diet also affects the health of infants, children, and adults. Easy access to cereal grains enabled the production of soft baby pap foods that made earlier weaning of infants possible. Young children fed high-carbohydrate diets without adequate protein and specific nutrients are vulnerable to nutritional disorders such as kwashiorkor and micronutrient deficiencies. Dental caries become a problem.

Increased sedentarism in villages, coupled with the dietary changes noted previously, led to fertility increases and population growth. Menarche in young girls occurred earlier because of increased fat stores in youth. Shorter breast-feeding duration and early introduction of supplementary infant foods reduced the natural child-spacing anovulatory intervals among postpartum women. Children were born closer together in families, and larger numbers of children were desired to provide household agricultural labor. The net effects of these demographic changes were larger family size and population increase.

Case study: Culture change, malaria, and sickle cell disease. The most significant public health consequence of the Neolithic Revolution was the creation of more densely settled populations, which could sustain the presence of infectious diseases. In addition, agricultural land clearing often led to environmental changes that affected the concentration of disease vectors such as insects. One such case that is cited often as a classic example of such linkages is the introduction of agriculture in sub-Saharan Africa 2,000 years ago, including its impact on the emergence of more lethal forms of malaria and the evolution of sickle cell disease in that area.

Prior to the domestication of food crops, foraging groups subsisted through traditional hunting and gathering of edibles within the thick rain forests of the region. Then Bantu-speaking horticultural tribes began moving into the forest zones, gradually clearing the land for planting, and in the process removing the trees and shady canopy that had heretofore blocked out the tropical sun. The reduction of tree cover left many wet areas exposed to the warm rays of the sun, just the right conditions for breeding *Anopheles gambiae* mosquitoes, the vectors for a severe form of malaria. Although malaria was present in the preagricultural populations, it was the introduction of the strain caused by *Plasmodium falciparum* that led to markedly increased mortality from this parasitic disease. The proliferation of the mosquito vector, coupled with the closer proximity of more numerous human hosts, led quickly to a serious problem. Mortality from the disease was high, often killing 25% of infected individuals. Caused by a protozoan that reproduces in red blood cells, malaria not only causes extreme debilitation from fever and chills, it greatly increases the incidence of low birth weight, miscarriage, and stillbirths in pregnant women, and it is particularly lethal among young children.

The malaria situation might have had even more devastating consequences had it not been for the opportune presence of a genetic mutation in the population that protected heterozygous human hosts from the most devastating effects of the disease. The anomaly in question is the abnormal hemoglobin condition we know today as the sickle cell trait. Unlike normal hemoglobin (A), sickle cell hemoglobin (S) molecules cannot carry oxygen well and tend to clump together and distort the red blood cells into their characteristic "sickle" shape. Individuals with the sickle cell gene produce fewer red blood cells that allow Plasmodium organisms to complete their full life cycle, so these people are spared the most severe effects of malaria.

Because human beings are born with a pair of chromosomes for each gene (one from each parent), this makes it possible to have three different hemoglobin combinations in the population (AA, AS, and SS). In the normal form (AA), individuals do not have impaired red blood cells but they remain vulnerable to malaria. In the heterozygous form (AS), the sickle cell trait remains recessive yet still confers significant immunity to malaria, and the homozygous form (SS) leads to sickle cell anemia and a short life expectancy. Thus, the heterozygote has selective advantage over both homozygous forms of the gene. In heavy malaria zones, a "balanced polymorphism" between the two genes has evolved within the population, so that the proportion of each hemoglobin type is maximally advantageous for survival of the group.

Thus, what began as a large-scale culture change in Africa had profound biological repercussions involving complex disease-genetic adaptations. The social ecology of malaria in Africa illustrates dramatically the interaction of physical environment and culture in the production of disease patterns. Yet, the story has a more recent chapter that highlights the consequences of other social changes for the sickle cell trait. The forced migration of African slaves to the New World has led to a situation in which, in North America today, the sickle cell gene persists in the African American population in a setting where malaria is now eradicated and the genetic anomaly confers no health advantages, only serious risks. Homozygous sickle cell individuals, like their African counterparts, suffer anemia and a high risk of early death. Heterozygous "carriers," on the other hand, face discrimination in employment opportunities within occupations requiring high altitude or physically demanding work. They also face difficult fertility decisions when the risk of conceiving a sickle cell child is present (Reese & Smith, 1997).

3. Preindustrial Cities (1200-1700 C.E.)

The public health problems that first emerged in settled village life became intensified in preindustrial cities as a result of even denser populations in urban areas. The Middle Ages are marked by the demands of food, water, shelter, and waste management, as even larger numbers of people had to live together in confined spaces. For the first time, pollution became a serious public problem. Food security, water supply, and sanitation became a challenge for local municipalities, as the state increasingly assumed responsibility for social welfare. This was also the age of exploration, and expanded trade contacts with the outside world introduced new diseases into European populations. Many infectious diseases reached the endemic state in medieval societies, with constant transmission among new hosts. Devastating epidemics also coursed through the population regularly during this age of the great pandemics. The Great Plague alone wiped out one third of the world's population in the 14th century.

Focus: Early public health practices. Organized public health actions have roots in the ancient cities of Greece and Rome. There, under the authority of government regulation, complex systems of water supply and waste disposal were built and operated to meet the municipal needs of urban populations. An awareness of the concept of community health was evident in the early medical texts, most prominently in the Hippocratic book *Airs, Waters and Places.* This classic work outlines the environmental conditions believed to affect human health at that time, most notably the noxious vapors emitted from fetid swamps and marshes, a view sometimes described as the *miasma theory of disease*. The book also introduced the notions of *endemic* and *epidemic* disease and laid out guidelines for public health practice that remained largely unchanged until the end of the 19th century.

During the Middle Ages (500-1500), understanding of health and disease was closely intertwined with religious dogma. When a person became ill, the misfortune was attributed to moral or spiritual transgression, a form of punishment from God. Likewise, epidemics were assumed to manifest the wrath of the deity hurled down on people for their depraved and evil ways. However, it was believed that the human body, the vessel of the soul, could be fortified against the work of the Devil by hygienic practices. Efforts to promote community health, too, were common in medieval cities, particularly the enforcement of codes designed to keep the waterways clean and prevent the accumulation of waste. A huge amount of refuse was produced in the preindustrial cities, which often housed livestock within their borders, and where all food and material goods were prepared from raw materials. Dirt streets thick with mud, trash, animal dung, household sewage, rotting food waste, and foul-smelling water were commonplace. Marketplaces were particularly important centers for the enforcement of sanitation measures, such as disposal of rotten food and contaminated goods.

Among the diseases that menaced the population were bubonic plague, tuberculosis, typhus, diphtheria, leprosy, smallpox, measles, influenza, anthrax, and scabies (Rosen, 1993). Organized responses to two of these diseases, leprosy and plague, helped shape the medieval emergence of a basic public health strategy—the use of isolation and quarantine. The Christian church took the lead in the isolation of lepers, based on scriptural prescriptions to avoid the contagious impurity of spiritually unclean, diseased persons. Lepers were cast out of their communities to protect the healthy members and forced to live in segregated areas outside the cities. They were required to wear special identifying clothing and to announce their approach to other persons.

Efforts to protect cities from plague, on the other hand, led to the institution of quarantine. First noted in mid-14th century Venice, the practice consisted of a time-limited sequestering of people and goods suspected of being infected. Ships coming into the harbor from Asia, believed to be the source of plague, were kept at bay for an interim to allow the sick to die. Persons who came in contact with a plague victim were quarantined for 2 weeks in their homes or special facilities. Later, the period of sequester was extended to 30 days, then 40 days, the latter being the Italian derivative of the term "quarantine." Organized efforts involving observation stations, isolation hospitals, and disinfection procedures laid the groundwork for this public health practice, which remains important today.

4. *Industrial Cities (1750-1950 C.E.)*

The Industrial Revolution transformed human society in dramatic ways, with profound repercussions both life-saving and hazardous to health. Many forces underlie the complex changes involved in the transformation process, including the mechanization of work, the emergence of the factory, mass production of goods and services, increasing urbanization, rapid transportation, and the enlarged role of government in public welfare. European colonization of the New World, Africa, and other areas laid the groundwork for present-day geopolitical issues. The modern era brought the demise of feudalism, the promise of human progress through technological innovation, the advent of Western medicine, and improvements in the standard of living and the life expectancy of the population.

Urban life was still fraught with the ongoing problems of food, water, shelter, and sanitation, which only intensified with the growth of large cities and metropolitan areas. Epidemics remained common, and endemic diseases held on tenaciously. Added to this were new sources of pollution from industrial wastes unregulated by government legislation, now contaminating air and land as well as water. Beginning in the 19th century, however, the sanitary reform movement in Europe sparked the beginning of organized public health efforts to improve health. Improvements in living conditions, not the emergence of scientific medicine as is sometimes assumed, accounted for most of the decline in mortality that began during this period. Most important, infant and child mortality from infectious diseases declined, improving overall life expectancy. As people began to live longer as well, chronic diseases emerged as the major public health problems.

Focus: Cholera epidemics of the 19th century. By the 19th century, the major cities of Europe and North America had been transformed by industrialization into teeming centers of commerce and manufacturing, home to large populations of factory workers, merchants, and tradesmen. Sanitary and living conditions in the cities had improved dramatically from medieval times, with organized waste disposal services and access to drinking water from municipal pumps. Such improvements made a significant impact on the morbidity and mortality of the urban residents. It was an era of enlightened thinking and optimism about addressing social problems through progress and reason. Officials believed that the health of the populace could be protected through environmental controls and healthful living conditions. The prevailing explanations of disease continued to be miasma theory and contagionism, with the corollary that people living under oppressive conditions (poverty, crowded housing, overwork, inadequate diet, and intemperance and immorality) were especially vulnerable to the deleterious effects of miasma and contagion. Outbreaks of infectious disease were controlled through public health measures such as isolation of the sick, quarantine, and hygienic procedures.

Against this backdrop, the cholera epidemics of the 19th century in Europe and the United States caused great consternation because the disease did not conform to prevailing views of contagion. A swift-acting bacterial infection spread by water contaminated with human feces, cholera causes severe diarrhea, dehydration, and death in a large percentage of its victims. Most perplexing was the fact that the epidemics affected diverse and geographically dispersed populations, including middle-class neighborhoods and communities far removed from miasmatic conditions. Moreover, traditional efforts to control the epidemic such as quarantine of vessels and seaports seemed to have little impact on its spread.

The cholera riddle challenged medical thinking and led to the physician John Snow's famous epidemiologic studies of the London public water supply. He was able to show that cases of cholera were highest among people whose drinking water derived from the most polluted sections of the Thames River. In particular, his investigation of the Broad Street pump provided confirmation of this theory that cholera was transmitted through water infested with the excreta of cholera victims. He published his thesis in an 1849 pamphlet titled *On the Mode of Communication of Cholera* (Rosen, 1993). He also showed that cholera could be transmitted from person to person through soiled hands, food, and clothing. His ideas were accepted by some people and repudiated by others. However, in 1883, Koch successfully isolated and cultivated the cholera pathogen, *Vibrio cholera*, proving the correctness of Snow's ideas. The discovery of waterborne diseases led to important improvements in sewage disposal and control of water pollution in the late 19th century.

5. Postindustrial Society (1950-present)

Following the end of World War II, tremendous changes took place in the industrial regions of the world. Improvements in sanitation, disease prevention, medical care, and overall quality of life have reduced mortality at all ages. Most of the infectious diseases that contributed to mortality in the past have been controlled by large-scale immunization programs and an array of antibiotic drugs (although some are reemerging). People are living longer and healthier lives, and the health needs of elderly people have emerged as a new public health concern (see Chapter 14, this volume). Chronic degenerative diseases have replaced infectious diseases as the main health problems, although the AIDS epidemic of the late 20th century dispelled the notion that global pandemic diseases were a thing of the past.

Pollution from industrial manufacturing and massive reliance on automobile transportation continue to pose threats, but government regulation of waste and emissions is much tighter than before. Maintaining an adequate and safe water supply is an increasingly troublesome challenge for local and regional jurisdictions. We are running out of space for disposal of solid waste, and toxic chemicals threaten our land and waterways. In addition, we now live in the Atomic Age, in which radioactive contamination is a serious risk, not to mention the possibility of mass destruction from nuclear weapons.

Our extremely sedentary lifestyle, coupled with a diet that is high in fat and low in fiber, has contributed substantially to the chronic disease burden of our times, including obesity, cardiovascular disease, and diabetes. Tobacco use constitutes a major threat to health, either directly or indirectly contributing to the leading causes of death such as lung, breast, and other cancers; heart disease; stroke; and chronic obstructive pulmonary disease. Mental illness and substance abuse are highly prevalent. Accidents and violent behavior are rampant, accounting for major proportions of deaths in certain age groups. Chronic stress and an unrelenting accelerated pace of life take their toll on the emotional and physical well-being of the population.

Industrialization turned agriculture into a large-scale business enterprise requiring large amounts of capital and energy. It relies heavily on fossil fuels rather than human labor, making it energy-intensive and technologically complex. For example, in the United States, more than 500 million gallons of gasoline are used annually to move fresh vegetables and produce to market, and 1.3 billion gallons are needed to move manufactured food products from processors to warehouses and supermarkets. Many scientists question the ability of intensive agriculture to feed the world's population without damaging the earth's ability to produce food for future generations. Industrialized agriculture also relies heavily on mechanical equipment, chemicals, and a complex system of food distribution. Chapter 12 discusses in greater detail the effects of industrial food systems on diet and nutritional status.

The same sociocultural influences that contribute to our sedentary lifestyle and high rates of obesity also make us highly reliant on vehicular transportation to get about in our daily lives. In the next section, we highlight some of the public health consequences of widespread automobile transportation, particularly resulting from the high rate of motor vehicle accidents.

Focus: Motor vehicle injuries and deaths. Motor vehicle crashes are the leading cause of injury and death in the United States and the third leading cause of significant years of life lost (Christoffel & Gallagher, 1999). Motor vehicle crashes are also the leading cause of death in American men under the age of 21 (Gillert, 1999). In 1995, more than 42,000 people in the United States died in motor vehicle crashes, making the traffic accident fatality rate higher than that for suicide, homicide, and all other types of accidents combined (NCHS, 1999). Although most of these deaths occur among motorcyclists, automobile, and truck occupants, thousands of pedestrians and bicyclists are also killed or seriously injured by motor vehicles each year.

Death rates from motor vehicle crashes vary by age, gender, ethnicity, and income. The highest fatality rates are found among boys and men aged 15 to 24 years of age. People in this age group are three times more likely to die in motor vehicle crashes than are girls and women their age. Elderly people are also at increased risk; due to their increased fragility, they are more likely to die in motor vehicle accidents than are younger people. Also, more people die from traffic injuries in rural areas than in cities or suburban communities (Christoffel & Gallagher, 1999). With respect to ethnicity, the highest death rates from motor vehicle injuries are experienced by Native Americans, followed by whites, blacks, and Asians (National Committee for Injury Prevention and Control, 1989). Whites have the highest death rates for motorcycle injuries, but Native Americans have higher death rates as motor vehicle occupants and pedestrians. Although the age-specific fatality rates for Hispanics is similar to that for whites, a higher percentage of Hispanics are killed at younger ages than of other ethnic groups (Sainz & Saito, 1997). The death rate also varies inversely with per capita income: People with higher incomes are less likely to die than those with lower incomes.

Historically, motor vehicles caused injuries and deaths long before automobiles were used widely. The first recorded incident of a motor vehicle death occurred in 1899, when a 68-year-old pedestrian was struck by a passing car in New York City. By the next decade, automobiles caused more deaths than the horse and buggy. Between 1910 to 1985, more than 2.5 million people died in motor vehicle crashes—more than the number of people killed in all of the nation's wars combined (National Committee for Injury Prevention and Control, 1989).

As with other widespread public health problems, a variety of factors contribute to traffic fatalities. The move toward lighter-weight, smaller vehicles to conserve fuel has created vehicles that are not as safe as larger, heavier ones. Many people do not properly maintain their vehicles, further increasing their chances of being involved in a fatal accident. In a society that enjoys a continuous stream of visual and auditory stimulation from advertising and new forms of technology, it is not surprising that speeding and other dangerous driving maneuvers are common. Other driving habits also place people at increased risk, such as the practice of carrying people in the back of pick-up trucks, especially common among the poor, rural, or immigrant populations. However, driving while intoxicated is the most serious problem; two fifths of all motor vehicle deaths are alcohol-related (Christoffel & Gallagher, 1999).

One of the most popular conceptual frameworks for understanding and preventing deaths from motor vehicle and other types of injuries is the Haddon Matrix (Haddon, 1980). Haddon developed a nine-cell matrix that classifies factors relating to an injury by the phase of injury (pre-event, event, and post-event) and the type of factor (those relating to the victim, the vector, and the environment). Examples of factors that affect motor vehicle accident fatality rates during each phase are listed in Table 2.5.

Public health professionals have attempted to lower the injury rate in this country through a combination of consumer education, policy development, and improved engineering strategies. For many years, professionals believed that most injuries were due to human error and, thus, relied heavily on consumer education to improve driving skills. Although concern shifted to traffic laws and conditions in the 1920s and 1930s, most changes were not introduced until the 1950s.

Today, educational messages promoting seat belt use and discouraging people from driving while intoxicated are commonplace. However, public health professionals have had greater success by developing new laws (e.g., stiff penalties for driving while intoxicated, mandatory seat belt laws) and enforcement mechanisms (sobriety checkpoints), working with car manufacturers to improve the engineering of motor vehicles (e.g., airbags, modified front ends), and improving road design. Unfortunately, one effective measure, the reduction of speed limits, has been reversed in many areas, accompanied by a 40% increase in serious injuries and a 20% increase in traffic fatalities (Barss, Smith, Baker, & Mohan, 1998).

Other strategies for decreasing traffic injuries that could be used more effectively include high taxation of alcohol, large registration fees for hazardous modes of transportation, redesign of urban spaces, increasing the age of licensure, establishing curfew laws to restrict teenage driving, and establishing other restrictions for driver's licenses (Barss et al., 1998). Even with these measures, it is unlikely that motor vehicle transport will cease to be a major contributor to morbidity and mortality in the United States. As long as Americans remain dependent on automobiles, trucks, and motorcycles, motor vehicle injuries and deaths will demand the attention of public health professionals.

TABLE 2.5   The Haddon Matric for Motor Vehicle Injuries

Type of Factor

Phase	Personal	Vehicle	Physical and Social Environment
Pre-Event (Factors that influence whether an event occurs)	Alcohol consumption, driving skills, eyesight and motor coordination, compliance with traffic laws	Quality and condition of tires, brakes, headlamps, etc.; load characteristics, ease of control	Road conditions, lighting, signage and signalization, speed limits, enforcement mechanisms (e.g., sobriety checkpoints), attitudes about drinking and driving
Event (Factors that influence whether an event results in injury)	Seat belt use, physical condition (e.g., bone density)	Weight and height of vehicle; design and condition of seat belts, air bags, and child constraints; load containment	Guard rails, recovery areas, type of road surface, roadside embankments, speed limits, laws and attitudes about safety belt use
Post-Event (Factors that influence the severity of the injury's consequences)	Age, physical condition (e.g., smoking and lung capacity)	Emergency kit	Response time and skill level of emergency medical service personnel, support for trauma care facilities, training of EMS personnel

SOURCE: Adapted from the National Committee for Injury Prevention and Control (1989) and Haddon (1980).

44

CONCLUSION

Taking a historical perspective on population and disease, as we have done in the foregoing chapter, enlarges our understanding of the complex interaction of human culture and social organization with the technological and physical environment in shaping disease patterns and societal responses to health threats. Population dynamics underpin demographic features that affect disease epidemiology, nutrition, and reproduction. Classic public health concerns, such as waste disposal, water supply, food security, and control of infectious diseases emerged with the first demographic transition, the shift from foraging society to settled village life and food growing. These issues remain important today, as do new problems created by the processes of industrialization and urbanization. Although technological developments have enabled profound advances in medicine and areas such as food production, technology also has created new health risks. Contemporary industrial nations face challenges posed by high rates of injury, violence, and chronic disease.

There are many lessons to be learned from human history, both in the general sense of understanding issues within a larger time frame and more specifically through specialized areas of study such as evolutionary medicine. Knowing where we have come from can help us envision the constellation of old and new problems that will encompass the public health agenda of the 21st century.

3

Social Epidemiology

The core discipline of public health is *epidemiology*, the study of disease patterns in defined populations. Epidemiologists investigate the distribution of health conditions across time, space, and social groups, analyzing factors associated with the incidence and prevalence of disease. *Incidence* is defined as the number of new cases of illness occurring within a certain time period, usually per 100,000 persons over a year's time, and *prevalence* refers to the total number of cases in a population at a particular time. Epidemiological research seeks to identify the factors associated with the causes or etiology of disease, which often are referred to as *risk factors*. For example, currently recognized risk factors for heart disease include genetic predisposition, diet, use of alcohol and tobacco, exercise habits, and distribution of body fat.

The aims of epidemiologic research in public health are usually very pragmatic. By identifying correlates of disease, studies can be designed to test hypotheses about causal mechanisms, which then can guide the design of interventions to prevent illness or reduce the burden of disease. Knowledge of epidemiologic patterns is also useful in planning health services and formulating public health policies to meet the needs of various populations (Friis & Sellers, 1999).

Social epidemiology is a more recently developed subfield concerned with the social characteristics or psychosocial risk factors associated with patterns of disease within and across populations (Berkman, 1981; Cassel, 1976). Even newer is the field of behavioral epidemiology, which focuses on the specific behaviors that contribute to the etiology of disease (Kolbe, 1988). Although social epidemiologic research often poses questions about differences in morbidity and mortality by gender, age, socioeconomic status (SES), and ethnicity, behavioral epidemiology usually targets lifestyle factors such as sleep habits, stress management, risk taking, and other health-related behavior. In this chapter, we use the more general term social epidemiology to include behavioral studies.

Some of the most common factors investigated as independent (etiologic) variables in social epidemiology include sociodemographic characteristics (e.g., age, education, income, occupation), cultural traits (ethnicity, religion), behavior patterns (diet, exercise), and social environmental factors (family structure, neighborhood, racism). Dependent or health outcome variables studied, on the other hand, often include measures of morbidity, mortality, incidence, and prevalence, usually expressed as a rate or ratio. Whereas the foregoing variables typically are disease-specific, more generalized health indicators such as overall mortality and life expectancy are also used. Health status measures sometimes include quality of life variables, such as ability to function in everyday life, and include indicators such as loss of workdays due to illness. Finally, risk behaviors such as looking at the predictors of smoking or seat belt use also can be studied as dependent variables.

CASE STUDY: THE YOUTH RISK BEHAVIOR SURVEILLANCE SYSTEM

Many of the leading causes of death and disability in adults are linked to behavior patterns acquired early in life. Much evidence shows that a limited number of these behaviors contribute markedly to today's major killers. They include tobacco use, unhealthy diet, inadequate physical activity, substance use, unsafe sexual activity, and behaviors that increase risk of violence or injury. Until the 1990s, little was known about the prevalence of these health-risk behaviors among young people. The Youth Risk Behavior Surveillance System (YRBSS) was initiated in 1991 to provide systematic information on specific health-related practices among young people aged 15 to 24 years. Developed by the Centers for Disease Control and Prevention (CDC) in collaboration with federal, state, and private-sector organizations, this initiative involves annual national, state, and local school-based surveys.

There are five broad purposes of the YRBSS:

- Determine the prevalence and age of initiation of health-risk behaviors.
- Focus the nation and relevant agencies on specific health-risk behaviors of young people.
- Assess whether health-risk behaviors increase, decrease, or remain the same over time.

- Provide comparable national, state, and local data.
- Monitor progress toward achieving national health and education goals.

To illustrate some of the findings of the surveillance system, consider the 1997 data for marijuana and cocaine use among high school students (CDC, 1998). Among all high school students in Grades 9 to 12, 47.1% had used marijuana during their lifetime, and 26.2% had used it during the previous month. For cocaine use, the lifetime use rate was 8.2%, and recent use was 3.3%. Male and Hispanic students were significantly more likely than black or white students to report current cocaine use.

State and local health and education officials can use the YRBSS data in several ways. They can set program objectives, monitor progress toward goals, create awareness of risks, promote school health education curricula, and support the need for funding intervention programs. For example, several states have used the data to improve teacher training programs, and others have designed comprehensive plans targeted at specific problems such as sexually transmitted diseases or drug use. Researchers also can access the data to conduct more refined analyses of psychosocial determinants of health-risk behavior.

THE CAUSALITY CONTINUUM

In Chapter 1, we presented two general frameworks for conceptualizing social and behavioral factors in health—the Social Ecology of Health Model and the Health Impact Model. Here, we introduce a third general framework—the Causality Continuum—which is particularly relevant for social epidemiologic research. Borrowing the terminology of social science research methods, the Social Ecology of Health Model can be seen as a kind of "cross-sectional" or synchronic view of interacting factors, and the Health Impact Model can be described as a more diachronic representation of the same phenomena. In contrast, the Causality Continuum (see Figure 3.1) is based on differing degrees of directness of effect for various etiologic factors affecting health. Variables that have a close, direct influence on health and illness are considered *proximate* in their effect, whereas *distal* variables are more removed and affect problems more indirectly, that is, through the linkages and pathways of *intermediate* and ultimately proximate variables. Proximate variables have the most direct effects on biological processes or situational events that precipitate ill health or other undesirable outcomes. Distal variables, on the other hand, derive from the macrolevel sociocultural and environmental context, and they often are described as background factors that predispose people to greater or lesser health risks. Intermediate variables can serve as buffers for distal factors, thereby mitigating their potential impact, or they can operate as intervening variables that channel the negative influence of distal factors through specific mechanisms.

Various categories of risk factors can be positioned at different points along the continuum, depending on the relative directness or indirectness of their impact on the health outcome under investigation. Of course, etiology never involves such a simplified linear chain of causality, and current epidemiologic models use more complex schema, such as the "web of causation" (Duncan, Gold, Basch, & Markellis, 1988) and the "scaffolding and bush" configuration (Krieger, 1994). Here, we intentionally use a simple model to highlight the relative directness of effects of different categories of factors. As noted previously, distal determinants include macrolevel sociodemographic and ecological factors, such as urban residence, poverty, or educational level. These kinds of factors are sometimes discussed as *structural* or *fundamental* causes, because they operate through large-scale social structural processes that affect large groups of people in complex ways (Link & Phelan, 1995). Intermediate determinants of illness correspond to what we would categorize as local or community-level risk factors, such as occupation, social support, and health care resources. Proximate

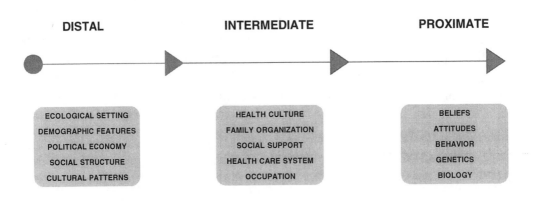

Figure 3.1. Causality Continuum Model

determinants, on the other hand, tend to fall mainly in the realm of behavioral epidemiology and involve specific activities linked to biological mechanisms (e.g. eating, sleeping, use of drugs).

When we consider the use of models like the Causality Continuum for planning prevention programs, it is worth noting that the further one moves away from the proximate factors, and the closer one moves toward the distal determinants, the more difficult it is to intervene in the chain of causality. The reason for this is that structural determinants tend to have very low changeability. For example, factors such as urban residence, SES, and gender, at the population level are, practically speaking, not amenable to change. Intermediate factors tend to have greater modifiability, but the easiest risk factors to change are behavioral patterns involving individual choice. This is one reason why many public health interventions focus on individual behavior change. It also helps explain why so few programs focus on changing the social conditions that are the fundamental causes of illness.

To illustrate how the Causality Continuum model can be applied to a specific health problem, we turn to the case of breast cancer. In the United States, incidence rates for breast cancer have been increasing at a rate of nearly 2% per year since 1973. Better detection through improved screening accounts for some of this increase, but the specific causes of the rise in breast cancer remain unclear. On the distal end of the causality continuum, we note that high SES is associated with an increased incidence of breast cancer (in contrast to most other diseases). Possible mediating factors for SES might include delayed marriage and therefore late age at first full-term pregnancy, breast-feeding experience, and fat consumption affecting age at menarche and hormone levels. The larger physical and social environment, also distal in level, includes technological aspects that affect type of and age at exposure to exogenous carcinogens through the workplace, community, and home (intermediate). A variety of socially mediated factors ultimately may affect dietary patterns, which can have a more proximate effect on disease risk.

CASE STUDY: APPLYING THE PRECEDE MODEL OF PROGRAM PLANNING

As noted in the previous section, selection of risk factors as focuses of public health interventions entails some form of appraisal of the significance, causal linkage, and changeability of relevant etiologic determinants. Health promoters use a variety of approaches to this assessment task; the most widely applied framework is the Precede Model (Green & Kreuter, 1991). Originally developed as a health education planning model, it was later expanded to include both program design and evaluation and renamed Precede-Proceed. In this section, we focus on the original Precede Model, which provides a systematic approach to selecting risk factors for intervention.

Through a series of steps, the Precede model guides the planner through a process of identifying behavioral and environmental determinants for the focal health problem. A core feature of the behavioral and environmental diagnosis phase is the appraisal of the *importance* and *changeability* of different etiologic factors. Determination of importance includes both the strength of the causal effect (how big of an impact it has on the problem) and the prevalence of the factor (what proportion of the population is affected by the risk). Changeability refers to the degree to which the factor is capable of being changed. Many distal factors, in terms of the Causality Continuum, as well as some proximate determinants, are not amenable to change. For example, ethnicity and gender (distal factors), and age and genetic predisposition (proximate factors), cannot be changed. The goal of Precede is to prioritize behavioral and environmental risk factors according to importance and changeability.

The next phase of Precede is the educational and organizational diagnosis, in which the etiologic determinants of the risk factors themselves are specified to guide program design. This process is analogous to behavioral epidemiology. The educational and organizational diagnosis categorizes risk determinants into *predisposing, reinforcing,* and *enabling factors.* Predisposing factors include knowledge, attitudes, beliefs, values, and perceptions that either support or inhibit a behavior. Reinforcing factors are things that occur after a behavior that reward it or provide some kind of incentive to continue it. Enabling factors are antecedents to behavior that facilitate action, such as having the economic resources to perform an activity or having access to health services. The goal of the intervention itself, then, is to influence the predisposing, reinforcing, and enabling factors in a specific way so that behavioral and environmental risks are reduced.

A good illustration of Precede is offered by its application to the design of a program to reduce noninsulin-dependent diabetes mellitus (NIDDM) in a Canadian aboriginal community (Daniel & Green, 1995). Like other Native American populations, the Okanagan Indian Band, located in the interior of British Columbia, has an elevated morbidity and mortality rate for NIDDM compared to the general population. Apart from the genetic predisposition shared with other native people, the most important risk factors are obesity, physical inactivity, and improper diet. Although all three risk factors may be interrelated, research suggests that exercise has an independent protective effect against diabetes. Other risk factors include female gender, older age, and family history of the disease.

To select specific behavioral and environmental risk factors associated with the prevention and control (treatment) of NIDDM in the population, the researchers systematically rated a list of potential factors according to importance and changeability (see Table 3.1). They did not consider family history, age, and gender, because these were not amenable to change. The results of the diagnosis identified exercise and dietary practices, as well as treatment behaviors (e.g., decreasing missed appointments) that qualified as focuses for intervention. The diagnosis also identified a number of environmental factors that facilitate effective treatment, including culturally sensitive education programs and increased availability of traditional foods.

The next step involved identifying predisposing, enabling, and reinforcing factors for each priority intervention focus. For example, for the behavioral priority to promote regular physical activity, a predisposing attitude is that exercise is important to health in general, an enabling factor is the opportunity for exercise in daily living, and a reinforcing factor is peer influence supporting physical activity. The systematic appraisal of risk factors and their influencing determinants allowed the planners to develop specific objectives with corresponding program components.

EXCESS MORTALITY AMONG MINORITY GROUPS

Many minority and socially disadvantaged groups experience a higher mortality rate than is found in the general population. The concept of *excess mortality* refers to the difference between the number of deaths actually observed in a minority group and the number of deaths that would have occurred in that group if it experienced the same death rates for each age and gender group as the majority population. Figure 3.2 graphically depicts the ratio of minority to white death rates for ages 1 to 65 and older in 1997. What is interesting about these data are the contrasting patterns observed for different ethnic groups at different ages. At the youngest ages, African Americans and Native Americans have excess mortality, and Asian and Pacific Islanders are advantaged. In young adulthood, Hispanic mortality is notably high compared to excess mortality at other ages. African Americans have the highest overall mortality across the life span, with the exception of the older age cohort, which is slightly below that of whites. Likewise, elderly Hispanic and Native American populations have lower mortality than do whites. An interesting phenomenon called the *crossover effect* is observed in mortality trends, in which disadvantaged minority populations that fare poorly at younger ages experience relative mortality advantages in relation to the refer-

TABLE 3.1   Application of the Precede Model to Noninsulin-Dependent Diabetes Mellitus in a Canadian Aboriginal Community

Behavioral or Environmental Factor	Importance		Changeability		Total Score
	Causal Effect	Prevalence	Evidence	Theory	
Behavior priority					
Maintain or attain a reasonable level of regular physical activity					
Predisposing					
Regular exercise may prevent or control diabetes (belief)	3	3	3	3	12
Exercise is important to health (attitude)	2	2	3	3	10
Lack of exercise increases risk of diabetes (perception)	2	2	2	3	9
Regular exercise is the right way to live (value)	3	3	2	1	9
Enabling					
Flexible goal-setting to increase adherence to exercise (new skills)	3	3	2	3	11
Opportunities for exercise in daily living (availability)	2	3	2	3	10
Social networks and resources supportive of physical activities	2	2	2	2	8
Forms of exercise can be adapted to individuals' lifestyles (tailoring)	1	3	2	2	8
Reinforcing					
Quality of, and satisfaction with, feedback from health professionals	3	3	3	2	11
Satisfaction from participation in development of exercise programs	2	2	3	3	10

Factor					
Congruence between knowledge, exercise, and health benefits	1	1	3	3	8
Peer influences supporting physical activity (exercising with friends)	1	2	2	2	7

Environmental priority

Develop culturally sensitive education and control programs

Enabling

Factor					
Coalitions to lobby for intersectoral cooperation and alliances with external health and education resources	3	3	3	3	12
Skills in community organization, to develop and implement strategies for researching common goals	2	2	3	3	10
Develop environmental supports in the form of policies, regulations, and organizational arrangements for program sustainability	3	2	2	2	9
Skills to achieve consensus and understanding on priorities for collective action	2	2	2	2	8

SOURCE: Daniel and Green (1995), reprinted with permission from the American Diabetes Association.

Note: Key for ratings: 1 = low; 2 = moderate; 3 = high; maximum overall score is 12 points.

a. Importance is based on causal effect and prevalence; ratings of causal effect and prevalence are of the negative form of the factor stated.

b. Changeability reflects evidence and formal theory, in which ratings indicate supportive evidence and applicable formal theory.

ence majority in later years. Greater robustness of overall health among survivors of early health threats has been suggested as an explanation for this phenomenon.

Such variable trends in mortality patterns surely reflect social environmental conditions, in addition to biological factors. For example, high rates of accidents and injury among young adults contribute significantly to the excess mortality among Native Americans aged 15 to 24. The mortality advantage of some groups at older ages has been linked to *selective survival*, which hypothesizes that under conditions of social disadvantage, the more biologically robust individuals tend to avoid earlier health risks and survive to old age. Analysis of mortality trends for specific causes of death can reveal an even clearer picture of the social risks affecting particular populations. For example, the largest factor contributing to the

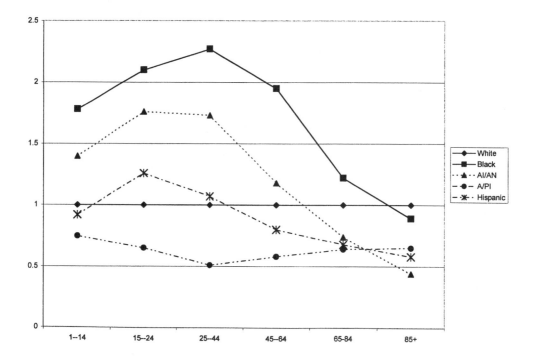

Figure 3.2. Ratio of Minority-White Death Rates Among Males Aged 1 to 65 and Older, 1997

SOURCE: *U.S. Department of Health and Social Services (1999b)*

NOTE: AI/AN = American Indian and Alaskan Native; A/PI = Asian and Pacific Islander.

excess mortality among African American boys and men is composed of homicide and unintentional injuries, reflecting the social context in which many young black men live. Recently, researchers also have argued for greater attention to the historical influences and ongoing racism and social discrimination in explaining the epidemiologic profile for African Americans.

POVERTY AND HEALTH

People who lack the money and material resources to meet the basic needs of living are said to live in poverty. Obviously, poverty can be defined only in relation to normative standards of living in a particular society. For example, in the United States, a family of four that had a total income of less than $16,700 in 1999 was considered to fall "below the poverty line." In Haiti, however, such a family income could provide a middle-class standard of living and would certainly meet basic living needs. Although acknowledging that deprivation is relative, it is worth noting that poverty is one of the most pervasive risk factors for ill health in all countries.

Despite the documented far-reaching health effects of poverty, however, the U.S. government does not routinely report health statistics by income level. For example, the National Center for Health Statistics provides periodic reports on mortality rates from all causes for the nation. These data are routinely broken down by age, race, and gender, but rarely by income or educational level. Although SES data are more difficult to obtain than basic demographics reported on death certificates, specialized surveys could be used to complement the vital statistics data by analyzing the impact of poverty, but such analyses are seldom performed. Consequently, racial disparities tend to be overemphasized and economic influences downplayed in official reports. In the absence of economic breakdowns, race becomes a proxy for SES, thereby reinforcing stereotypes about African Americans.

One reason for our society's reluctance to address the relation between poverty and health is our discomfort with social class differences (Dutton, 1987). We do not like to acknowledge openly the extreme differences in wealth that underlie many social problems. Instead, we substitute proxy measures of social disadvantage, such as race and ethnicity, and this practice tends to reinforce negative stereotypes of marginal groups.

The lack of good data on SES and health makes it difficult to formulate health policies that adequately address the effects of poverty (Farmer, 1999). For example, epidemiologic data document excess rates of HIV and AIDS among African

Americans and Hispanics. Closer analysis of intervening variables reveals that most of this excess is related to intravenous drug use in these populations. Drug use, in turn, has been linked to lack of opportunity for occupational and economic success in marginal populations, as well as perceptions of deprivation relative to the majority.

Research from industrial countries on the relation between life expectancy and income has revealed some interesting findings regarding the distribution of income within societies. Several cross-national comparative studies have demonstrated a robust, statistically significant relation between income inequality within a single society and its overall life expectancy rate, which is linked to mortality. Countries with a more egalitarian income distribution have a higher life expectancy than do countries in which there is a wide gap between the upper and lower income range (Wilkinson, 1992). Surprisingly, overall per capita income does not appear to affect life expectancy, so that in the developed world there is no linear relation between the wealth of a nation and mortality. Rather, health is adversely affected when the gap between "rich" and "poor" is large. The negative health effects of income inequality also are seen in rates of infant mortality. Among wealthy industrial countries, relative poverty within countries has a stronger impact on infant mortality than does variation in the level of economic development between countries. Moreover, public policies related to family welfare, such as medical care and family leave benefits, also affect infant mortality (Wennemo, 1993).

The intervening variables that may account for the impact of relative wealth on health are not entirely clear; however, some interesting hypotheses have been suggested. First, because of market forces, there is a tendency for the material infrastructure and organization of society to be geared to people close to the average income. For this reason, people with lower incomes are often unable to afford the goods and services that would allow them to manage day-to-day tasks without a lot of additional effort, which could affect health. Second, one's income must be adequate to maintain self-respect and to participate in the social life of a society in which most people are much better off. Consequently, poor people often skimp on food, heating, and even use of health services to maintain the publicly visible symbols of acceptability, such as clothing and participation in social activities. A related issue here is the notion of *financial stress* among both low- and middle-income people who constantly strive to support a costly "normative" lifestyle that is skewed toward the wealthier end of the income spectrum. Third, relative wealth deprivation has been shown to be socially isolating (Townsend, 1979), so that the health benefits of social support may be enjoyed less by lower-income groups. Fourth, relative poverty is widely understood to be a demeaning and devaluing experience that can affect one's sense of self-worth and, indirectly, health status. Taken together, these hypotheses suggest a relation between perceived relative deprivation and psychosocial stress, which contributes to ill health and mortality. Alternative hypotheses suggest the possible role of social ordering or "dominance status" within groups. Hierarchical position may have direct effects on physiological processes and neuroanatomic structures that may increase biologic vulnerability to disease (Adler et al., 1994).

FOCUS: SOCIOECONOMIC STATUS AND HEALTH

Public health professionals long have recognized the relation between SES and health. SES is one of the strongest and most consistent predictors of morbidity and premature mortality. Everywhere, poor people suffer disproportionately from most diseases and die younger than their wealthier counterparts. SES has been associated with infant mortality, cardiovascular disease (CVD), many types of cancer, arthritis, diabetes, and numerous infectious diseases. Particularly puzzling is the fact that this relation runs across the entire population, so that people who enjoy the greatest wealth live longer and experience lower rates of many diseases than do those in the middle class.

As early as the 1840s, Chadwick reported significant differences in the life expectancy of the gentry (36 years), tradesmen (22 years), and laborers and servants (16 years) (Committee for the Study of the Future of Public Health, 1992). More recently, four large population studies found similar health disparities between people in lower and upper socioeconomic brackets. The first Whitehall Study (Marmot, Shipley, & Rose, 1984) was conducted among British civil servants employed in white-collar jobs between 1930 and 1982. A follow-up study of these same employees—Whitehall Study II (Marmot et al., 1991)—examined these employees between 1985 and 1988. The Wisconsin Longitudinal Study (WLS) (Marks, 1996) studied men and women who graduated from Wisconsin high schools in 1957 and were followed until the early 1990s. The National Survey of Families and Households (NSFH) (Sweet, Bumpass, & Call, 1988) was conducted among a national sample of adults living in the United States, including people who were extremely poor. Despite differences in samples and methodologies, all four studies found a strong association between social position and mortality rates. In the first Whitehall Study, for example, mortality rates were three times higher among men working in the lowest civil service grades than among those in the highest classifications. More important, social differentials in mortality were discovered in most of the major causes of death. The follow-up study of these men revealed that socioeconomic differences in health persisted even into retirement (Marmot, Bobak, & Smith, 1995).

These four studies also documented significant differences based on SES and a variety of other health indicators, including self-reported health status, depression, and psychological well-being. For example, SES was strongly correlated with research participants' answers to a three-question self-esteem measure used in the NSFH, a question about finding "little meaning in life" in Whitehall II, and a seven-question purpose of life scale used in the WLS (Marmot, Ryff, Bumpass, Shipley, & Marks, 1997).

Although the association between SES and health status is well established, the factors at work in the relation are poorly understood. Why do people who live at the top of the socioeconomic ladder enjoy a longer and healthier life than those below them? How do income, occupation, and education—the major components of SES—affect health? A variety of answers to these questions have been vigorously debated. A brief summary of the most popular explanations follows.

Limited Resources

A common explanation points to the obvious health risks that accompany poverty. As a family's income drops, they have an increasingly difficult time obtaining clean, safe housing needed to maintain good health. Crowding, rat and insect infestation, leaky roofs, and lead paint are among the many health hazards associated with low-income housing. Poor people also have difficulty purchasing an adequate diet. In fact, notions of a "poverty line" date back to the turn of the century, when nutrition surveys revealed that no matter how wisely very poor families managed their budgets, they did not have enough purchasing power to consume an adequate diet. Since that time, many countries, including the United States, have calculated an income level, known as the *poverty threshold*, below which malnutrition eventually will result. This amount is adjusted for household size and then used to determine eligibility for federal assistance programs and to estimate poverty rates.

No one argues against the proposition that absolute deprivation leads to poor health. However, lack of resources only explains the relation between health and the social standing of people living on the lowest rungs of the SES ladder. If lack of material resources were the key factor, an income threshold would exist below which people would have poor health but above which there would be no detectable effect. However, this threshold does not exist. As mentioned previously, a gradient runs across the entire population, with people at each position better off than those immediately below them, and worse off than those immediately above them. It is easy to understand why someone in the middle of the SES scale has better health than someone at the bottom, but why is a corporate executive who makes $250,000 healthier than managers in the same organization who make $100,000?

To answer this question, we must consider other factors that affect health and may help to explain the gradient that exists between health and SES—for example, health selection, factors operating early in life, health care, health behavior, and the social ecology of inequality.

Health Selection

Another popular explanation is that health determines social position rather than the reverse—also known as the *health selection theory*. This theory posits that people who are unhealthy are less productive and drift down the socioeconomic gradient, and those who are healthier are more productive and migrate up. As people drift downward socially and economically, a disproportionate number of unhealthy people end up at the bottom.

This theory has received some support from studies of people with specific diseases, such as schizophrenia, and studies of children who are ill before their education has been completed who subsequently enter the labor market (Marmot et al., 1995; Wadsworth, 1986). Both groups are more likely to experience downward social mobility than their healthier counterparts. However, the effect of these cases is limited and does not account for the more general relation that exists in adulthood (Marmot et al., 1995; Wadsworth, 1986; West, 1991). As a result, this theory has largely rejected as the major cause of social inequities in health, forcing us to search further.

Factors Operating Early in Life

Another explanation posits that factors operating early in life, such as genetic and other biological factors, education and cultural advantages, and psychosocial factors affect both social standing and health status in later life. Known as the *indirect selection* theory, this explanation claims that the relation between SES and health status is actually an artifact of the other forces that affect them both.

It is difficult to test this hypothesis because it is so hard to separate early child factors from those operating in adulthood, and both types of factors may affect mortality and morbidity risk. Not surprisingly, little evidence has been accumulated to support this proposition. None of the four major studies described previously followed people from early childhood into adulthood and, therefore, could not test this theory directly; however, each study was able to control for measures of early childhood disadvantage to determine if it influenced the SES-health gradient. The Whitehall II study, for instance, found that the gradient did not change when the social background of parents was taken into account. The WLS found that the strength of the relation between health and SES was reduced, but only slightly, when parents' education, whether the person grew up in an intact family, and IQ measured in high school were controlled. Finally, the NSFH showed that the association between SES and mortality remained the same after parents' education and nonintact family composition during childhood were accounted for (Marmot et al., 1997).

Health Care

A third explanation for the SES-health gradient is differential access to health care between people in the different socioeconomic strata. In the United States, people who cannot afford health care are at a greater risk for a wide variety of health problems that could be treated, if not prevented all together. Early detection of cancer and other diseases, for example, greatly improves the odds of cure and extends survival time. Poor people are less likely than more affluent people to have health insurance and the means to pay for drugs and medical procedures not covered by their insurance policies.

Although this argument explains the difference between insured and uninsured people's health status, it, too, provides an insufficient explanation for the socioeconomic gradient that runs across the broader SES scale. How do we account for differences between insured people in the middle- and upper-income brackets? Can the rich really buy medical care that is so much better that it gives them lower morbidity and mortality than those with slightly less income and social standing? Most scholars do not think so.

Evidence suggesting that more is at work than differential access to health care coi ies from nations that offer their citizens universal access to health care yet still show the same SES-health gradient as found in the United States (Adler, Boyce, Chesney, Folkman, & Syme, 1997). The United Kingdom offers one of the best illustrations: During the 30 years after universal health care access was granted to British citizens, inequalities in health status actually widened.

Finally, this theory fails to account for socioeconomic differences that exist in rates of diseases not amenable to medical care, again suggesting that other factors are at work (Marmot et al., 1995).

Health Behavior

Another common argument is that poor people behave in ways that make them more likely to get sick and die than do affluent people. Advocates of this view point to well-known socioeconomic differences in rates of smoking, alcohol consumption, physical activity, seat belt use, fat intake, and other health behaviors that place the poor at greater risk than affluent people (Frankish, Milligan, & Reid, 1998). Again, no one would argue that health behaviors are not an important pathway between SES and health outcomes. But again, this explanation alone cannot account for the linear relation between SES and health status (Adler et al., 1997). In the Whitehall II study, for example, the strength of the relation between SES and health was reduced only slightly when smoking and other health behaviors were held constant. When looking just at nonsmokers or just at smokers, a gradient still existed between SES and health (Marmot et al., 1997).

The Social Ecology of Inequality

To explain the relation between SES and health, many scholars are now turning to an ecological model, one in which health status and social standing are linked to a combination of interrelated social, cultural, and psychological factors. Although each of the factors already mentioned plays a role in explaining this conundrum, other social, psychological, and environmental factors also must be taken into consideration.

An important additional factor is *relative deprivation*. When income disparities are pronounced and highly visible, citizens feel deprived relative to those who have more than they do. Even people who have abundant resources to meet their subsistence needs and maintain good health may feel resentful and frustrated when they cannot share the riches they see others enjoying. In societies like the United States that view competitive achievement and economic affluence as the result of personal qualities, relative deprivation also may lead to feelings of failure and hopelessness. Relative deprivation also may trigger hostility, depression, and other psychological reactions that adversely affect health. The impact of prolonged depression, stress, and hostility on disease vulnerability is now widely recognized. Although most people realize that those in the lowest SES brackets experience higher levels of stress and less support needed to cope with absolute deprivation, only recently have researchers begun to consider the impact that relative deprivation can have on health.

Support for the psychological effects of relative deprivation comes from studies of the relation between hypertension and ability to achieve a socially normative material style of life. Using cultural consensus analysis—a technique for measuring the degree to which individuals achieve in their own behavior a culturally shared model of lifestyle indicative of "success"—researchers (Dressler, Balieiro, & Dos Santos, 1998; Dressler, Bindon, & Neggers, 1998) found a strong association between the latter measure and arterial blood pressure among African Americans living in the southern United States and among Brazilians living in urban areas. The researchers described the observed level of lifestyle concordance as "cultural consonance." Interestingly, cultural consonance was a stronger predictor of hypertension than were conventional indicators of SES, including income, education, and occupation. The investigators interpret these findings as evidence that feelings of deprivation relative to cultural norms play a role in the link between poverty and health.

In addition to psychological responses associated with relative deprivation, the social environment responds in ways that affect health. In societies with wide gaps in income levels, people's comparison with others and their sense that they have failed to achieve enough can lead to discontent, distrust, and strained social relationships. The society becomes less cohesive and people have access to less social support—changes known to affect health adversely (Patrick & Wickizer, 1995). Relative deprivation also has been linked to another health hazard—violent crime (Kawachi, Kennedy, & Wilkinson, 1999). Meta-analyses of 34 studies of crime found that places with large income gaps experienced significantly higher crime rates than did more egalitarian communities (Wilkinson, 1998).

Further evidence that relative deprivation affects health status comes from studies comparing life expectancy and income distributions between and within nations and other geographical units. As one would expect, life expectancy is lower in poorer nations than in wealthier ones. However, once countries have attained a certain level of wealth (e.g., about $5,000 per capita in 1990), the relation between the absolute income level as measured by income or gross national product (GNP) per capita disappears. In more affluent countries, the size of the income gap replaces GNP as the predictor of life expectancy. Countries with large income disparities have shorter life expectancies than do more egalitarian countries (Wilkinson, 1996). Also, when changes in six nations' income disparity were examined (Wilkinson, 1992), Japan experienced both the greatest increase in equality of income dispersion and the greatest increase in life expectancy. In contrast, the United Kingdom experienced declining equity in income distribution and the smallest gains in life expectancy. Looking at the 50 states in the United States, Kawachi and Kennedy (1997) documented a strong association between mortality rates and income inequity. Americans living in relatively egalitarian states outlive citizens living in states with large income gaps.

Implications for Public Health Professionals

No one explanation can explain adequately the persistent and perplexing relation between SES and health. Most likely, multiple factors are at work, with different combinations exerting the most influence at different points along the gradient (Marmot et al., 1997). For the poorest families, inferior health status may be due to limited resources, an inability to purchase preventive or curative medical care, and increased stress associated with poverty and unhealthful lifestyles. In contrast, the health differentials between families in the middle and upper reaches of society may be largely a result of relative rather than absolute deprivation, with associated differences in stress, frustration levels, and social cohesiveness.

If health disparities result from multiple factors, public health professionals must be prepared to combat the problem with a multifaceted approach. Universal access to health care may be an attractive strategy, one that helps many uninsured families achieve better health status; however, it should not be seen as the only solution. Public health professionals also must be prepared to raise standards of living among the poor so that they can purchase adequate housing, a nutritious diet, and other essentials for healthy living. And they must be prepared to deal with more affluent citizens' perceptions of acceptable standards of living and their sense of well-being relative to others. To counter social disorganization, public health professionals should be familiar with community organizing approaches that allow them to strengthen social network ties, build trust, and increase communities' collective efficacy. Finally, public health professionals need to enact policies to reduce income inequality and to give citizens in all socioeconomic strata access to the resources needed for a long and healthy life.

HISPANICS AND THE EPIDEMIOLOGIC PARADOX

Somewhat contradictory to the foregoing discussion of the relation between poverty, social disadvantage, and poor health, the health status of Hispanic populations in the southwestern United States stands out as an anomaly. Mostly of Mexican origin, southwestern Hispanics have a sociodemographic profile much closer to that of African Americans than that of European Americans. Compared to the majority population, they are less wealthy and less educated, and they have linguistic and cultural differences that tend to marginalize their position in society. Despite these social disadvantages, for several decades it has been noted that the health profile of Mexican Americans appears to be comparable to, and in some cases better than, their Anglo counterparts. First noted in relation to mental health, this phenomenon has been called the Hispanic "epidemiologic paradox" (Markides & Coreil, 1986).

Supported by evidence on such key indicators as infant mortality, life expectancy, mortality from CVD, mortality from major types of cancer, and measures of functional health, the paradox remains a puzzle, although numerous explanations have been proposed to explain various findings. For example, the favorable infant mortality rates experienced by Hispanics have been linked to low incidence of prematurity and low birth weight in newborns (see the following sections). But these factors are also health outcomes, so the question remains why Hispanic mothers produce such healthy babies. Some propose that the high value placed on children and the strong tradition of care for pregnant and parturient women contribute to favorable birth outcomes in this ethnic group. For other health advantages, hypotheses posit the influence of cultural practices, family supports, selective migration, diet, and genetic heritage. Untangling the causal factors in such anomalous epidemiologic patterns can expand our understanding of the complex links between social factors and health. Investigations of situations in which you find people experiencing more positive outcomes than would be expected is sometimes referred to as *positive deviance analysis*. It contrasts with the more usual approach to deviance as a negatively sanctioned social problem (see Chapter 7, this volume).

CASE STUDY: INFANT MORTALITY AND LOW BIRTH WEIGHT

Infant mortality is generally considered one of the most sensitive indicators of the general health status of a population, and it is also reflective of societal-level standard of living. The *infant mortality rate* (IMR) is defined as the number of deaths among infants during the first year of life per 1,000 live births. In this chapter, we are concerned with cross-ethnic differences in IMRs and what such comparisons reveal about social and behavioral risk factors for this outcome. Figures 3.3 and 3.4 present data on rates of infant mortality and low birth weight for various ethnic groups in the United States during the 1990s. Low birth weight—weights of less than 2,500 grams or 5.5 pounds at birth—is the single greatest cause of infant mortality in the United States. Not surprisingly, then, the rate of both infant mortality and low birth weight is consistently highest for African Americans and is notably high compared to other ethnic groups. However, although infant mortality is high among Native Americans (American Indians and Alaskan Natives), their rates of low birth weight are comparable to those of whites, Hispanics, and Asian Americans.

Low birth weight, in turn, is heavily influenced by preterm delivery rates, which are also about twice as high among African Americans. Both preterm delivery and low birth weight can be reduced by early appropriate prenatal care, good maternal nutrition, and adequate weight gain. On the other hand, living in stressful neighborhoods, single-parent families, lack of social support, and high prevalence of drug use and HIV/AIDS increase the risk of preterm birth and low birth weight. But these structural factors are difficult to change, as already noted.

Not surprisingly, more recently, increased attention has been given to the role of bacterial vaginosis in increasing risk for preterm labor, and interventions based of prophylactic antibiotic treatment have gained interest (Paige, Augustyn, Adih, Witter, & Chang, 1998). This relates to the greater changeability of the more proximate factor of vaginal infection, but it also reflects core aspects of the culture of Western medicine, including reliance on (particularly pharmacologic) technology and an emphasis on individual-focused, single-cause, quick-fix treatment modalities (see Chapter 8, this volume).

Ironically, the United States has the best technology in the world to save the lives of premature babies, but it has the worst track record in preventing its occurrence. What is lacking is the political will to provide universal access to care,

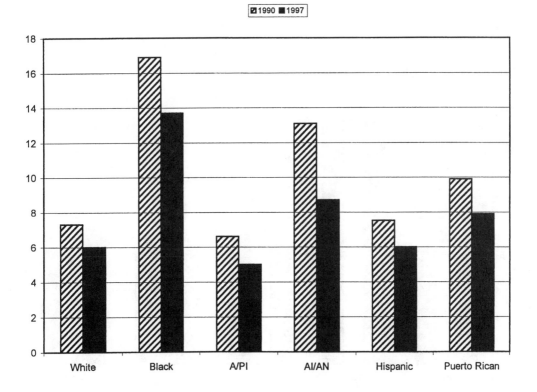

Figure 3.3. U.S. Infant Mortality Rates by Ethnicity of Mother

SOURCE: U.S. Department of Health and Human Services (1996).

understanding women's perceptions of prenatal care, the ability to motivate women to use maternal services, and helping women to avoid drug addiction. Nevertheless, noteworthy progress has been made in lowering infant mortality during the 1990s, and special initiatives have been sponsored at the federal and state level to reduce ethnic disparities in this important health indicator.

THE RISK FACTOR APPROACH: PERSONALITY AND CARDIOVASCULAR DISEASES

Personality

Each person is a combination of traits, talents, past experiences, qualities, and behaviors. Personality traits are styles of relating to and thinking about the

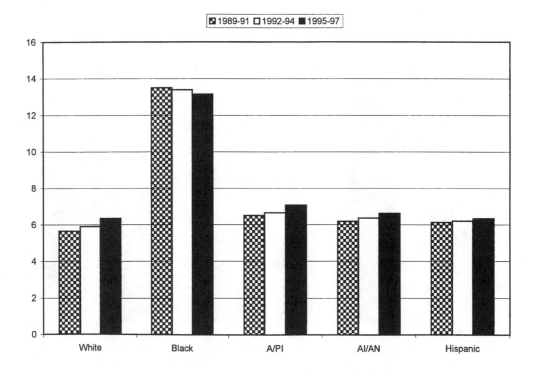

Figure 3.4. Percentage of Low Birth Weight Live Births in U.S. Ethnic Groups, 1997

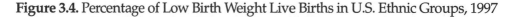

SOURCE: U.S. Department of Health and Human Services (1999a).

world, representing consistent ways of representing thoughts, feelings, and behaviors. The sum of these unique characteristics results in our personalities. The
field of personality psychology plays a central role in understanding health behavior. Early personality theories proposed that individuals with certain personality types were predisposed to developing specific illnesses (Dunbar, 1943;
Menninger, 1935). For example, arthritis was thought to be associated with per-
fectionism and competitive behavior (Moos, 1964). It is now believed that the direction of causation is reversed: The illness causes a person to display a certain
type of personality characteristic or emotional problem.

Although there are hundreds of personality characteristics that may have
bearing on health behaviors, numerous personality theorists have argued that
personality can be characterized along five basic dimensions (Flay & Petraitis,
1994):

1. Behavioral control (e.g., behavioral constraint, impulsivity, task persistence, hyperactivity, aggressiveness, and motivation to achieve);

2. Emotional control (e.g., psychological adjustment, emotional stability,
neuroticism, and emotional distress);

3. Extroversion/introversion (e.g., social activity, social adaptability, and assertiveness);

4. Sociability (e.g., likability, friendliness, compliance, and conformity);

5. Intellect or general intelligence. (p. 31)

Previous research has revealed many links between personality type and
health-risk behavior (e.g., Jessor, 1977; Shedler & Block, 1990). Personality traits
are believed to contribute to people's health behavior. For example, adolescents
who score high on sensation-seeking behavior scales are less likely to use contraceptives and more likely to drive drunk (Arnette, 1990a, 1990b). Research also
suggests that adults who commit crimes are more likely to be impulsive, have
high rates of aggression, and lack a sense of social responsibility (Zuckerman,
1989).

Personality traits also affect the behavior change process. People who have
the will to control their behaviors, strong self-determination, and social competency should be more likely to decide to adopt health-promoting behavior skills
and have the skills needed to follow through with their decision. Although it is
difficult to modify personality traits over a short period of time, understanding
the impact personality traits can have on behavior is helpful in matching behavior change strategies with personality types.

Social Epidemiology of Cardiovascular Diseases

The social epidemiology of CVD is distinctive in that, more than any other major public health problem, research has emphasized psychological risk factors in addition to sociocultural variables (Jenkins, 1988). The leading cause of death in the United States since about 1930, CVD has been a central national concern since the mid-20th century. Research has documented a number of behavioral factors that predispose individuals to hypertension, cardiac arrest, stroke, and other circulatory problems. Most of these behaviors cover the usual broad-spectrum health risks, such as age, SES, race, cigarette smoking, alcohol consumption, dietary fat consumption, sedentary lifestyle, blood lipids, and obesity. However, in addition, research has focused on personality factors such as the Type A Behavior Pattern, hostility, and anger expression. First described in the 1950s, the classic features of the Type A personality include competitiveness, intense striving for achievement, easily provoked hostility, a sense of urgency, quick actions, punctuality, impatience, abrupt and rapid speech, emphatic gestures, and concentration on self-selected goals to the exclusion of other aspects of the environment (Prokop, Bradley, Burish, Anderson, & Fox, 1991). Numerous studies from 1960 to 1980 showed strong associations between Type A symptoms and coronary heart disease in diverse populations. After 1980, however, the empirical results became more inconsistent, and researchers began investigating the effects of specific components of the behavior pattern, including chronic anger and hostility (King, 1997). Depression and anxiety also have been suggested as important risk factors, although it is not clear whether Type A personality and anger led to depression and anxiety or whether the latter are independent risk factors for disease. A person who is anxious about meeting deadlines and feels in competition with others may begin to view the world in a hostile and cynical fashion and eventually may become emotionally exhausted by the struggle. Some have suggested that chronic arousal associated with confronting the world as an enemy is the common thread among psychological risk factors for CVD.

Given the complexity of factors that interact in the process of chronic disease development, it is not surprising that studies attempting to isolate individual-level risks have found inconsistent results. For example, the characteristics of Type A personality are reinforced by the environmental demands of many work settings of modern industrial societies, where there is unrelenting pressure to produce more, faster, and with fewer resources. In contrast to predictions that people would spend less time working as technology changed the workplace, the opposite has occurred, with people spending more and more time on the job and less time in leisure activities. Not surprisingly, work overload has been linked to increased risk of coronary heart disease. This association holds for white-collar jobs as well as assembly line work, and it seems to be particularly strong for occupational stress related to conflicting demands and low flexibility and control over the organization of work. The Japanese term *Karoshi* has been applied to describe this phenomenon of death from overwork. It has been implicated in 30,000 deaths per year in that country, and it has served as the basis for some wrongful death suits filed against employers (Bowman, 1999). Chapter 5 takes a closer look at the interaction of individual factors and environmental stress, including occupational setting.

Some critics have argued that if there is a "coronary-prone behavior pattern," it is not a personality defect but a conditioned way of acting that is embedded in social relationships (Radley, 1994). For this reason, it has been suggested that the Type A Behavior Pattern is a "culture-bound syndrome,"—a disorder that occurs primarily in and can be understood only within the context of a particular culture, in this case Western culture, with its inexorable time urgency and capitalist competitiveness.

CONCLUSION

Like the central position that epidemiology holds in public health, social epidemiology constitutes a core component of the subject matter of this book. Understanding the ways in which health problems are differentially distributed among social groups helps to clarify the etiology of such conditions and can inform policy development and intervention design. Behavioral epidemiology applies the risk factor approach to identify determinants of lifestyle behaviors that affect health. In this chapter, we present a third organizing framework, the Causality Continuum, as a way to depict the relative effects of distal, intermediate, and proximate determinants of health status. We illustrate the applicability of the model to problems such as breast cancer etiology, excess mortality among minority groups, and determinants of low birth weight. Special attention is devoted to the economic factors that hold such prominence in public health, poverty, and SES, exploring the links that mediate the effects of these more distal determinants on proximate causes of illness. Despite common trends in the social epidemiology of disease, some anomalous patterns are noted, such as the overall positive health status of Mexican American populations. Finally, the risk factor approach to social-epidemiologic studies is discussed in relation to the coronary-prone behavior pattern commonly known as Type A.

We present the Causality Continuum as a simplified representation of the concepts of distance and directness of effect in etiologic processes, recognizing that current epidemiologic approaches incorporate more complex models of causality. In the real world, the impact of multiple factors at different levels of the ecosystem is not linear, as the continuum might suggest, but multilinear with complex causal pathways. Nevertheless, it is helpful to view social and behavioral determinants of health in terms of their relative proximity to the outcome of interest, particularly because this relative position is so significant in evaluating the "changeability" of the factor, as noted in the overview of the Precede model.

II.

Conceptual Foundations

T he next set of chapters outlines the basic concepts that guide much of current-day research on social and behavioral aspects of public health. It begins with an examination of the determinants of health-related behavior, organized into three broad categories of preventive, illness, and sick-role behavior. Widely used models of health behavior change are described and illustrated through case examples. This domain of inquiry corresponds with the "Antecedents" dimension of the Health Impact Model. Chapter 4 also covers the "Responses" dimension of this model in its discussion of factors that influence illness and sick-role behavior.

Chapter 5 addresses in greater depth aspects of the social environment, which were introduced in Chapter 1. We discuss the ways in which concepts such as social roles, gender, stress, social support, and family systems help explain variability in who gets sick and the consequences of illness for different people. The chapter represents an elaboration of the ecosocial approach that provides the foundation of the book.

Building on previously introduced concepts from social epidemiology and social environment, Chapter 6 critically analyzes public health issues related to social differentiation and cultural diversity. It deconstructs the concepts of race and ethnicity by examining the underlying social structural and economic processes that shape societal attitudes toward disadvantaged groups. Social differentiation is further discussed in terms of subsistence, religion, and minority status. It concludes by introducing the concept of intercultural influence as a means to inform a more balanced public health practice based on respect for diversity.

4

Health and Illness Behavior

Gwendolyn P. Quinn and Jeannine Coreil

HEALTH-RELATED BEHAVIOR

In Chapter 1, we discussed the Health Impact Model, which conceptualizes the illness process in terms of antecedents and responses to health problems. We noted that both antecedents and responses are influenced by a wide range of social and cultural factors, such as ideological, behavioral, social structural, and technological determinants. In this chapter, we take a similar approach by examining factors that influence the different kinds of *health-related behaviors* (HRB), differentiated by where they occur in the illness process. Sociomedical scientists traditionally have distinguished three types of HRB (Gochman, 1997). *Health behavior* refers to actions taken in the absence of observable illness and includes primary prevention such as diet and exercise as well as some secondary prevention such as screening for specific diseases. The term *illness behavior* is used to designate help-seeking behavior and diagnostic testing for obvious or suspected illness and includes consulting health care providers and engaging in self-care activities. The third type of HRB is *sick-role behavior*; this category encompasses all the things people do in response to a diagnosed illness. Although the behavioral response can be very broad, including missing work and cutting back on other responsibilities (see Chapter 7, this volume), in the context of HRB, most attention has focused on what researchers call *compliance with medical regimens or adherence to treatment*.

Historical Behavior Theories

To understand fully the etiology of health and illness behaviors, we must review those factors that are believed to influence human behavior. Human behavior is a complex and intricate field of study. Attempts at understanding human behavior may have originated with Hippocrates and his proposition that "humors" in the body governed behavior. At that time, it was believed that individual temperaments corresponded to an overabundance of one of these four types of humors: sanguine (those who had an excess of blood); melancholic (those with an excess of black bile); choleric (an excess of yellow bile); and phlegmatic (an excess of phlegm). There was even a period of time in which "phrenology," the study of bumps on the skull, was given credence in explaining people's behavior.

Behaviorist Theories

Closer to modern times, psychologists credit Ivan Pavlov (1927) and his salivating dogs as identifying some of the true origins of behavior. Pavlov's experiments in classical conditioning showed that animals and humans can learn behaviors, based on the presentation of stimuli in connection with innate behaviors or with those behaviors we are born knowing how to do, such as salivating or feeling hunger in the presence of food or its aroma. We learn to anticipate danger at the sound of a gunshot. Initially, we are programmed from birth to react to a loud noise, but our environment shapes our behavior to the extent that we may run or cover our head if we hear a noise that sounds like gunfire. Like Pavlov's salivating dogs, we learn to anticipate consequences based on past experience.

Pavlov's experiments gave way to B. F. Skinner (1953) and his work with operant conditioning. The theory of operant conditioning is based on the repeated pairing of a targeted behavior with a reinforcement or punishment to either strengthen the association with the former or weaken or extinguish the behaviors with the latter. For example, a child who behaves well at the doctor's office may get a lollipop. The lollipop is meant to strengthen the behavior (behaving or cooperating during the visit). This is an example of positive reinforcement. Conversely, if you are caught speeding, the police officer may give you a ticket. The ticket is meant to extinguish, or stop, your speeding behavior. This is an example of a punishment. There are other key factors in operant conditioning, such as the timing and types of punishments and reinforcements.

Skinner's research showed that brand-new behaviors could be learned or shaped based on intentional or unintentional consequences. Students learn to raise their hand if they want to be called on in class. The ability to express yourself, or "being called on," is the reinforcement for exhibiting the desired behavior of hand raising. Presumably, students are punished by being ignored or not called on if they do not follow the correct procedure.

Not all behavior is developed through intentional consequences. If you win a softball game while carrying a penny in your pocket, you may develop the idea that the penny was somehow related to your success. Although superstitious behavior is only a small part of learned behavior, it illustrates the fact that humans are influenced by their perceptions of antecedents and consequences.

Pavlov and Skinner fall into a category known as *behavioral psychologists.* Behaviorism is centered on the idea that behavior is learned and maintained external to the learner, that is, the learner does not put conscious effort into the process. To some extent, this is very true, but it is probably more relevant to young children and animals. However, if you want to try it out, see if you can engage your neighbors in a small experiment of behavior modification. The next time you are at a social function, try to reinforce the behavior of a friend or colleague who is talking while standing up. For example, when your friend is sitting down, you should look very bored, yawn, or act disinterested. When your friend is standing up, you should maintain eye contact, nod your head, and smile. Notice how quickly you have shaped the behavior of your friend. You probably will find that he or she is talking to you almost exclusively from a standing position—most likely without any knowledge or conscious thought as to why he is standing continuously.

Cognitive Theories

Recent philosophies on human behaviors bring into play the idea that cognition—thinking—also has a significant role in behavior. Humans are more than a series of responses to external stimuli. We expect thought to govern most of our activities, no matter what the life form. Cognition refers to "those personal thought processes that serve as frames of reference for organizing and evaluating experiences" (Gochman, 1988, p. 21).

The term *health cognition* refers to beliefs, attitudes, and perceptions that provide a frame of reference for organizing and evaluating one's health (Gochman, 1997). The traditional social and behavioral theories of health behavior—for example, Social Cognitive Theory—are derived from behavioral and cognitive theories of psychology. These approaches include those that center on how health and illness are represented or organized within the cognitive structure of the individual (Gochman, 1997).

It is difficult to talk about health behaviors or behavior in general without talking about learning, even though they are distinctly different terms. Health behaviors, like other behaviors, are a combination of actions and thoughts, perceptions and feelings, past experiences and future predictions. Some of the things we do regarding our health may be deeply ingrained from things learned in childhood, such as eating chicken noodle soup when we feel sick. Other behaviors may be the result of newly learned information, such as the need to protect oneself against HIV infection.

Just as there are a multitude of ways to learn new behaviors, existing behaviors are influenced by an equally immense variety of situations. Some of these opportunities affect individuals from an internal perspective while appealing to thoughts, beliefs, hopes, and fears. Other behavioral influences come from external sources such as the environment through microcultures like family and friends, or macrocultures like national norms or policy. Several of the predominant theories of explaining and predicting health behavior incorporate these external and internal influences. In this next section, we examine the social psychological models for studying health behavior

HEALTH BEHAVIOR

Health Belief Model

In the 1950s, despite widespread publicity, a large proportion of the population failed to take advantage of important screening and prevention programs, most notably tuberculosis screening (Rosenstock, 1974). The Health Belief Model was developed by social psychologists at that time to attempt to explain this perplexing behavior.

The Health Belief Model is based on four central health beliefs that govern an individual's perceptions of their unique relationship to the disease or prevention in question. The first of these beliefs is the individual's perception of his or her personal susceptibility or vulnerability to a disease. For example, a man who, based on family history, believes he is a likely candidate for heart disease is more likely to pay attention to an advertisement for a program to reduce the risks of heart disease. This man perceives he is vulnerable to the disease, and his beliefs will influence the decisions he makes regarding his health.

The second belief is that of severity of the disease or condition. This belief operates on two levels. On the individual level, a person has a perception of how severe the condition is or could be in his or her own life. A person newly diagnosed with diabetes may not be likely to make major life or diet changes if he or she is not experiencing any symptoms. This person perceives the severity of diabetes to be "overblown" and perhaps regards his physician as overcautious. The second level of this belief is the reality of the disease in those who are afflicted. How severe is the condition in the lives of those experiencing the disease? A person may look at others experiencing diabetes and conclude it is not a serious health risk. This has been a central supposition in complying with flu shot programs (Glanz, Resch, Lerman, & Rimer, 1996). People tend to believe that "coming down with the flu" is not a severe condition and therefore does not warrant the extra time and possible pain to obtain a flu immunization.

The third component of the Health Belief Model is the perceived efficacy of the behavior in dealing with the condition. Does it really work to use deep breathing techniques as a substitution for smoking? If an individual perceives that adopting a new behavior will be efficacious in preventing disease, that person is more likely to attempt or maintain the behavior. Men and women involved in a smoking cessation program who believed that breath holding was an effective way to reduce their craving for a cigarette were more successful in quitting smoking (Hajek, Belcher, & Stapleton, 1987)

The fourth key belief is composed of the perceived barriers to adopting the behavior. To what extent does the individual believe there are barriers preventing him or her from conducting the behavior? These barriers may take many forms: financial, cultural, language, attitudes of family members, and others. A woman who has the primary responsibility for preparing meals for the family, especially on a limited budget, may perceive the barriers to weight loss to be too great. If her family complains about the low-calorie meals she prepares or if she is unable to purchase low-cost fruits and vegetables, she is likely to perceive the barriers to attempted weight loss to be too great.

The Health Belief Model is one of the most widely used theoretical models in the field of public health. In the early days of HIV/AIDS research, the Health Belief Model was used to explain the health-related behaviors of homosexual men. A significant relation was found between perceived susceptibility and perceived efficacy and benefits of behavior change. Susceptibility was found to be weakly associated with self-reported efforts to reduce the number of sexual partners. Susceptibility was negatively correlated with avoidance of anonymous partners, that is, the Health Belief Model assisted researchers in determining those beliefs that had direct effects on behaviors. Men who felt they were moderately at risk for HIV/AIDS were somewhat likely to attempt to reduce the number of partners with whom they engaged in sexual activity. However, men who perceived their risk level to be high were highly likely to engage in sexual activity with an anonymous partner, fearing an intimate relationship and not fearing the risk of infecting a stranger. The majority of respondents reported high levels of efficacy for behavior change (Emmons, Joseph, Kessler, & Wortman, 1986). These results suggested that the understanding of beliefs and the strengths and directions of these beliefs could assist in the development of interventions for behavior change.

A follow-up study with this cohort group conducted 6 months later showed that perceived efficacy was significantly lower and that perceived susceptibility was only negatively associated with avoidance of anonymous partners. Only normative behavior—the sense that peers were changing their behavior—was significantly related to behavioral intentions (Joseph, Montgomery, Emmons, & Kirscht, 1987). The results of this case study of the Health Belief Model suggest that perceptions about severity, risk, and efficacy may change over time and that only beliefs held immediately before a behavior are likely to influence it (Joseph et al., 1987).

Case study: Health Belief Model. Senior citizens tend to believe they are not at risk for some diseases typically associated with younger people, such as HIV and AIDS. Because there is a low perception of risk for HIV/AIDS and no fear of pregnancy, seniors tend to engage in risky sexual behavior without being aware of the potential consequences (Rose, 1995). A survey of American adults aged 50 and over showed that the majority did not use condoms and had never been tested for HIV (Rose, 1995). Most of the advertising regarding the prevention of HIV is aimed at teens and young adults, so it is not surprising that older people do not consider it an issue with which they must contend.

Researchers at the Allegheny School of Nursing decided to use the Health Belief Model to examine the effect of an HIV/AIDS education program that was designed specifically for people at senior meal sites. The education program was preceded by a test to determine if the adults were aware of HIV/AIDS (knowledge), considered themselves to be at risk (perception of susceptibility), and what their perceptions were of the prevalence of HIV/AIDS in the general population of older Americans (perception of severity).

The researchers predicted that seniors' beliefs about susceptibility and severity would predict their health behavior. Their predictions were mostly accurate. Although most of the seniors knew about HIV/AIDS, they did not consider themselves to be at risk nor did they think that AIDS was prevalent among people their age. The seniors behaved in a manner consistent with their beliefs, that is, they took few or no precautions.

An educational program was introduced to the seniors. This program taught them more facts about HIV/AIDS, gave statistics on the numbers of HIV-infected older people, and promoted the need for HIV antibody testing within the senior populations. In addition, the program promoted the idea of sharing this information with grandchildren, relatives, friends, and neighbors.

The results of this study showed that education did increase the seniors' perceptions of their risk and the severity of HIV/AIDS among people their age.

Posttests showed they learned new information. The authors report that a significant benefit of the study was the seniors' willingness and desire to share this information with grandchildren and young adults. The possibility of intergenerational HIV/AIDS education programs shows promise based on this study.

Theory of Reasoned Action

The Theory of Reasoned Action and its extension, the Theory of Planned Behavior, focus on individual motivation as a determinant of the plausibility of an individual engaging in a specific behavior (Fishbein & Middlestadt, 1989). The focus of this theory is on the attitudes, beliefs, and intentions regarding the behavior. Ajzen and Fishbein (1980) assert that behavioral intentions are the key determinant in predicting health-related behavior. However, one's beliefs and attitudes often shape intentions.

In the previous section, we discussed the Health Belief Model and the relation between the four central beliefs thought to influence behavior. The Theory of Reasoned Action incorporates those belief systems, combined with the affective domain of attitude.

Attitude is defined as the tendency to react negatively or positively to an object, person, or situation. Individual attitudes have great influence over behavior. With health behaviors, attitudes are strongly linked to consequences. How a person feels about adopting a health behavior is related to his or her perception of the outcome. A man who is contemplating reducing his alcohol consumption is likely to have a positive attitude toward the decision if he immediately begins to feel better after he has stopped drinking. Conversely, if his decision to reduce alcohol proves to be difficult, in that it affects his ability to socialize, he is likely to develop a negative attitude. The perception of positive consequences for performing health behaviors creates positive attitudes. The more barriers one experiences or perceives, the greater likelihood for the development of negative attitudes.

The expansion of the Theory of Reasoned Action—the Theory of Planned Behavior—takes into account the effect of "perceived behavioral control," a concept similar to the notion of "self-efficacy" (see the next section). In addition to this factor, intentions are determined by health beliefs, attitudes toward the behavior, self-efficacy, personality factors, social norms, and motivation to comply with those norms. Because intentions are derived from multiple beliefs, values, and norms, it is difficult to study them in isolation.

Studies of the relation between intentions and health behavior have yielded mixed results. For example, Rise, Astrom, and Sutton (1998) categorized a group of adolescents as *intenders* and *non-intenders* when studying dental floss use.

Teens in the intenders category were more likely to actually perform the behavior (flossing) based on the belief it would result in positive outcomes. However, intentions often are led astray. Several studies of adolescent sexual behavior have shown teens may state that they have no intention of engaging in sexual activity, only to find themselves being sexually active one night, without contraception (Guttmacher Institute, 1999). Chan and Heaney (1997) also found a relation between intentions and participation in a work site smoking cessation program. Workers who intended to participate were more likely to actually attend the sessions than were those who had not expressed intentions. However, the perceived stress levels of the employees in that case mediated the relation between the intentions and the behavior. Those individuals who perceived their jobs to be high-stress were likely to believe they needed to participate in a smoking cessation program. In contrast, a study of pregnant women's intentions to breastfeed showed that predelivery intentions were not significantly correlated to postpartum behavior (Wambach, 1997). This was particularly true with first-time mothers, who were not able to predict what their life would be like with a newborn.

Motivation and ability mediate the perception of intentions and individual control. Thus, the teen who perceives that he is capable of using an asthma inhaler correctly and is motivated to do so in order to participate in athletics has a high degree of perceived control. This teen is likely to have strong intentions to follow the prescribed regime for managing his asthma.

Case study: Theory of Reasoned Action. Taplin and Montano (1991) used the Theory of Reasoned Action to predict women's likelihood of participating in a mammography screening program. Their research question sought to examine the correlation between attitude, intention, beliefs, and the actual behavior of obtaining a mammogram. Their research found mixed results. In older women (65 and over), their beliefs and attitudes were highly correlated with their behavior—the more they believed mammograms were good tests for discovering cancer early, intended to get a mammogram, and felt positive about getting one, the more likely they were to actually get a mammogram. However, this did not hold true for younger women. Although many younger women expressed similar beliefs, attitudes, and intentions as the older women, their behaviors often were not correlated. In other words, they did not participate in the mammography screening. For younger women, the variables of time and transportation tended to mediate their behavior. For some women, the belief that mammograms are good tests and the intention to get one is not enough. If transportation to the mammography clinic is a problem or if they lack time in the day to attend, then they will not go, no matter how strong their intentions.

This research has implications for program development. It would be unwise to think that older and younger women face the same barriers in seeking health care. Younger women may still be caring for children or grandchildren. Older women may have greater access to public transportation or the ability to get a ride from a friend. This study shows that intentions and beliefs do not provide the total picture in determining who will use health care services. Sometimes the "unexpectancies" of life get in the way.

Social Cognitive Theory

The concept of perception in relation to motivation and ability overlap with Social Cognitive Theory. The theory has made important contributions to understanding behaviors related to health care. One of the primary components of social cognitive theory, or social learning theory, is the idea that many of our thoughts and beliefs are rooted in the observational learning experiences that have occurred in our environment. These experiences, in turn, are related to our attribution of our abilities and our sources of motivation.

Focus: Behavior modeling. Social cognitive theory is rooted in Alfred Bandura's (1986) early career research on observational learning. Bandura was not satisfied by Skinner and Pavlov's explanation of behavior that focused on people learning only by doing. Bandura felt there were times when humans learned by watching what others do and what happens to them when they do it.

In a classic experiment, Bandura used a large inflatable doll known as the "bobo doll" to demonstrate that children who observe violent, aggressive behavior are more likely to demonstrate this behavior than are children who do not observe it. Bandura and his team also studied the "models," those people who demonstrated a behavior that others may later follow. He discovered that age, gender, the perceived status of the model, and the perceived similarity of the model to the observer all influenced whether the behavior was duplicated.

Imagine you are walking out the door of a large office building. You see a newspaper stand near the front door. Several of the employees who obviously work in the building are helping themselves to today's paper. You'd really like to have one too but you are not sure if it is free or only for employees. Do you take the newspaper? Chances are you will wait to see what happens to those who do. Do the people taking the paper hide it in their briefcase or openly walk by the guard? What if you see someone you know who does not work there and she takes a paper? You are probably likely to take one too, perceiving they are of similar status to yourself.

Now imagine you are in a restaurant and a famous celebrity is helping herself to the dessert tray without ordering. Will you follow suit and do the same? Probably not; you are likely to perceive that the celebrity has a higher status than you and may be deserving of special treatment. You may think to yourself, "They'll throw me out if I do that, but the celebrity will probably get that and her dinner free."

Think about the implications of modeling and some of the advertising we do for healthy behaviors using celebrities. Is it effective? Are you likely to follow what a celebrity model does? Do you think if you exercise each day you will get the same results as Cindy Crawford or other fashion models? Chapter 10 discusses in greater detail the use of models in social marketing of healthy behavior.

The term *attribution* attempts to explain behavior on the basis of the perceived causes that an individual might use to account for success or failure in performing a behavior or attempting or avoiding the behavior (Weiner, 1980). How do people determine the cause of their successes or failures in behavior? Weiner (1977) proposed that there are five determinants of this decision-making process. The first is previous history. A good indication of the likelihood of an individual adopting a new health behavior is to examine the behaviors that he or she currently is exhibiting. A woman who exercises and follows a healthy diet is likely to maintain those behaviors, and perhaps even increase her adherence to diet and exercise, during pregnancy. A consistent record of success breeds the idea that one has the necessary ability to adopt or maintain healthy behaviors. Conversely, failure or negative outcomes may cultivate ideas that one is not capable of or does not have the ability to perform a specific behavior. It would be unrealistic to expect an overweight woman with a history of diet failure to adopt and maintain new health behaviors suddenly, even though she may be highly motivated at a specific time in her life, such as during pregnancy.

The next determinant of attribution is the performance history of others. Have most of your coworkers failed to attend the on-site exercise classes after work? It is likely you will view their performance as being similar to your own. On the other hand, do your coworkers turn out in droves to donate blood? If they do and you see this has been a positive choice for them, you are likely to donate as well.

The third source is effort. If it is very convenient for you to stay after work to attend an exercise class, that is, if there is little preparation and it does not prevent you from doing other things, you are likely to continue to go, even if your coworkers do not. If your efforts pay off, if you feel better and have more energy, this can be an additional source of motivation for you. Conversely, if your efforts do not manifest in a positive experience, you may decide the effort outweighs the benefits.

A fourth source of attribution within Social Cognitive Theory is the extent to which assistance is required to perform the behavior. Attempts at behavior that result in positive experiences and for which an individual feels confident that these experiences were based on his or her own efforts are more likely to be repeated than are those that require assistance. A diabetic who maintains her blood sugar at normal levels through the help of a home health aide's daily glucose monitoring and insulin injections is less likely to perceive that she was responsible for her own health outcomes. This woman may perceive the health outcomes to be related to external sources, such as the assistance she received, rather than her own efforts.

The final source of causality relates to the randomness of the outcome. A person who receives an appointment for a mammogram at the local clinic via a lottery is less likely to perceive that she is responsible for maintaining her own health. A woman who saw an advertisement for free mammograms, called the clinic to make an appointment, and arrived at the proper time may be more inclined to perceive the success of the process as due to her own behavior.

Although attributions are good indicators of the likelihood of behavior occurring, behavioral therapists tell us the single most influential factor in predicting whether behavior will occur is the extent to which the individual feels the new behavior is rewarding (Michelson, 1985). Another key factor in predicting health is rooted in the individual's experience with actually attempting the behavior. For example, suppose you are not sure you can run a mile in less than 5 minutes. The best way to find out is to actually attempt to run the mile. If you do run the mile in 5 minutes and you feel good or rewarded by your accomplishment, chances are you will consider yourself capable and will probably repeat the behavior.

Social Cognitive Theory is expansive and complex, and we have just touched briefly on its chief aspects. Individual processing of information mediates observational learning and attributions about success and failure with a behavior. The concepts of self-regulation and reflection, the act of thinking about one's experiences, and applying a developed set of criteria to one's behaviors are also essential to understanding behavior through this model. It is through this self-reflective behavior that the concept of self-efficacy is developed. Self-efficacy often influences the extent to which we feel capable of attempting or continuing a new or learned behavior. *Self-efficacy* is defined as a self-judgment about a person's ability to perform a task or goal successfully.

Self-efficacy can determine whether someone attempts a new behavior, such as following a weight loss program. A woman who has low self-efficacy for the task and who does not believe that she is capable of successfully following a weight loss program is much less likely to try than is a woman who believes she will be successful. Although a woman with low self-efficacy may attempt a weight loss program, when it becomes difficult to continue she is likely to use reflection to say to herself, "I never stood a chance, I could never follow a program that had so many restrictions."

Strategies that attempt to boost the sense of self-efficacy for individuals attempting behavior change tend to be more successful than those that do not take this internal source of behavioral influence into account (Glanz, Marcus, Lewis, & Rimer, 1997). In fact, self-efficacy is second only to the Health Belief Model in its use by health researchers as a central construct in predicting health behavior (Glanz et al., 1997 p. 29).

Case study: Social Cognitive Theory. Learning by watching others can be a powerful determinant in shaping behavior. Younger children tend to imitate the behavior of their parents and older siblings, and teens tend to imitate the behavior of those they admire. Drawing on this concept of observational learning, researchers in California developed a program to prevent substance abuse among Hispanic youth. The program was aimed at middle school students in a community that was fraught with crime, high incidences of substance abuse, and school dropout. The researchers discovered that preteens were highly influenced by their peers, and that few positive role models were present within this population.

Armed with this knowledge, they set out to create a bilingual program that provided positive peer models for substance-free living. Included in the program was a skill-building component that taught teens how to say no to situations in which they were encouraged by peers to use drugs or engage in other illegal activity. The program provided social support for "drug-free" teens who often felt they were "the only one not doing drugs in my school." Finally, the program created social norms within the community showing that following the law, not using drugs, and staying in school were acceptable and common ways to live.

Although the program was not evaluated formally, participants felt it had a tremendous impact on their lives. Teens said they now had a supportive environment to be open about their lack of drug use, whereas previously they felt the need to hide their "drug-free lifestyle" in order to appear "cool" to their peers.

Transtheoretical Model

The three theories covered in this section so far have dealt with predicting behavior based on beliefs (Health Belief Model); attitudes, beliefs, and intentions (Theory of Reasoned Action); and observational learning, attributions, and self-efficacy (Social Cognitive Theory). A fourth theory, the Transtheoretical

Model (TM), aims to define the stages individuals go through as they attempt behavior change. The TM theory considers behavioral change to be a process that an individual progresses through in a series of six stages (Prochaska, Redding, & Evers, 1997). Originally developed to explain the development of behavior change in addictive behaviors, it recently has been applied to the broader context of health behavior, including head injury rehabilitation (Lam & Shaw, 1997) and help-seeking in psychotherapy (Prochaska, 1989).

As in the Theory of Reasoned Action, intentions are a key element in Prochaska and DiClemente's (1986) TM and in their definition of the six stages of change that serve as the organizational framework for the theory. These stages are precontemplation, contemplation, preparation, action, maintenance, and termination (Prochaska & DiClemente, 1986).

Focus: Stages of change. The first stage, precontemplation, is a stage in which the individual has no intention to attempt behavior change. For example, Dawn, a heavy smoker, may have no conscious sense that her smoking behavior is harmful and may require change. The precontemplation stage may encompass those who are uninformed as well as those who are in denial about their health.

The second stage, contemplation, is a period of time in which the individual is thinking about behavior change but is in the process of weighing the benefits and costs of such action. This is a crucial time for behavioral intervention, but individual commitment to the change is the key element in determining whether the person moves on to the next stage.

You probably have heard the joke "How many psychologists does it take to change a light bulb? Only one, but he has to really want to change." The serious side of this illustration is the idea that the individual must be prepared to weather the challenges that come with change. For Dawn, this stage may include a series of challenges framed in questions such as "Will I gain weight? Do I have the willpower to quit? Do I need a nicotine patch or should I do it cold turkey?"

The preparation stage is characterized by intention to take action in the very near future, usually 1 month or less (Prochaska, Redding, et al., 1997). People in the preparation stage typically have taken some form of action to arrange for their behavior change. In the case of our heavy smoker, Dawn, she may have begun to cut down the number of cigarettes she consumes each day and checked into smoking cessation classes at the local hospital.

The action stage of the TM theory involves observable behaviors currently conducted in relation to behavior change. For Dawn, this will mean she has actually stopped smoking. For those seeking mental health therapy, this could mean attending a session with a therapist.

The next stage of TM is maintenance. In this stage, the individual's behavior is centered on preventing a relapse into the old behavior. Dawn may avoid having coffee in the morning or engaging in other behaviors she associated with smoking. She also may begin a diet to prevent the weight gain she initially feared with smoking cessation.

The importance of the TM theory is its emphasis on the temporal nature of behavior and its recognition of the varying cognitive processes a person engages in as he or she attempts behavior change. At each stage, there are decisions one must make—Do I believe my health is at risk? Do I believe I have the ability to change my behavior? How likely am I to be successful if I attempt change? Will the results of my efforts be worth the time and resources involved?

Individuals in the precontemplation stage have no intention of changing their behavior within the near future. Individuals in the contemplation stage intend to change in the foreseeable future, usually measured as the next 6 months. During the preparation stage, people intend to change in the immediate future, usually measured as the next month, and they may have attempted to change during the past year. Action is the stage in which individuals overtly change their behavior, environment, and other related factors to alter the health behavior in question. Maintenance is the stage in which individuals avoid relapse and continue to integrate the behavior change into their life for a minimum of 6 consecutive months (Prochaska et al., 1992). The sixth stage, termination, refers to the period when individuals no longer experience temptations or doubts about their ability to maintain the new behavior (Prochaska, Redding, et al., 1997).

Progression through the stages is not a linear process; rather, there are opportunities for individuals to regress back to earlier stages. For example, smokers tend to "quit" smoking several times before they are actually able to be classified as being in the maintenance stage, thereby demonstrating the potential for regressing back to either the contemplation or preparation stages after reaching the action stage (Prochaska et al., 1992; Prochaska & Velicer, 1997). The realization that relapse "is the rule rather than the exception" led to a modification of the original linear descriptive model to a "spiral pattern of change" that allows for behavioral and intentional regression (Prochaska et al., 1992, p. 1104).

One of the critical assumptions underlying the TM is that most people will remain stuck in the early stages of the change process if directed change strategies are not employed. Moreover, studies of people who progress through the process suggest that the factors that influenced progression during the early stages are different from the factors that help people move through later stages (Prochaska, Redding, et al., 1997). Because the factors that determine people's movement from one stage to another vary throughout the change process, the researchers recommend that interventions be matched to an individual's stage of readiness to change (see Prochaska et al., 1992; Prochaska & Velicer, 1997).

Case study: Transtheoretical Model. Pregnancy is often seen as an ideal time for women to initiate healthy behaviors and cease risky or adverse behaviors. Motivated by the thought of doing what is best for her unborn child, women tend to make extreme changes in their health behavior during pregnancy. It is not uncommon for women who rarely see a physician to become diligent about keeping their prenatal care appointments. Many women begin to exercise, develop healthy eating habits, and give up vices such as caffeine and alcohol to help ensure their child will be healthy. However, some of these newfound behaviors do not become lifelong. Some women make these changes to their health care and lifestyle routine only for the duration of the pregnancy.

A study sought to examine if smoking cessation behaviors in pregnancy were similar to those experienced by nonpregnant women. Using the stages of change theory, the researchers reasoned that pregnant women had greater self-efficacy and more motivation to quit smoking than did their nonpregnant counterparts.

The study showed that pregnant women stopped smoking at greater levels, more quickly, and with less coping skills than did nonpregnant women. However, longitudinal follow-up with these women showed that women who quit smoking during pregnancy tended to perceive themselves as "stopping" smoking for a period of time rather than making a commitment to a lifelong behavior change. Because they considered themselves to be quitting for a time-limited period, they did not develop coping skills or other behaviors to assist them in breaking the habit.

The implications of this study are twofold. It reconfirms the idea that pregnancy is an ideal time to promote behavior change among women. It also highlights the fact that promoting healthy babies solely for the purpose of having a healthy baby undermines the potential for long-term behavior change. Women should be encouraged to adopt healthy behaviors for the benefits they will experience in addition to the health of the baby. If not, behaviors such as smoking, substance abuse, and alcohol abuse may resume after the baby is born. Health educators should promote the idea that "you've come a long way, baby" means longer than 9 months.

Each of the theories presented thus far has introduced varying aspects of the key influences of behavior. The Health Belief Model places heavy emphasis on the social context of behavior as implied through belief systems. The Theory of Reasoned Action and the Theory of Planned Behavior emphasize the cultural-environmental context of behavior in relation to attitudes and expectancies. The Social Cognitive Theory is rooted in biological and personality perceptions based on self-efficacy and social competence. However, despite the uniqueness and varying origins in their explanations of behavior, these theories when operating together provide a better sense of human behavior than when operating alone.

ILLNESS BEHAVIOR

When people experience bodily sensations, they often go through a process of appraising the symptoms as a possible sign of sickness. Then, they react to what they perceive in a variety of ways. Some consult their doctor at the first sign that something might be wrong, whereas others put off seeking help until it is absolutely necessary or until others pressure them into taking action. Between the initial event of symptom recognition at the start of the illness process and being prescribed a treatment by a health care professional, many steps and sequences may take place. Social scientists have devoted considerable attention to the complex pathways through which sick persons evaluate and manage their health problems, for better or for worse. They have found that these pathways tend to follow predictable courses, and they have developed conceptual models to explain the influence of factors at different points along the way. Central to all the models is the assumption that illness behavior is a culturally and socially learned response pattern.

Researchers have approached the study of illness behavior from two general perspectives. One approach focuses on the process that unfolds over the course of the illness, including the appraisal stage, self-care activities, and patterns of help seeking. The unit of study is the entire illness episode. Studies of this type tend to be more subjective, descriptive, and qualitative in nature. The other approach focuses on identifying objective factors that predict utilization or choice of health services. The unit of study is a specific outcome or event, such as consultation of a physician, the amount of health services used, or therapeutic choice among alternatives. The goal of such studies is to specify which variables predict the behavior in question. More often than not, quantitative analysis is used, guided by conceptual models of health service utilization.

The Illness Episode

We look at the illness process approach first. When someone experiences troubling bodily sensations, the illness appraisal process usually begins with some kind of evaluation of the symptoms based on personal experience and culturally shared knowledge. Different disciplines use various terminology to describe this interpretive process of attributing meaning to the sensations. For example, psychologists refer to illness *representation* (Leventhal, Leventhal, & Contrada, 1998) to describe the interpretation and elaboration of meaning assigned to somatic sensations. This occurs at an early stage in the appraisal process and may involve consultation with others in one's network or watching to observe changes in the sensation over time. The person may decide the sensation is not a real symptom of illness and end the appraisal process without taking action. However, once a symptom is identified or "recognized" and a tentative diagnostic label applied, a patterned response typically ensues, involving further assessment of the cause, duration, consequences, and appropriate remedial action. Some theorists, mostly from psychological backgrounds, use the term *attribution* (Lewis & Daltroy, 1990) to describe this evaluative process, and anthropologists have favored the term *explanatory model* of illness (see Chapter 8, this volume). Psychologists tend to emphasize the subjective and emotional dimensions of attribution, such as self-assessed level of health and the effects of mood states, depression, stress, and anxiety on symptom interpretation. A good illustration of this approach is the study by Haug, Musil, Warner, and Morris (1998) of older U.S. adults to identify the effects of external stresses, psychological factors, health attitudes, and contextual variables on three types of illness representations (applying an illness label, consulting a physician, and engaging in self care). Taking a different approach, anthropologists more often frame the appraisal process issue in terms of how people apply cultural models to recognized symptom constellations. For example, a study of Mexican American causal models of diabetes (Hunt, Valenzuela, & Pugh, 1998) identified the importance of *provoking factors* such as self-indulgent behaviors and life crisis events in the shared cultural models of the disease.

The illness episode process can be examined further with regard to multiple phases and evaluated outcomes of sequences of therapeutic action. Here again, there can be different emphases. Sociologically oriented investigators tend to focus on social network interactions such as feedback from significant others and movement through lay and professional referral systems. For example, Pescosolido (1992) applies a type of social network model to identify eight distinct *strategies* of health care use involving different combinations of consulting family, friends, coworkers, classmates, physicians, nonprescription drugs, home remedies, and no action. Anthropologists, on the other hand, have identified *hierarchies of resort* (Romanucci-Ross, 1969), such as self/traditional/modern health care and other structures in the help-seeking process.

One of the most well-developed formulations of illness behavior is sociologist David Mechanic's (1978) General Theory of Help-Seeking. Starting from the premise that illness behavior is grounded in perceptions and coping resources, Mechanic identifies 10 determinants of help seeking, which he groups into four categories. The first category includes the perceived salience and evaluation of symptoms, which are shaped by one's sociocultural background. This category includes the visibility, recogniziability, or perceptual salience of deviant signs and symptoms; the extent to which the symptoms are thought to be serious; and available information, knowledge, and cultural assumptions and understandings of the evaluator. The second category of determinants concerns the disruptive and persistent nature of the symptoms and includes the extent to which symptoms interfere with family, work, or other social activities; the frequency of the appearance or recurrence of the symptoms; and the tolerance threshold of those who are exposed to and evaluate the deviant signs and symptoms. A third group of factors addresses the competing needs of those affected and alternative interpretations of the situation. Included here are basic needs that can lead to denial, other needs that may compete with illness responses, and other possible explanations of the symptoms once they are recognized. The fourth category encompasses available coping resources, including treatment options, accessibility of care, and psychological or monetary costs of taking action.

Mechanic (1978) acknowledged that the determinants of illness behavior operate at both the level of self-defined illness and other-defined problem situations. In the case of other-defined illnesses, the sick person may not recognize that a problem exists or may resist being labeled as "ill." In such instances, others may have to take charge of the situation and exert pressure or even coercion to get the person into care. Children, for instance, because of their lack of knowledge and experience, must be helped by others through the illness process. Adults, on the other hand, must be persuaded to seek care or involuntarily forced to through legal actions. Anthropologists have developed the concept of the "therapy managing group" to describe the coordinated actions of significant others in the case of illness (see Chapter 8, this volume).

A number of theorists have developed stage-models of the help-seeking process (e.g., Chrisman, 1977; Romanucci-Ross, 1969; Suchman, 1965). A recurrent feature of these models is the notion of *therapeutic networks*, the interconnected linkages people have with others who provide advice or give suggestions about managing an illness. The term *lay referral networks* has been applied to those segments of therapeutic networks that include family, friends, colleagues, and others who are not medical specialists. The *professional referral system*, on the other hand, involves the advice of medical specialists who may recommend consultation of other types of practitioners. Typically, the movement through therapeutic networks begins with self-directed care, then proceeds to lay referral networks, and then to professionals operating in the formal medical system. However, the sequence is not always unidirectional, because sick persons continually monitor the situation themselves and may seek information and advice from lay sources throughout the process.

More recently, research on the illness process has shifted toward a narrative approach, that is, viewing the episode or experience in terms comparable to a story. This approach borrows many aspects from life history and life story research. The account might be told or written by the person or persons directly involved, or it may be constructed through interaction with the primary parties. The focus is on understanding the meaning of the illness for those affected (Kleinman, 1988; Lieblich, Tuval-Mashiach, & Zilber, 1998). When interviewing is used to elicit the illness narrative, an attempt is made to allow the story to develop with minimal direction from the researcher, in a "collaborative" fashion, in which the interviewee is actively involved in the process. For example, Kolker (1996) gave a first person account of her experience with health care rationing when her insurance company refused to pay for a bone marrow transplant recommended by her oncologist for treating the author's breast cancer. A slightly different perspective on breast cancer is provided by Matthews, Lannin, and Mitchell (1994), who elicited illness narratives from African American women about their breast cancer experiences. Comparison of narratives across women showed contrasting patterns of illness behavior that are relevant to the problem of delay in seeking treatment for breast cancer in this population.

Health Care Utilization

We now turn our attention to the second general approach to health behavior, the study of health care utilization. By far the greatest attention in research on illness behavior has been focused on utilization of formal medical services. There are probably many reasons for this, including the interests of research funding agencies, concern for economic aspects of health services, and a bias toward giving priority to "official" or "orthodox" therapy as opposed to self-help or alternative care. Wolinsky (1988) groups the various types of health service utilization models into seven types. In this scheme, *demographic models* use variables such as age, gender, marital status, and family size as proxy measures of life stage position, based on the assumption that health care needs vary as individuals move through the life course. *Social structural models,* on the other hand, emphasize variables such as education, occupation, and ethnicity, which reflect the individual's position in the social system: People who share similar social statuses tend to have comparable health service utilization patterns. However, the explanation researchers attribute to these commonalities may vary considerably; for instance, explanations for why people of low educational status use services less often than do better-educated people might cite factors such as social inequality, common life experiences, barriers to care, or a combination of reasons. Wolinsky's third category is that of the *social psychological models,* which focus on the individual's attitudes and beliefs regarding the illness; one such model is the Health Belief Model, previously discussed in this chapter. *Family resource models* give primacy to the ability to obtain needed services and often focus on household income, health insurance coverage, and access to a regular source of care; as managed care has increasingly become the dominant mode of health service provision, family resource models have gained prominence. Likewise, *organizational models* also have attracted increased attention as researchers seek to compare different forms of service delivery (e.g., fee for service, salaried, prepaid). *Community resource models,* in contrast, focus on the macroeconomic supply side of service accessibility and are particularly relevant to public health and its concern for population-based health care planning.

Most researchers recognize that, ideally, a comprehensive model of health service utilization should combine aspects of all these models. Such a combined framework Wolinsky (1988) describes as a *health systems model*—the seventh type of health service utilization model. The difficulty of using a health systems model lies in collecting data on many different variables within a single study. The most widely used health systems model over the past few decades has been Ronald Andersen's Behavioral Model of Health Services Use (Aday & Andersen, 1974; Andersen, 1968, 1995). Originally devised to explain individual utilization of health services, the model identified three categories of influence: predisposing, enabling, and need characteristics. Over time, the model has been expanded to encompass health care system variables as well as external environmental characteristics in explaining service utilization, and it has been applied as an intervention framework to promote equitable access to care. In applying the model to improving access, the concept of *mutability*—the degree to which a factor can be intentionally modified—becomes important. For example, demographic and social structural variables are very difficult to change, whereas health beliefs and resources are much easier to modify, as seen in Chapter 3. The most recent formulation of the model also incorporates feedback from the perceived outcome of service use, such as evaluated health status and consumer satisfaction. In this version, the focus is on evaluating medical care system performance (Aday & Awe, 1997).

Although sociological models of health service utilization have focused on formal health services, anthropological models have emphasized choice among pluralistic health options, including home-based and folk sector care, as well as bureaucratic medicine. This is not surprising given the continued reliance on nonprofessional therapy in developing country settings where many anthropologists continue to work. Early anthropological work on treatment choice applied a hierarchical model to explain the sequence of help seeking from home therapy to traditional healing and then modern medicine. As Western medicine became increasingly available and accepted, treatment choice patterns were better explained by applying decision modeling to individual episodes of illness. A good example of such decision models is Young's (1981) ethnomedical choice-making approach, which applied the four criteria of illness gravity, knowledge of a home remedy, faith in the efficacy of a treatment, and accessibility of a service. The utility of the model was assessed by comparing actual treatment choices with those predicted by the four criteria for a sample of illness episodes.

Case study: Illness behavior. An important difference between a health systems model of service utilization, such as Andersen's (Aday & Andersen, 1974; Andersen, 1968, 1995) sociobehavioral model, and a decision theoretic model, such as Young's (1981) ethnomedical choice-making approach, is the focus of the study. In a health systems model, the focus of the study is the aggregate population, and it typically involves multivariate regression modeling of factors that "predict" aggregate patterns of health service use. The statistical model can be used to develop a conceptual model identifying which set of factors predict use of services. With a decision theoretic model, on the other hand, the focus of study is the individual illness episode, in which the goal is to determine whether a particular case of help seeking correctly fits a predetermined set of decision criteria. In a sample of cases examined this way, the researcher can calculate the proportion of episodes "correctly" classified by the decision model.

Typically, researchers select a utilization model based on the goals of the study; however, in some instances, they are interested in comparing the relative utility of different models. Such was the case in Weller, Ruebush, and Klein's (1997) investigation of treatment-seeking behavior in Guatemala. Illness case histories ($N = 736$) were collected from a random sample of 270 households in six villages. Using the same data set, two predictive models—Andersen's health systems model and Young's decision theoretic approach—were compared to determine which model better predicted health care choices among four main categories: home or store-bought remedies, pharmacy medicines, health post services, or physician/hospital care. In this study, the sociobehavioral model of health systems use better predicted illness than the decision theoretic approach. The systems model correctly classified 60% of cases, which was 23% better than chance, whereas the decision model correctly classified 48% of cases, only 9% better than chance. The authors noted that both models identified similar predictor variables (e.g., illness severity and loss of work), and that the two approaches have different strengths and weaknesses.

SICK-ROLE BEHAVIOR

Once a person has been diagnosed with a specific illness and prescribed an appropriate treatment regimen, he or she is expected to follow the medical advice given. Failure to comply with treatment is socially disapproved and may even lead to negative sanctions, such as loss of the privileges associated with the sick role (see Chapter 7, this volume). Given such consequences, you might expect that patient compliance is usually very high, but in fact it often is not. It is estimated that 30% to 60% of patients fail to comply fully with treatments, and only about 50% of patients adhere to long-term care regimens. About half of all patients also do not take medications properly, and for asymptomatic conditions, noncompliance rates rise to 75% (Becker & Maiman, 1975, 1980).

Concern for improving patient compliance was an important impetus for the early involvement of social scientists in medical settings. Seeking answers to questions such as "How can we get more patients to follow regimen X appropriately?" or "Why don't more people in the target population use our services?" a huge body of literature has been generated on patient compliance, or adherence to treatment. Between 1960 and 1995, close to 12,000 articles were published on this topic (Trostle, 1997). Studies have identified consistent determinants related to illness characteristics, patient variables, aspects of the medical encounter, and regimen factors. However, the concept of "compliance" and the literature focused on it have been the targets of critical deconstruction in recent years. Central to this critique is the need to expose an implicit ideology of hierarchical power relations in compliance-oriented conceptualizations of patient behavior (Kotarba & Seidel, 1984; Trostle, 1997). In response to such criticisms, some researchers have adopted less authoritarian terminology such as *acceptance* of medical therapy, which accords greater latitude for patient agency in responding to recommended advice. In this section, we use the traditional terminology of *compliance*.

Research on patient compliance has identified several types of problems. To begin with, there are those individuals who fail to fill their prescriptions or begin treatment. More commonly, it is the interruption of the medication or regimen before completion that is problematic. Then there are those who take an incorrect dosage, do not follow the right schedule, or ingest medicines improperly. Finally, there is the problem of "supercompliance" with prescriptions received from multiple caregivers (Griffiths, 1990).

Compounding the compliance problem is the fact that clinicians overestimate the extent to which their patients follow recommended treatment. When clinicians do recognize noncompliance, they tend to see it as a problem residing with the patient and having little to do with their own interaction or communication with the patient. This view is reinforced by the fact that compliance research has emphasized patient variables and has neglected aspects of the medical encounter (Svarstad, 1987). Also, there are persistent methodological difficulties involved in monitoring patient compliance both in clinical practice and research.

Most studies have relied on patient self-report or physician estimation to measure compliance, but both of these approaches are subject to bias. Likewise, indirect assessments, such as measuring the remaining contents of medication supply, also can be unreliable because they can be manipulated. The most objective approach is measurement of a medication or its metabolites in body fluids, but this technique only can be used with certain kinds of drugs and has limited applicability for behavioral regimens.

With regard to illness characteristics, compliance has been found to be lower for chronic illnesses, asymptomatic or minimally disruptive disorders, less severe disorders, socially unacceptable conditions, and incorrectly diagnosed problems. Less compliant patients tend to be at the older or younger extremes in age, have low health motivation, and to perceive as slight both their own susceptibility to the illness or its sequela and the seriousness of the illness. The types of regimen factors that lower compliance are not surprising: prolonged adherence to a treatment, use of multiple medications or therapies, frequent administration of a drug or performance of an activity, costly treatment, side effects, and interference with one's usual lifestyle (Sclar, 1991).

In recent years, increasing attention has been given to the dynamics of the medical encounter as sources of influence on patient compliance. For example, effective communication between practitioner and patient, as well as the degree of concern and supportiveness demonstrated by the clinician, improve patient adherence (Svarstad, 1987). Other findings point to the importance of the opportunity and encouragement for patients to ask questions and express feelings. The extent to which patient expectations are met also affects compliance, as does the level of congruence between the patient and clinician's explanatory models of the illness.

Efforts to use the previous findings to devise strategies for improving patient compliance have generated several successful approaches. One such strategy is tailoring the regimen to the patient's daily activities so that following the treatment is less disruptive. Another technique is to introduce graduated regimen plans that start out at a minimal level and then slowly build to full strength. With some patients, written or oral contracts have been found to be effective incentives, whereas with others the use of environmental cues works well. Attention to social environment, such as enlisting family support and involvement in the patient's regimen, also has proved beneficial. With the specific problem of multiple medications, the use of fixed-ratio combination drugs can simplify the number and schedule of pills (Becker & Maiman, 1980).

In keeping with the medicocentric bias of compliance research, the dominant perspective of this area of study has been largely that of clinical practice. Problems of adherence have been accorded greater attention in medicine than in public health, because the latter is more concerned with prevention than treatment. However, there are a few exceptions to this general rule. Throughout the 20th century, public health authorities have focused attention on chronic conditions and communicable diseases that require sustained therapeutic regimens to control effectively. Among the chronic diseases that have been targeted for improved management are hypertension and diabetes, and communicable diseases of concern have been sexually transmitted diseases and tuberculosis. In the following highlight section, we take a closer look at the history and current issues in tuberculosis control, a problem once considered a worry of the past. Midcentury optimism about the elimination of infectious diseases, thanks to an ever-expanding arsenal of antibiotic drugs, has been replaced with a more sober realization that infectious diseases will always be part of the human condition, with the most marginal social groups suffering the brunt of them. Moreover, we now recognize the alarming development of drug-resistant disease strains, a problem directly exacerbated by incomplete treatment of persons with the disease. The story of tuberculosis is instructive on all these issues.

Focus: Tuberculosis control. During the 18th and 19th centuries, tuberculosis occupied a similar role in society as HIV / AIDS does in the late 20th century. It was the leading cause of young adult mortality, it killed people slowly, available treatments were not very effective, and its victims were shunned and stigmatized within their communities. "Consumption" affected all classes of society, but then, as now, the poor and disadvantaged segments were disproportionately burdened with this disease. The discovery of microorganisms at the end of the 19th century, along with the development of effective antibiotic drugs, revolutionized the treatment of infectious diseases such as tuberculosis in industrial countries. In the 1940s, the new drug streptomycin was found to act particularly effectively against *Mycobacterium tuberculosis,* the agent responsible for tuberculosis.

In 1900, the mortality rate from tuberculosis in the United States and Europe was more than 200 per 100,000 population. Like other infectious diseases, incidence rates declined in the early part of the 20th century in response to improved health conditions and better nutrition. Following the introduction of streptomycin therapy, incidence rates declined further after 1950, reaching a low of 9.1 during the early 1980s (Wilson, 1990, cited in Morisky & Cabrera, 1997). Since the mid-1980s, however, new cases of tuberculosis have increased dramatically worldwide. The World Health Organization (WHO) reports that, by 1998, more than 8 million new cases of tuberculosis were occurring each year, with close to 3 million deaths annually from the disease (WHO, 1998). The resurgence of tuberculosis has been attributed to several factors: its association with immuno- suppression in HIV infected persons, the emergence of drug-resistant strains of the bacillus, a deteriorating public health infrastructure, increased immigration from high-prevalence countries, and conditions associated with higher rates of homelessness and drug abuse in disadvantaged populations.

Despite the multifaceted nature of the "reemergence" of tuberculosis, however, many discussions of the problem tend to focus on issues of "noncompliance" within the active patient population. The weight given to this issue is reflected in the fact that "directly observed therapy" (DOT) has been accepted as the standard regimen for treatment of tuberculosis patients considered to be at high risk for not maintaining or completing the typical 6-month course of multiple drug therapy. DOT involves daily or biweekly doses of medication, a demanding schedule for any person.

In their review of research on compliance with tuberculosis treatment, Morisky and Cabrera (1997) discussed a broad range of contributing factors. They apply a psychosocial model of behavior, which organizes the factors into three categories: cognitive, environmental, and reinforcing. The types of cognitive factors that have been investigated reflect the early influence of the Health Belief Model on research in this area. As noted previously in this chapter, the Health Belief Model originally was developed to guide research on behavior related to tuberculosis control, although the primary focus was screening behavior, not treatment. Not surprisingly, cognitive factors investigated in research on compliance with tuberculosis treatment include knowledge about the disease, perceptions of severity and personal susceptibility, and the costs and benefits of treatment.

A wide range of environmental factors, both physical and social, have been linked with adherence to tuberculosis regimens. Among these are availability and accessibility of care—including location and facilities, physician competency, follow-up, and referral systems—and both direct and hidden costs. It is important also to note aspects of the sociocultural environment that influence behavior in this area, such as how tuberculosis fits into the health culture of the group affected (Rubel & Garro, 1992), and the degree of stigmatization from the health care system, family, and community (Hunt, Jordan, Irwin, & Browner, 1989). Because of its insidious transmission to close associates and its high prevalence among people who are poor and socially marginal, tuberculosis long has been viewed with dread and disdain by society. This is evident in the low status traditionally accorded to people who work in tuberculosis treatment programs. It also underlies public perception that tuberculosis is no longer a serious health problem, because the populations who continue to be affected lack power and influence (Third World people, the poor, immigrants, drug-abusers, HIV/AIDS cases, the homeless, prisoners).

Thus far, we have addressed negative influences, or "barriers," to compliance with tuberculosis treatment. Determinants of successful therapy also have received attention. Such positive or reinforcing factors, according to Morisky and Cabrerra's (1997) psychosocial model, include material, social, and organizational resources. There is considerable evidence that a successful treatment program must provide tangible incentives, such as food, cash, transportation vouchers, and other forms of direct compensation (Fugiwara, Larkin, & Frieden, 1997). Likewise, as is true for all types of sick-role behavior, a strong supportive network of family, friends, and health care providers and links to community services are important. In particular, the quality of patient-provider interaction, including communication of respect and caring, and attention to patients' basic welfare needs are fundamental to the therapeutic process.

Because of the lengthy and frequent treatment involved in tuberculosis control, regimen failure tends to be high, which poses risks to the patient, close contacts, and the wider community. One of the most serious risks is the emergence of drug-resistant strains of tuberculosis; a high rate of such resistant strains in a community usually reflects an inadequate or poorly functioning local tuberculosis control program. The adoption of DOT as the standard regimen for tuberculosis treatment imposes strict standards of service delivery and organization within a control program. It also requires a great deal more resources and political support than has characterized tuberculosis control in developed countries for much of the 20th century. The history of the New York City tuberculosis control program is instructive in this regard.

Like that of many major cities of the United States, the New York City Department of Health had a robust tuberculosis control program in the first half of the 20th century, but public funding cutbacks and a deteriorating public health infrastructure eroded the program (among others) during the 1970s and 1980s. The surge in new cases of tuberculosis observed in the mid- to late-1980s, and continuing through the 1990s, sparked a vigorous response from national, state, and local health agencies. In 1992, the city health department initiated a large-scale control program emphasizing DOT, with both clinic-based and outreach components. In the outreach program, community health workers visit patients at home, work, a local hangout, or some agreed-on secluded location and "observe" firsthand the patient taking the medication. In the clinic-based version of DOT, observation of treatment by staff takes place at the clinic. Although many programs reserve DOT for patients judged to be at risk for noncompliance (homeless, drug user, HIV-infected, or previous history of noncompliance with tuberculosis treatment), New York City made DOT the standard procedure for management of all patients. Local commitment to such an intensive program was backed by a city ordinance that allowed mandatory treatment of infected persons and detention of individuals who could not be properly supervised to follow treatment. These individuals were kept on a locked hospital ward for the course of their treatment. Between 1992 and 1995, the New York City program had reduced the number of cases of tuberculosis cases by 34% and the number of multidrug-resistant cases by 75% and was commended by WHO (Fugiwara et al., 1997).

Despite the success of DOT and other coercive measures, some critics reject the framing of the issue in terms of patient compliance altogether, arguing that locating the problem within the patient population diverts attention from the root cause of the resurgence of tuberculosis, widespread "structural violence" against the poor and disenfranchized (Farmer, 1997, 1999). The critics fault the public health establishment for ignoring the fundamental social conditions that conspire to inflict disease scourges—tuberculosis being just one of many—upon the world's poor. In the terminology of the Causality Continuum presented in Chapter 3, defining the problem in terms of compliance directs the focus to very proximate behavioral factors related to the sick role, and the critical perspective emphasizes more distal social structural influences.

CONCLUSION

Of the topical areas covered in this book, the study of health-related behaviors is notable for having generated a theoretically rich body of research, including widely applied conceptual models and constructs. Many of these were presented or mentioned in the foregoing discussion of HRB. Among the three types of behavior addressed, contemporary public health research, in large part because of its focus on prevention, tends to emphasize health behavior, with less attention to illness and sick-role behavior. Hence, concepts and models of health behavior change have gained increasing popularity in many fields. Other social science traditions give greater attention to health care systems as the unit of study, including critical perspectives that locate problems within social structures as opposed to individual behavior.

In discussing the theoretical underpinnings of various approaches to HRB, we noted the disciplinary roots of key concepts, models, and perspectives. For example, health behavior research has been very influenced by the behavioral school of social psychology, as reflected in different predictive models integrating concepts related to cognition and learning. In contrast, illness behavior research draws from both sociological and anthropological traditions of help-seeking and health system analysis, with systematized models for studying illness episodes and service utilization. Research on sick-role behavior has emphasized heavily compliance with therapeutic regimens, itself an area that, like health behavior, is theoretically grounded in behavioral psychology. These lines of influence illustrate the distinguishing features of the major social science disciplines applied to public health outlined in Chapter 1.

5

The Social Environment and Health

As we discussed in Chapter 1, the social environment constitutes an important component of the human ecosystem that frames our understanding of health and illness. In this chapter, we take a closer look at specific aspects of the social environment, such as gender and family systems, and the ways in which these domains affect both the illness process and coping responses. Simply stated, the social environment is made up of all the human groups, social systems, and institutional settings that we belong to and interact with in our lives. It includes both the microlevel environment, such as family, work groups, friends, and community organizations, as well as the macrolevel environment, such as professional associations, government agencies, social institutions, and society at large. The core discipline from which we draw concepts and theory to study the social environment is sociology, the discipline that studies the relation between the individual and larger social systems, as well as relationships among social entities.

A great deal of writing about the social environment has been based on the concept of *social roles*, that is, the behavioral norms and expectations associated with a defined status or position in the social structure. For example, people fulfill multiple roles in their lives, including that of spouse, parent, employee, club member, and citizen, each role influencing their personal health situation in distinct ways. The kind of influence one's role may have on health has been conceptualized in various ways, such as the notion of health risks associated with a role, or how role demands affect help seeking and the recovery process. Mothers' competing roles in child care and employment have been studied as a possible barrier to seeking health care for their children. In the sociomedical sciences, there has been considerable research on the roles of health care providers, the patient role, and the role of family members in medical care. Studies of role strain in nurses, for instance, examine the multiple demands on the job for efficiency, caring, and technical expertise. In recent years, however, interest in role theory as an explanatory framework for the social environment has waned somewhat. Attention has shifted to *social construction* and *political economy* as theoretical frameworks for social relations. These shifts are illustrated by the following review of research on gender and health.

GENDER AND HEALTH

Conceptual Frameworks for Studying Gender and Health

As an introduction to this section, let us begin by presenting some of the major conceptual frameworks that have been applied to issues of gender and health (Brown, 1997). First, there is the *biological* perspective, which emphasizes the genetic and physiological differences between men and women that contribute to gender differences in health. Examples of such differences are presented in the next section, such as sex differences in brain function and reproductive processes. This category includes "sociobiological theories" of sex differences. Sociobiological theory applies principles of natural selection and evolutionary adaptation to explain social and behavioral natural phenomena. For example, a sociobiological explanation of gender differences in mating patterns posits that women tend to be monogamous and men polygamous because the two patterns differentially favor reproductive success for each sex. By mating with many women, a man "maximizes" his chances of producing offspring, whereas a woman's reproductive success depends on her safely nurturing a growing fetus for 9 months and then maintaining an adequate support system for the infant's early years. Having a stable partner, particularly one with social ties and obligations to the offspring, is advantageous to the mother. Hence, men are said to be biologically "wired" to be promiscuous, whereas women are programmed to favor single unions. This type of biological explanation is often invoked in public health discussions of sexually transmitted diseases, such as the difficulties of changing men's sexual behavior.

A second conceptual framework for understanding gender and health is the *epidemiologic perspective*. This approach examines gender differences in patterns and rates of diseases and health problems (Gove, 1984; Verbrugge, 1989). Such an approach is often used to target different risk factors and to assess the need for different kinds of health services and programs for men and women. Interest in gender differences within public health often takes an epidemiologic approach, to set population-based health goals, and to help design gender-focused prevention programs. However, epidemiologic analysis can be taken a step further to suggest hypotheses based on other explanatory frameworks. For example, explanations of the higher mortality rate among men often rely on sociological concepts such as gender or occupational role demands (Waldron, 1995). Practical applications of such analysis might address social environmental changes such as improving family leave policies in the workplace for both men and women. Other examples of the *sociological perspective* include analysis of gender issues in the socialization of health professionals, differential treatment of male and female patients in medical settings, and health repercussions of the gender order in society (Lorber, 1997).

The concept of the gender order is closely linked to *political-economic perspectives* in health. This approach emphasizes the social structural relations that underlie unequal access to power and wealth in a society (Fee & Krieger, 1994). For example, a political-economic explanation of gender differences in health might highlight the effects of gender discrimination in education and employment or the exploitation of female sexuality in advertising and commercial marketing (Doyal, 1995).

The last two conceptual frameworks are somewhat related. One is the *anthropological perspective*, which takes a cross-cultural and evolutionary approach to gender differences. By making comparisons across cultures and time periods, insights can be gained about how much of what we think of as "gender" is basic human nature and how much is culturally constructed and therefore flexible. For example, Margaret Mead's (1935) early work on gender and temperament challenged Western notions of sex-based differences in personality characteristics such as nurturance and aggression, and subsequent cross-cultural studies document substantial variation in gender roles (Schlegel & Barry, 1991). Evolutionary perspectives on gender relations also have challenged assumptions about sex roles; for example, foraging societies are known to be more egalitarian than more complex societies regarding the division of labor between men and women. In a similar fashion, the *historical perspective* makes comparisons across different time periods to gain insights into how men's and women's life circumstances affected their health status (Leavitt, 1984). For example, contemporary gender issues are often analyzed in the context of previous centuries' situations, such as the effects of war and military duty on the lives and health of men.

Gender Differences in Health

Only in recent years we have learned much about health-related differences between men and women, largely because up until the 1990s women were systematically excluded from medical research (Hamilton, 1996). The rationale for exclusion of women from clinical investigations was that women's reproductive functions (e.g., pregnancy, menstruation, hormonal changes) might create health risks for female participants or (probably more importantly) might interfere with the study protocol and distort research findings. The creation of the national Office of Research in Women's Health in 1991 led to legislation mandating the inclusion of women and minorities in all federally funded research. Consequently, we are learning more and more about gender differences in physiology, metabolism, response to medication, organ function, and the progression of disease.

Research has shown that female brains have more neurons than male brains, and that men and women use their brains differently for the same tasks. For example, men doing rhyming exercises mainly use the left brain, whereas women use both sides of the brain. Women wake up significantly faster from anesthesia than men, and they have a higher heart rate than men, even during sleep. High blood pressure is two to three times more common in men than women, and aspirin reduces the risk of stroke in men with high blood pressure, but not in women. Women get heart disease at later ages and at lower rates than men, but males have a better chance of survival after a first heart attack than women. Men experience clinical depression at far lower rates than women, and they respond better to antidepressant medications. Men are less susceptible to certain carcinogens, such as those in tobacco smoke (Crose, 1997).

One consistent difference that has received considerable attention is the fact that women have higher overall morbidity, that is, they get sick more often, but men have higher mortality at all ages. A related pattern is that women utilize health services at a much higher rate than men, and they live longer than men across diverse societies. The pronounced discrepancy in mortality and longevity between men and women has been called the *gender gap*. A central question underlying much of the research on the gender gap asks to what extent these differences can be attributed to innate biological differences or to psychosocial factors, including gender roles (Rodin & Ickovics, 1990). This is another formulation of the old nature versus nurture question, only it is more complicated now because we no longer view biological and social influences as operating independently. Current perspectives seek to understand how biology and culture interact, which makes for interesting and complex research on gender and health (Waldron, 1997).

Earlier approaches to gender focused on *gender differences* and *sex roles* primarily from the standpoint of individual characteristics and behavior. Sex roles were defined in terms of individual psychology, incorporating concepts such as identity, personality, and socialization. It was assumed that much of the sex role distinctions found in a society derived ultimately from biological sex differences and reproductive role functions, although the social elaboration of the patterns was not necessarily considered to be determined by biology. This notion of sex roles increasingly has been replaced by the perspective of gender as a social institution, that is, a complex, organized system with associated ideology and structure, which permeates many aspects of human social life (Lorber, 1997). This perspective views gender as socially constructed—given meaning and substance through social relations. Our images and expectations of what "male" and "female" signify are produced through everyday interactions as well as social structural processes (e.g., what the "church" and the educational system say and do). Like other domains of culture such as kinship, religion, and technology, gender affects the lives of individuals, families, and other social institutions, and it is a separate entity as well. Gender ideology shapes the way we think about the world, and gender stratification reflects the hierarchical order of privilege and power one gender exercises over the other (Doyal, 1995). For example, gender ideology assigns certain characteristics to women, such as emotionality, which may result in differential diagnosis of men and women exhibiting similar psychiatric symptoms. Gender stratification, on the other hand, is reflected in the fact that occupations dominated primarily by women have less prestige and lower salaries than those associated with males.

The terms *sex* and *gender* have come to be used to refer to the biological and social aspects of maleness and femaleness, respectively. Thus, sex differences include anatomical, physiological, hormonal, and reproductive processes, whereas gender refers to socially defined attributes. A rephrasing of the old nature-nurture question, then, would be, "Is it sex, or gender, or both?" This age-old question is still very much alive in the field of gender studies. For example, take the phenomenon of the mortality gap. Around the world, women live longer than men in every society, a pattern that first emerged in the 20th century. The *sex gap* varies from 8.3 in Finland to 3.3 in Israel. In Western industrialized countries, there is an average of 6 to 7 years' difference between male and female life expectancy. Various hypotheses put forth to explain differential longevity between women and men have emphasized biological factors (Collins, 1993). First, there is the fertility hypothesis. As we have seen, in foraging and agricultural societies, women typically spent most of their lives either pregnant or lactating, which required a certain physiological robustness. In industrial societies, lower fertility makes fewer biological demands on women's lives, so they live longer. Also, lower maternal mortality in modern times contributes to overall gains in female life expectancy. A second hypothesis points to the importance of hormones. This theory begins with the fact that male sex hormones provide a favorable environment for the production of low-density lipoproteins, which increase risk of heart disease, whereas female hormones boost high-density lipoproteins, which are protective against coronary disease. Add to this men's less healthy life-style (diet, alcohol, tobacco) and you have a coronary-prone gender group. Finally, it has been suggested that chromosomes may hold the key: Men may be genetically programmed to live at a faster pace and therefore have shorter lives than women.

Greater understanding of gender effects in some cases has called into question whether some apparent epidemiologic differences are, in fact, real. The case of depression is a good illustration. The relative contribution of biological and social factors to women's higher rate of clinical depression has been debated for some time. As medical understanding of the disease has moved increasingly toward a chemical imbalance model, with treatment focused on medication, biological explanations of sex differences have gained favor. At the same time, political economic studies of gender have demonstrated how the health consequences of gender stratification and social disadvantage cannot be ignored in the social production of illness, including depression. Women's depression may be directly related to their disadvantaged position relative to men in society. This is consistent with the view that depression is higher across all groups that experience social discrimination, including the poor and uneducated who struggle to make a living. Women's systematic exclusion from the power structures of industrial society probably contributes significantly to their depression. However, there is also the view that the prevalence of depression may be more similar across the sexes than we think, because it is simply expressed differently in men and women. Men tend to express emotional problems to a greater degree through aggressive behavior, antisocial activity, and substance abuse, which accounts for the higher rate of violent crime and chemical addiction among men. In addition, women are socialized to talk about their feelings more openly than men, and in conversation they are more inclined to reveal feelings of sadness and other negative affects. Such gender differences may mask a large amount of depression in men that goes undiagnosed.

Gender politics shapes the social construction of public health problems in various ways. The significance accorded particular problems, as reflected in media attention, research funding, targeted programs, and the like, can be influenced by the way that advocacy groups frame the issue. For instance, breast and prostate cancer have similar morbidity and mortality in the United States; there are roughly 200,000 new cases per year and about 40,000 deaths annually. Yet, for many years, breast cancer has enjoyed a much higher profile in the public eye than prostate cancer. More programs and financial support for research and treatment of breast cancer exist, and it is common to see stories in the media about celebrities and public figures who faced this disease. In contrast, advocacy groups for prostate cancer have faced perplexing obstacles in getting the public interested in their cause. Screening for prostate cancer lags far behind early detection of breast cancer, insurance coverage for routine testing remains controversial, and comparatively little money goes into research. This can be partly explained by the lack of clarity and consensus regarding appropriate treatment of prostate cancer. However, some analysts also attribute the imbalance to our cultural preoccupation with the female body as a sex object, others to the greater organization around women's health issues because of the Women's Movement. Following the lead of women activists, men's organizations are beginning to organize politically to lobby for greater support for prostate cancer and other men's health problems.

It fits with the broader gender culture of Western nations that women's heath issues are portrayed in a sympathetic light, whereas men's health issues are often socially constructed to reflect prevailing negative stereotypes of men and their behavior. Feminists have portrayed the female condition in terms of women being victims of discrimination and subjugation, a narrative that fits with contemporary problems such as domestic violence and depression. Men's health issues, on the other hand, have been described in terms of the just consequences of unhealthy male behavior—their bad habits such as smoking, drinking, eating fatty food, getting into fights, driving too fast, and indulging in "couch potato" laziness. Headlines such as "Men's Health: Their Own Worst Enemies" (Williamson, 1995) place responsibility on the men themselves for their ills. This interpretation is consistent with gender ideology, which describes men as autonomous agents actively controlling their lives and health, even to the extreme of taking excessive risks and acting recklessly. Women, in contrast, are portrayed as passive subjects, often as victims, living out their lives at the mercy of outside influences. As men's health issues begin to receive increased attention, undoubtedly will come greater awareness of the social pressures that influence men's health.

Gender-focused research on the health care system has addressed a variety of issues related to occupational roles, professional socialization, communication in medical settings, and gender hierarchies in the health labor force. The latter topic, for example, has been addressed from a political-economic perspective by examining patterns of gender segregation and corresponding inequalities in income, status, and power. Although women make up 75% of the health labor force, they are concentrated in the lower status occupations in the health care hierarchy. Only 2% of all female health workers earn the higher levels of income realized by 46% of all male health workers. Also, women who enter traditionally male-dominated technical curative fields earn, on average, less than half what men do (Butter, Carpenter, Kay, & Simmons, 1994). Gender bias in the wage gap is partly explained by the fact that "women's work" tends to be devalued in a male-dominated patriarchal society.

Focus: Men's Health

As an area of specialized study and policy formulation, men's health, compared to women's health, is in an early stage of development (Sabo & Gordon, 1995). One reason for this lag is that for a long time, gender and health research was largely confined to women's health issues. The formative literature on men's health tends to emphasize epidemiologic and sociological perspectives on observed contrasts between men and women's health issues. For example, gender differences in overall mortality and by specific causes are often highlighted. Males across societies at different stages of development share the common pattern of dying at higher rates than their female counterparts, although the excess mortality observed among males is even more pronounced in industrialized countries (see Table 5.1). In market economies, the ratio of male to female mortality is greater than 2:1, whereas in developing countries the relative risk of death ranges from 1.17 to 1.39 for men. Much of this differential stems from the fact that men suffer from serious heart disease much more frequently than do women.

TABLE 5.1   Male and Female Mortality Ratio for Industrial and Developing Countries

	Ratio of Male and Female Mortality
Industrialized countries	
Market	2.31
Nonmarket	1.93
Developing world	
Asia	1.17
Latin America/Caribbean	1.52
Middle East/North Africa	1.17
Sub-Saharan Africa	1.19

SOURCE: Murray, Yang, and Qiao (1992).
NOTE: Participant ages ranged from 15 to 60 years old.

Explanations for male health disadvantages often invoke sociological explanations such as role expectations and occupational pressures. Scholarly writers still cite as relevant Brannon's (1976) early description of four aspects of Western male identity: "no sissy stuff," "the big wheel," "the sturdy oak," and "give 'em hell." Possible health effects of these idealizations of male identity might include their lack of preventive behaviors and greater risk taking (no sissy stuff), injury-related competitiveness and stress-related frustration (the big wheel), denial of symptoms and delay in seeking treatment (the sturdy oak), and the high rate of male-to-male violence, heavy drinking, and fast driving (give 'em hell).

Male gender-role identity, and notions of "masculinity" in particular, have been given greater attention in men's health studies generally, compared to the corresponding emphasis on "femininity" in women's health. For example, the use of steroids among male body builders, despite its serious health risks, has been linked to psychological attempts to achieve the masculine ideal of large size, strength, power, mastery of self and others, and bravery in the face of pain (Klein, 1995). Similarly, the differential health risks of African American males, including higher rates of homicide, suicide, drug use, HIV / AIDS, and other sexually transmitted diseases, have been explained with reference to black men's pursuit of the masculine mystique (Staples, 1995). Male patients' response to reproductive health problems, such as testicular cancer, also focus on self-image and masculinity as key influences (Gordon, 1995).

Somewhat ironically, biological factors have not been emphasized in discussions of men's health. In fact, the significance accorded to social and behavioral factors in men's health contrasts notably with biomedical explanations of other health phenomena. Whereas in nearly all biomedical reasoning it is assumed that there is a real biological cause beneath a phenomenon (and social and cultural factors are "noise"), in explanations of sex differentials in mortality, social and behavioral factors are clearly considered primary, and biological considerations are seen as residual (Brown, 1997).

Perhaps because women's health issues have been so politicized, men's health issues also tend to trigger political redefinitions of the problem, often in terms of gender equality and discrimination. For example, when the male impotence drug Viagra burst on the health scene, its rapid consumer demand and the ensuing debate about insurance coverage sparked pointed criticism from feminist camps who have long fought to get medical coverage of contraceptive pills by insurance companies. That male sexual function, which some interpreted as "pleasure," was considered a legitimate medical concern, but the need to practice birth control was not, struck many people as a blatant sexist double standard.

In the practice arena of men's health, the focus has been on health promotion and lifestyle change—getting men to live healthier lives and reduce specific risks such as substance abuse and cigarette smoking. In Britain, where the field of men's health is more evolved than elsewhere, the men's health and wellness clinic model has gained acceptance (Griffiths, 1996; Piper, 1997; Williamson, 1995), but specialized men's clinics are rare in the United States. Most writers support the position that men's health practice should be broadly defined to include psychosocial as well as physical dimensions of health (Rees & Jones, 1995; Robertson, 1995), including the less common issues for men such as sexual assault (Rentoul & Appleboom, 1997).

STRESS, SOCIAL SUPPORT, AND HEALTH

The notion that stress contributes to all kinds of illness is so well accepted within both the general public and professional circles that it is hard to believe that as recently as the 1970s researchers were just beginning to investigate the nature of this relation and were, in fact, still posing the question "Is stress a causal factor in disease etiology?" Thousands of studies later (between 1985 and 1995, more than 3,000 articles on stress and health were published in social science journals alone), we now take for granted the idea that not only is stress a significant factor in many chronic diseases, it is probably an underlying component of all kinds of health problems, from infectious diseases to mental disorders to family violence.

Although our understanding of deleterious effects of stress is a fairly new development within sociomedical sciences, early work in this area actually dates back more than a century to the work of French sociologist Emil Durkheim. In 1897, Durkheim published the now classic study of suicide in which he used population-based statistics to identify social groups at differential risk for suicide (Durkheim, 1897/1951). His comparisons of suicide rates in different countries revealed a link between level of social integration and suicide—the more alienated people are from the larger social system, the higher the suicide rate. At a more general level, the study demonstrated the profound impact of the social environment on both individual and group health.

In the 20th century, the experimental studies of Walter Cannon and Hans Selye made significant contributions to our understanding of the stress response. Cannon's (1929) work demonstrated how human beings respond physiologically to external threats in a patterned reaction he termed the "fight-or-flight response." When aroused by fear or anger, the body uses biochemical reserves to mobilize energy for defense or escape. Through learning and cognitive processes, we come to associate symbolic threats, such as an angry boss, with real danger, and we exhibit the same physiological response pattern (elevated blood pressure, sugar and fatty acids in the blood to enable strenuous exertion). Building on this early work, Selye's (1956) experiments revealed that the body goes through a predictable series of stages in response to all kinds of stress, which he called the "general adaptation syndrome," that, if prolonged, can lead to illness. In the first phase, an alarm reaction occurs in response to a stressor, which diminishes resistance to disease. In the second phase, or state of resistance, the body adapts to the stressor and resistance rises above normal. If adaptation is successful, a new level of equilibrium and functioning, the third stage, is achieved. However, if exposure to the stressor continues for a long period, exhaustion may set in, leading to illness or death.

An important milestone in the history of research on stress and health was the identification of *life change events* as measurable indicators of stress that could be empirically linked to subsequent illness. The Social Readjustment Rating Scale (Holmes & Rahe, 1967) was developed to measure the cumulative effects of an individual's multiple life stressors over a year's time, which could then be correlated with illness episodes. The life events items in the scale include both positive events, such as birth of a child, as well as negative events such as divorce, each item given a score representing its stress value. Numerous studies have shown a strong relation between high scores on the scale and illness. However, more studies have focused on the health effects of negative life events than total life change events. Some studies also have investigated the effects of *chronic strains* such as a disabling condition, caregiving burdens, or unemployment.

Other researchers have argued that although major life events are important stressors affecting health, what is more important are the "daily hassles" that wear us down and lower our immune threshold to illness. For example Kanner, Coyne, Schaefer, and Lazarus (1981) developed a 116-item Daily Hassles and Uplifts Scale that, in some studies, was more predictive of illness than major life changes. Criticisms of the daily hassle scale include the observation that some of the items are confounded with life events and the fact that a number of the items are correlated with social disadvantage. Thus, a person living in difficult economic circumstances might be exposed to more vexing situations than an affluent person, thereby confounding socioeconomic status (SES) with daily hassles. In fact, a consistent finding of the stress research in general is that socially disadvantaged groups (women, the elderly, the unmarried, and low SES individuals) are disproportionately vulnerable to stress, both in terms of exposure to specific stressors and from the standpoint of coping resources (Thoits, 1995). This reflects the fact that social stratification, marginalization, and discrimination are often the root causes of stress-related ill health, and it underscores the importance of this area of research for public health.

Not all stress is harmful, and in fact some stress can be beneficial (*eustress*); total lack of stress, which is analogous to sensory deprivation, can have serious deleterious consequences. The key seems to be finding the right balance between overload—distress—and healthy positive stimulation.

Social support can be defined as aid and assistance exchanged through social relationships and interpersonal transactions (Heaney & Israel, 1997). Like stress, social support can have both positive and negative dimensions. Although most research on social support has focused on its health-enhancing effects, there is a downside to too much support. For example, being enmeshed in a very dense network of social ties, such as is characteristic of people with deep bonds to extended family relationships, can generate undesirable social pressures (Rook, 1992). In such situations, social obligations for participation in activities and provision of support may outweigh the benefits gained from social integration. However, the vast majority of studies of social support investigate positive aspects.

The literature on social support typically distinguishes four different types: *emotional* (expressions of empathy, love, trust, and caring), *instrumental* (tangible aid and service), *informational* (advice, suggestions, and information), and *appraisal* (information that is useful for self-evaluation). Some researchers also have differentiated between direct and indirect social support, and between formal and informal social support (Pearlin & Aneshensel, 1987). *Direct support* refers to the provision of instrumental aid, information, or emotional sustenance, all of which may have immediate utility for the receiver. *Indirect support*, on the other hand, refers to individual enhancements such as self-esteem building and assertiveness training, which enable the recipient to take positive actions and manage situations that otherwise might have been more difficult to do. The distinction between formal and informal support is based on the nature of the relationship between the parties involved. *Formal support* occurs within a contractual relationship in which providing help is part of the defined role of the giver, and the receiver is in the role of client, such as that between psychotherapists and patients, or lawyers and their clients. The relationship is hierarchical, the direction of support is one-way, and the basis for the support is professional knowledge and expertise. Furthermore, the setting for the provision of support is usually an office, with fixed appointments and remuneration based on set fees. In contrast, *informal support* occurs in natural settings between people who have an ongoing primary social relationship, such as among family members, friends, and associates. The relationship is egalitarian, support flows both ways, and it occurs in the context of everyday interactions. Although many problems are best addressed by formal, direct support, such as needing legal advice in dealing with a lawsuit or requiring medical consultation for serious illness, the more everyday kinds of life problems are often best handled through indirect, informal support, such as receiving affirmation from close friends.

A variety of measures of social support are found in the literature. Social integration and its converse, social isolation, refer to the quantity, type (e.g., kin, nonkin) and frequency of contacts with other people. Network analysis focuses on social network structure, such as size, density, and dispersion of the complex of linkages to others. Other studies investigate the relational content of social support by looking at aspects such as the source, types of demands, conflicts, role expectations, and social regulation or control of behavior. For example, investigators have differentiated between direct and indirect social control of health behavior (House, Umberson, & Landis, 1988). Direct control would include immediate actions or facilitation such as limiting the kinds of foods served at the family table, and indirect control would include influences such as self-regulated conformity to peer expectations. The distinctions between direct and indirect social control of behavior are similar to those noted earlier for indirect and direct social support and their impact on health.

One of the earliest influential studies examined the relation between level of supportive relationships a woman had during pregnancy and the frequency of complications she experienced during labor and delivery. In that study, Nuckolls, Cassel, and Kaplan (1972) found that fewer supportive relationships, coupled with high stress, led to greater pregnancy complications. A large body of literature has addressed the health benefits of marital status. The consistency of positive effects of marriage are striking: Married people have lower morbidity and mortality at all ages and for both genders, and they exhibit higher levels of mental health than their unmarried counterparts. However, there is some question regarding the directionality of the relation between marital status and health. Much of the research relies on cross-sectional studies in which it is unclear whether mentally healthy people are more likely to marry (the *social selection hypothesis*), or whether marriage itself leads to health (the *social causation hypothesis*). This question is discussed further in Chapter 13.

Because of the limitations of cross-sectional studies, investigators have turned to prospective studies to measure the effects of social support on health outcomes. In a well-known study, Berkman and Syme (1979) interviewed 2,229 men and 2,496 women aged 30 to 69 living in Alameda County, California, in 1965. Four measures of social support were taken: marital status, contacts with family and friends, church membership, and other formal and informal affiliations. Over the succeeding 9 years, each of the four measures of social support independently predicted mortality at follow-up, with marital status and family contact having the strongest effects. A decade later, House, Robbins, and Metzner (1982) replicated and extended this study in Tecumseh, Michigan. These researchers conducted interviews as well as physical exams on 1,322 men and 1,432 women aged 35 to 69. Three measures of social support included inti-

mate social relationships, formal group affiliation, and leisure activities with social network members. Over a follow-up period of 10 to 12 years, significant
health benefits of social support were found.

Other replication studies in the United States and Europe confirm these findings linking social support to positive health outcomes. Furthermore, the evidence shows that the physical health impact of social support is nonspecific:
Overall morbidity and mortality are enhanced, but not the risk of particular
medical conditions. Also, rather than a dose-response type effect, social support
appears to have a curvilinear relation to health, especially for men living in small
communities. At very low levels, lack of support has a strong negative effect on

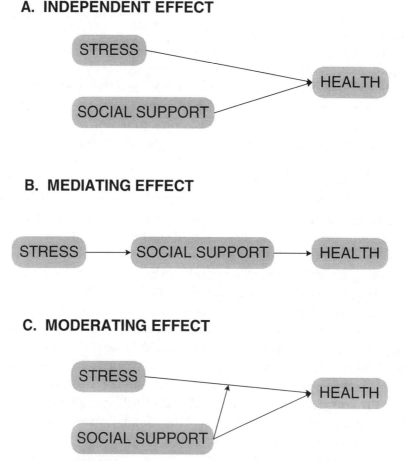

A. INDEPENDENT EFFECT

STRESS

SOCIAL SUPPORT

HEALTH

B. MEDIATING EFFECT

STRESS ⟶ SOCIAL SUPPORT ⟶ HEALTH

C. MODERATING EFFECT

STRESS

SOCIAL SUPPORT

HEALTH

Figure 5.1. Three Models of the Relations Among Stress, Social Support,
and Health

health. At moderate levels, it has a protective effect, but this impact decreases at higher levels.

Interestingly, the strength of the relation between social support and health seems to vary across different types of communities. Its effects appear to be strongest and most linear for men and women who live in urban areas. In small communities, on the other hand, the association is weaker for women and non-linear for men, as noted previously. Some observers suggest that this gender difference is probably due to the smaller variance and the fewer numbers of women experiencing the lowest levels of support among women in small communities (Thoits, 1995).

Overall, there is a notable gender pattern in the research findings for social support and health. The association with health benefits is much stronger among men than among women. This is consistent with studies of marriage and death of a spouse, in which being married is more beneficial for men and being widowed is more detrimental for men than women. Also, men tend to remarry sooner than women following divorce and widowhood. One explanation for this gender difference is that women benefit more from relationships with female friends and relatives and are less dependent than men on the support derived from marriage. Alternatively, older single men may be socially and demographically in greater demand than their female counterparts, making remarriage easier for them.

Despite the emergence of a rich literature documenting the nature of the association between social support and health, we still lack a good understanding of the biopsychosocial processes that mediate this association, and we know very little about the macrosocial processes that give rise to various social relationships and supports. For example, it is likely that large-scale social changes—such as women entering the workforce in record numbers, the insidious persistence of racial discrimination, and the increasing social isolation of urban environments—all contribute to the underlying phenomenon captured by individual measures of social support. A better understanding of the intermediate pathways of effect would give us a better handle on potential interventions to circumvent negative consequences.

Some of the hypotheses that have been advanced regarding the micro- and macrolevel effects for social support on health include biological, psychological, and behavioral mechanisms. At the biological level, it has been suggested that social support reduces cardiovascular and other arousal, thereby triggering the relaxation response that is conducive to adaptation. At the psychological level, social support is suggested to enhance cognitive appraisal of external stress, as when a potential stressor is perceived as nonthreatening. Finally, behavioral explanations posit that social support is associated with a healthier lifestyle through both direct and indirect regulation of health behavior.

Among the various hypothesized relations mediating stress, social support, and health, three basic pathways of effect have been suggested (see Figure 5.1). In the *independent effect model*, stress and social support are conceptualized as operating separately on health outcomes, so that it is the net combined effect that is observed. In this view, social support can be beneficial or detrimental in the absence of stress. In the *intervening effect model*, social support is positioned as occurring temporally after the appearance of a stressor, in which it protects against the negative effects of stress. This view considers social support to serve primarily as a buffer against stress, with little independent effects of its own. The *moderating effect model* combines elements of both independent and mediating conceptualizations. In this view, stress and social support can act both independently and in conjunction, and temporality is not important. Rather, the presence of support can affect health directly and attenuate the potentially negative effects of a stressor. Both the intervening and moderating models posit a "buffer effect" as the mechanism responsible for the interactive effect of stress and social support on health.

HEALTH-RELATED SUPPORT GROUPS

One of the most remarkable phenomena of recent times is the rapid proliferation of health-related self-help groups in Western society. There are literally thousands of different kinds of support groups for every imaginable life problem, more than 2,000, in fact, for illness conditions alone. There exist mutual aid entities for every disease recognized by the World Health Association, even the most rare and obscure. For example, have you ever heard of the Arachnoiditis Information and Support Network? No, it is not for people afraid of spiders; it is a self-help group for people affected by a condition that destroys the pia mater of the brain. In addition to groups that meet face to face, there also has been an explosion of electronic mutual interest groups through the Internet and cyberspace.

Some writers make distinctions between self-help, mutual aid, and support groups. The term *self-help* covers the efforts of both individuals and groups to help themselves, although it is used more often in the context of peer-led group behavior. *Mutual aid*, on the other hand, has the broadest reference and includes people helping others in a variety of domains such as fund-raising and political advocacy, as well as social support. The term *support group* is the most commonly used term to denote groups whose primary functions are supportive communication through group dynamics. Some organizations reserve the term support group for professionally led groups, whereas others use the label for peer-led groups or for any kind of self-help group regardless of leadership.

Despite the ubiquity and popularity of health-related support groups, surprisingly little scholarly research has been conducted in this area (Riessman & Carroll, 1995). Research from members' own perspective consistently shows that the most important benefit experienced by participants is the social support provided through interaction with others similarly affected by a health problem (Levine, 1988). Health care professionals' interest in support groups, in contrast, has tended to focus on the role that such groups can play in facilitating therapeutic goals, including adherence to medical regimens.

Self-help groups offer a unique setting for examining aspects of the broader social environment of health because they are like microcosms that frame larger, more complex social systems (Luke, Roberts, & Rappaport, 1993). The groups encompass not only the individual participants present but also the family systems of which they are a part, as well as their linkages to the health care system, gender structures, and other social institutions. They also represent an excellent example of community-based health resources that operate outside the expert-dominated "official" health services sector.

Probably the earliest, and certainly the most influential, health-related support group is Alcoholics Anonymous (AA). Established in 1935, AA has inspired an array of behavioral disorder self-help groups, all based on the "Twelve Step" model of spiritual self-awareness, behavior change, reconciliation with significant others, and sharing lessons learned with other members. Like many support groups, AA and other 12-step groups also stress the importance of regular participation in the group meetings. Likewise, Weight Watchers, the most influential and widespread weight-control support group, emphasizes the necessity of meeting attendance for long-term success with the "program." Another early prototype mutual aid group was the Paralyzed Veterans Association, founded in 1946. Still active today, this group exemplifies the advocacy-oriented organization, which conducts fund-raising and lobbies for legislative action and social policy.

Although a few groups such as those mentioned previously have been around for quite awhile, most support groups were started after 1975, and it was in the 1980s that an explosion of new groups appeared. This phenomenon occurred primarily in Western industrial countries, but especially in the United States, which places a strong value on self-reliance.

A number of lines of influence have been noted for the emergence of health-related support groups. First, there is the self-help movement in general, which dates to the 1970s and seeks to empower people to manage their own problems without recourse to professional services. Second, the community development movement, which emerged in the 1960s, focuses on the use of local, community-based resources to meet social welfare needs, and it shares with self-help the goal of nonprofessional citizen empowerment (see Chapter 9, this volume). A third influence was the popularization of group therapy as an approach to management of psychosocial life problems. Finally, the enduring importance of religious experience shaped the Western support group model, particularly the themes of finding new spiritual meaning through adversity and sharing one's insights through "testimonials" before an audience.

Although there is certainly a great deal of diversity across different kinds of support groups, most share a number of basic principles that give Western support groups their unique flavor. To begin with, there is a strong orientation toward member empowerment and participation, including a bottom-up orientation and antibureaucratic perspective. Most groups are nonhierarchical in structure and emphasize democratic group processes. Leadership is usually rotated among members, and if professionals are involved, they clearly play a consultant role only. Hand-in-hand with this antielitist perspective is the notion that knowledge should be shared freely among all members and not controlled by "experts." Groups are organized along lines of personal, informal, community, and neighborhood networks. Spiritual values are expressed in group philosophy, such as the importance of living a good life with personal meaning and helping others. Most groups espouse the helper principle that "helping others helps oneself." Learning is fostered through reflection on personal experience, with the goal of self-determination. There is an ethic of tolerance for deviance, such as acceptance of addictions as "illness" deserving sympathy and support. The entire process is geared toward decommodification of helping as a fee-based professional service to one of a freely shared interactive experience among peers.

Self-help groups have become particularly strong in the area of health-related problems. There are a number of reasons for this. In the late 20th century, we came to recognize the limits of scientific medicine in solving our health problems. At the same time, interest in alternative medicine and approaches grew and gained credibility. There was a backlash to the rampant commercialization of health care in an attempt to preserve the humanistic dimensions of care for the sick. All this fit in with the growing consumer movement, which stressed empowerment of lay persons to take control of their own health care. It was also the time when we realized that there would never be enough health care resources to meet all society's needs and that some kind of economizing would be needed. Support groups offer a low-cost alternative to expensive high-tech medicine. Increased focus on "prevention" as a more cost-effective approach gained attention. Finally, the Women's Movement influenced the health scene through its promotion of "consciousness-raising groups," self-care, and patient rights.

Health-related support groups help millions of people around the world, yet very little attention has been given this topic in the research or policy literature.

Moreover, the benefits of support groups are ignored in economic analyses of disability and quality of life. What factors might account for this? Powell (1994) cited the "culture of professional privilege" as underlying the widespread disregard for support groups. Support groups represent a competing power base within the medical community. Professionals tend to regard peer-led support groups with skepticism, suspicion, and sometimes outright antagonism. One survey found that 90% of professionals think their colleagues believe there are "serious risks" involved in joining a support group (Chesler, 1990). The perceived risks include misinformation, bad advice, and interference with recommended treatment regimens. Research conducted by professionals on the benefits of support groups has tended to impose an outsider's definition of success, such as "compliance with treatment," instead of members' own definitions, such as adopting a new "meaning" for their illness experience. There are also pragmatic reasons for the paucity of research on support groups. Funding agencies are interested primarily in research on client use of professional services because they are part of the business of selling these services to customers; peer-led support groups do not have market value.

Research on the components of "support" that participants find through self-help groups has identified several common dimensions (Levine & Perkins, 1987). The groups promote a psychological sense of community and an ideology that serves as a philosophical antidote to the problem members face. Often, this ideology is incorporated into "sacred writings" such as AA's "Big Book." The meetings provide an opportunity for confession, catharsis, and mutual criticism. Observing other role models and hearing their stories offer coping strategies for day-to-day living. Participants expand their social networks through ties with other members.

If we apply some of the concepts of social support discussed earlier in this chapter, we can say that self-help groups provide many different kinds of support to members: emotional, instrumental, informational, and appraisal. Participants receive empathy, practical assistance, advice, and a new way of thinking about their illnesses. These forms of support typically are experienced through informal and indirect means. Participation leads to changes in feelings, attitudes, and behavior as a result of members' internalizing and using a socially shared ideology that offers a useful interpretation of the person's situation (Levine & Perkins, 1987).

Generally speaking, support group participants tend to be female, white, well-educated professionals, although this sociodemographic profile varies with type of group. For example, men predominate in AA but are rarely seen at Weight Watchers. There are more support groups for women's health issues, such as breast cancer, than for men's health problems, such as prostate cancer.

The following highlight profiles the emergence in recent years of two somewhat competing support groups for prostate cancer.

Case Study: Prostate Cancer Support Groups

Participation in support groups for chronic diseases such as cancer has been particularly noteworthy in the past 20 years or so (de Bocanegra, 1992; Greener, 1991; Johnson & Lane, 1993; Slaninka, 1992). However, the existence of groups for exclusively male diseases is a fairly recent development. The case of prostate cancer support groups provides an interesting example of both gender and health care system influences.

In 1990, two different prostate cancer support group entities independently emerged. "Us Too" was cofounded in Chicago by a group of prostate cancer survivors and their urologist. The group obtained sponsorship of the American Foundation for Urologic Disease (AFUD), which provides administrative support and other assistance. "Man to Man" was founded by the late James Mullen of Sarasota, Florida, and, in 1994, it became a sponsored program of the American Cancer Society (ACS).

Both groups fit the typical model of the Western chronic disease support group in which members meet on a regular schedule, usually once a month, to participate in a group session involving educational and support components. The motto of Man to Man is "Knowledge = Survival," signaling the importance members place on keeping up with the latest scientific developments in prostate cancer treatment. Participants feel they do not always receive adequate information and counseling about the disease from their doctors. They would like to reach more newly diagnosed men to help with decisions about treatment. A survey of Man to Man members found that participants placed more value on instrumental knowledge gained at meetings than on emotional support from other members (Coreil & Behal, 1999). This appears to be a gender-related characteristic of the groups.

Whereas Man to Man aims to help more men choose the treatment best suited for their situation, Us Too views the role of the support group primarily as one of facilitating adherence to an ongoing treatment regimen (Porterfield, 1997). These two philosophies partly reflect the groups' affiliation with different sponsors, in the former case the ACS, which tends to support greater patient empowerment, and in the latter case the AFUD, which supports the health professional view of support groups as ancillary to treatment. Health professionals play a limited role in patient referral to Man to Man groups, and they express some skepticism about the benefits of the group. Likewise, urologists underestimate the social support benefits of Us Too groups (Crawford et al., 1997). There also appears to exist some turf protectionism in the prostate cancer support community, with Us Too and Man to Man groups each claiming to better represent the needs of patients. It will be interesting to see how the two groups evolve as prostate cancer support groups become more institutionalized.

HEALTH AND FAMILY SYSTEMS

Family systems can be defined as small, dynamic, semiclosed groups composed of members who have mutual obligations to provide a broad range of emotional and material support. Families have structure, functions, assigned roles, modes of interacting, resources, group culture, and a history that forms part of the developmental or life cycle of the group. Structurally, families are often categorized as nuclear, extended, or attenuated, that is, having more or fewer members than the basic nuclear core of parents and children. Many of the functions performed by families are societal processes that must be achieved to ensure the survival of the species: reproduction; socialization of children; social control; and provision of food, clothing, shelter, security, social support, and identity. In some societies, families also function as units of economic production, such as in agricultural populations. Contemporary families tend to be viewed more as consumption units, although interest in the household production of health has grown in recent years.

Like biological organisms, families grow and develop through predictable stages, and the needs and problems they face at different stages vary across the life cycle. This is certainly the case with public health problems affecting families. For example, social concern about adolescent childbearing derives in part from the fact that it departs from the normative pattern by age and marital status, that is, progression to young adulthood, when conjugal bonding and coresidence are the expected preliminary stages to reproduction. Infertility can be a problem for couples in the early stages of family development. During the childbearing years, public health concerns fall within the realm of maternal and child health: pregnancy complications, including premature labor and low birth weight; infant health, which is heavily focused on preventive care such as immunization, developmental disabilities, and childhood injury; and, eventually, adolescent health issues, such as substance use and suicide. In the middle years of the family cycle, children have left home, and adult health issues rise to the fore. For example, women's health issues such as those related to menopause gain attention, and both men and women begin addressing chronic health problems such as hypertension, heart disease, and cancer. In the later years, elderly health issues are often infused with family considerations, such as one spouse taking on the role of caretaker for a partner, or the long-term care needs for aging parents who cannot live with family members. Some have noted, however, the limitations of the developmental cycle model for family dynamics stemming from the complications of divorce, remarriage, stepfamilies, childless families, and same-sex couples.

Many aspects of health status are closely linked to the family environment in which people live. To illustrate some of these, we draw on findings from a study of health and U.S. families conducted by the National Center for Health Statistics (Collins & Leclere, 1996). As previously noted, married persons enjoy many health benefits that unmarried people do not. For example, married men and women of all ages are less likely to be limited in activity due to illness than single, separated, divorced, or widowed individuals. Moreover, middle-aged adults who live alone have higher rates of doctor visits, acute conditions, and short- and long-term disability. It has been suggested that persons living with a spouse are likely to have better health profiles because of lifestyle differences, such as better eating habits and having someone with whom to share a problem, and because of higher income. The confounding of family composition with income can be problematic. Children living with a single parent or adult report a higher prevalence of activity limitation, disability, and hospitalization, and they are more likely to be in fair or poor health than are children living with two parents. However, children living in the poorest families also report a higher level of activity limitation, poor or fair health, and hospitalization than do those in families with higher incomes. Thus, it is difficult to disentangle family structure from economic factors in studies of health impacts.

Household Production, Maternal Employment, and Child Health

One of the most profound changes in family organization of the 20th century has been the increased numbers of mothers who work in the paid labor force. In 1995, more than 76% of married women with children between 6 and 18 years of age were employed outside the home, compared with only 39% in 1960 (U.S. Census Bureau, 1996). This change has prompted researchers and policymakers to focus attention on the impact of maternal employment on child health and well-being. Studies have investigated a wide variety of outcome variables, including children's cognitive abilities, school achievement, psychosocial development, emotional adjustment, behavior problems, and health and nutritional status. However, few consistent effects of maternal employment have been found (Hoffman, 1989; Kamerman & Hayes, 1982; Rosenfeld, 1992).

The framework of household economics, or household production, allows us to look at how certain desirable "commodities," such as children, prestige, and well-being, are produced by the selective investment of family resources, including money, time, and energy (Berk & Berk, 1983; Berman, Kendall, & Bhattacharyya, 1994; England & Farkas, 1986). Conversely, an economic approach can be applied to study household factors that influence negative health outcome, such as child illness and malnutrition. The kinds of variables studied in household production research include household composition, parental employment and time availability, the competence of child caregivers, and various health-related practices in the home.

A number of studies have used a household economic model to analyze the relation between maternal employment and child behavioral outcomes, such as school performance and cognitive abilities (Desai, Chase-Lansdale, & Michael, 1981; Greenstein, 1993, 1995; Parcel & Menaghan, 1994). Some studies have gone beyond looking at money and time resources and have considered the mediating effects of nonmarket commodities such as maternal attention, affection, emotional support, and companionship on child well-being. Here, too, both positive and negative effects have been found.

Of particular interest to public health is the relation between maternal employment and preventive health behavior. A study conducted in Pinellas County, Florida (Coreil, Wilson, Woods, & Liller, 1998) applied a household production model to look at the relation between the number of hours mothers worked and preventive child health practices. Using data from a longitudinal study of children who entered kindergarten in 1989, the study analyzed a sample of more than 5,000 families. Children of mothers who worked 20 hours per week or more outside the home were compared with children of women who worked less than half-time or not at all. Three measures of preventive health behavior were used: immunization status at school entry, use of automobile seat belts, and use of bicycle safety helmets. All analyses controlled for maternal age and education, household income, ethnicity, and number of siblings. Only children's use of bicycle helmets was significantly associated with maternal employment; children whose mothers worked half-time or more were less likely to wear helmets at least some of the time than were children of nonworking mothers.

Possible explanations for the negative effects of maternal employment on helmet use include the fact that employed mothers are not able to supervise and enforce directly the wearing of helmets during work hours. Also, at the time of the study, bicycle helmet use was not the norm in the study population, in contrast to seat belt use, which was not affected by maternal employment. Furthermore, children ride in cars with adult drivers, who are able to enforce seat belt use, but they often ride their bikes on their own, making it more difficult to enforce helmet use, particularly without direct parental supervision.

CONCLUSION

In this chapter, we focus attention on selected aspects of the social environment that affect health, namely gender, social support, and family systems. Many other topics could be addressed under this rubric; indeed, in a sense, the entire book relates to the social environment in one way or another. Thus, the chapter amplifies certain dimensions of the Social Ecology of Health organizing framework, from the microlevel of the family, to intermediate systems such as support groups, to macrolevel societal structures such as the gender order. The discussion also illustrates the applicability of the Health Impact Model in that all of the topics cover both antecedents and consequences of health problems. Gender, social support, and family organization affect epidemiologic patterns of illness, and they also influence how people respond to problems that arise.

6

Social Differentiation, Cultural Diversity, and Community Health

Human communities are among the most amazingly complex phenomena that scientists can hope to understand. People, as individuals, are often enigmatic and sometimes even bizarre. Groups of people produce incredible and always changing interrelations of values, behaviors, interactions, religions, economics, politics, and health patterns. The dynamic mix of human belief and behavior challenges the success of even the best public health efforts designed to induce healthful change.

This chapter delineates crucial aspects of the complex nature of human communities so that public health practitioners can better conceptualize and implement effective interventions. Without appropriate attention to the dynamic and diverse nature of communities, even the best plans may fail miserably.

The nature of communities is examined here from an ecological framework in which interrelated human social systems are connected to fundamental biological systems that, in turn, reconnect to social and cultural systems. Human communities are comprised of groups of people defined in ways that differentiate them from each other. These groups are numerous, overlapping in membership, formally organized, informally recognized, and constantly changing in composition. For example, although the parameters of "family membership" can be specified in biogenetic terms, it simultaneously can be specified in sociocultural terms. "Blended families" resulting from remarriage, in addition to changing the basic group membership, may bring together varied religions, languages, family histories, and many other cultural processes that cause "the family" to exist in multidimensional forms. If a community health intervention that pivots on aspects of family membership is being planned, the planners must understand the multiple variations of family membership found in that potential subject pool or community. Otherwise, the unit of analysis will be wrongly conceptualized. Because the initial conditions of the intervention plan are seriously flawed, the subsequent stages of the intervention plan and, possibly, its outcomes, can be undermined completely.

Because communities are dynamic, there is a need to understand how such a constantly shifting social entity can have any organization to it. At first, it may seem that explaining community social and cultural diversity is simply a matter of identifying the basic social and cultural traits that different groups in the community express. This produces a list or inventory of traits that a certain group can be expected to possess. For example, whites are highly individualistic, competitive, and live in drab-colored houses in the suburbs. However, it easily can be seen that the putative "white traits" may not be fundamentally valid and certainly do not apply to all whites. Yet, the concept of trait listing still serves too often as a guiding principle used in public health interventions. It should be remembered that the concept of trait listing or its actual use leads to the wrong belief that understanding cultural diversity in a community simply requires that public health agents go out and learn a smattering of "quaint" beliefs and behaviors of the "target" group. Such approaches lead to the erroneous notion that public health agents can amass enough traits to show that a community group indeed possesses a "strange" culture that interferes with "normal" uptake of their intervention. Then the error cascade continues with the belief that they have become culturally competent on group X and can go on to neutralize the "problem" traits. If this superficial level of understanding of group X is used as a guide to understanding cultural diversity in this community, the effort certainly will fail. It fails because the crucial part of community diversity is the *process* of how people relate to each other using a multitude of symbols.

In the classic work of Anthony F. C. Wallace (1970), the transformation of the complex dynamics of community diversity into a thriving system of cultural relationships is labeled the *organization of diversity*. The organization of diversity concept is a counterpoint to the *replication of uniformity* approach commonly found in flawed public health interventions. The replication of uniformity perspective is the notion that society and culture are highly patterned with near-perfect correlation of expected cultural traits to behavioral manifestations. Examples of this type of model are found in commonly used aphorisms, such as, "African American community organization revolves around churches." Embedded in this statement is a host of unrealistic assumptions. For example, the implication is that "all" African American communities exhibit this trait. Also, and more subtle, is the assumption that it is possible to adequately define *African*

American. Who is an African American by whose terms? Such definitional foundations, if not fully considered, can introduce problems in service interventions, ranging from participant recruitment to eligibility criteria for use of the intervention.

Conversely, rather than a static view of behavior patterns ascribed to some community group, the organization of diversity approach assumes that substantial intragroup variation exists not only normally but of necessity. In any one social situation, people may participate for numerous individual reasons, but they tacitly share an expectation of some predictable outcome. For example, people at a public health service nutrition site may have very different reasons for being there. One may really want the nutritional product, whereas another may be there as a participant mainly because the nutritional product saves money on the total household food bill. Both expect and get the nutritional product outcome, albeit motivated by highly divergent reasons.

It is not necessary for all people of the community or group to hold exactly the same values, beliefs, or perceptions to interact successfully, that is, everyone does not have to adhere to the same inventory of cultural traits purported to describe them. In fact, such uniformity is highly undesirable, because such a fictional and philosophically frozen group of people have lost their adaptability to new problems because no one with alternate views would exist who could "push the envelope" to imagine new solutions to inevitable problems. Examples of highly variant viewpoints clashing and then producing new outcomes abound in politics and research. Imagine how meager politics would be if there were truly only one perspective on life. In essence, the organization of diversity concept is supported by the notion that culture is a writhing knot of convoluted, tangled, and constantly mutating values, beliefs, and perceptions that must exist to provide variability of lived experience. Experiencing diverse living conditions helps to provide a dynamic wellspring of viewpoint for adaptation to ever-changing biocultural conditions.

Finally, there is a need to define *community*. As with most efforts to place conceptual boundaries on cultural entities, defining community is more a product of asserting one's biases explicitly than of finding a single, "correct" definition. For most public health issues, community is defined as a place or portion of a place in which some phenomenon is occurring. However, community can be a Standard Metropolitan Statistical Area or a ghetto. Similarly, community can be an age-segregated care center for children or older adults. Also, community can cut across geographic place and exist as professional organizations. Within any of these stated community types, there will also be found intracommunity variation. For example, the Latin communities in southern Florida are composed of people of different immigration political eras and different reasons for immigrating. Also, these Latin communities are composed of people with variable connections to European Spanish, west African, Chinese, and native Caribbean descent. The multidimensional nature of communities makes it necessary to state clearly how community is defined in a given intervention or, perhaps more important, how the people living in some community define their community themselves.

Regardless of the definition of community, analyses of societies worldwide show the presence of universal systems of human organization that are highly germane to public health work. For a roster of the most typical societal organizational systems, simply scan the table of contents of introductory anthropology and sociology textbooks. Here will be found a set of biosocially determined adaptations for group survival. These include categories such as subsistence, kinship, religion, economics, education, and communication. For example, all people must survive by extracting sustenance from the earth and/or participate in economic systems that allow for acquisition of basic necessities of life. This is referred to as *subsistence* and *subsistence technology*.

People also have settled into communities of varied population densities, commonly termed *rural* and *urban*. It is also true that all people have developed some form of religious belief, although extremely variant, about a nonempirical environment. Furthermore, people have organized themselves into ethnic, age, gender, and socioeconomic groups, to mention only a few. For public health intervention in communities to be optimally successful, a detailed understanding of these parts of communities and their interrelations must be understood.

In the next sections, a selected set of important and universal exemplars of human community organization is described briefly in the context of public health issues. The set is comprised of (a) subsistence activities with specific examples from agricultural pursuits relative to health behavior and morbidity due to chemical exposures; (b) interacting religious and sexual-conduct values relative to cervical cancer prevalence; (c) influences of socioeconomic status (SES) on community health; and (d) constructs of race, minority status, and ethnicity in public health interventions.

SUBSISTENCE

Community health can be intimately tied to the subsistence technology of its region. The concept of occupational medicine was derived from observing injuries and deleterious exposures from the nature of work done to make a living. When such work is related to the community's food and water supply, maintenance of workers' health is critical to the population of the area.

Although agricultural pursuits are among the most dangerous jobs done to sustain communities, injury prevention is not the only connection to community health. For example, in a wheat farming belt in the U.S. Midwest, a family medicine clinic experienced not only medical/injury morbidity as a consequence of the wheat growing season but a multitude of nonmedical problems, as well. The nonmedical problems that affected the area included missed physician appointments to work the fields, increased negative stereotypes of the "ignorant farmer" due to neglect of their health, physician frustration with being unable to "reach" the recalcitrant farmer, lost days of school for children to help "bring in the wheat," and increased anxiety of the farmers at critical seasonal times (Stein, 1982).

To understand the community health of this region, the agricultural cycle and its associated uncertainties must be delineated as a part of an annual cycle system. Health interventions must be inserted into this system in ways that work with it and not against it. For example, preventive health visits or health fairs should be held at times prior to major agricultural necessities, such as harvesting. Vaccinations for children and adults likewise would precede times of relative quiescence compared to planting or harvest times. Preparations to meet the needs of certain injuries or toxic exposures could be made by emergency medical settings.

Industrial pursuits are also commonly associated with health risks. Probably no other hazardous substance has resulted in as much disabling disease as has asbestos. Asbestos is employed in building materials, brake linings, textiles, insulation, paints, plastics, caulking compounds, floor tiles, cement, roofing paper, radiator covers, filters in gas masks, ironing board covers, and so on. A useful and diverse material, asbestos nonetheless represents an occupational hazard of phenomenal proportions. In this country alone, there are 8 million to 11 million current and retired workers who have experienced exposure to this substance; of these, 30% to 40% will die of cancer. Inhalation is the primary mode of exposure for these workers (Nadakavukaren, 1995).

Also implicated in exposure within the community are families of industrial workers. Mesothelioma has been diagnosed in the families of workers. The route of exposure was the clothing that the worker removed at home; the asbestos fibers became part of the domestic environment, and thus there was a 24-hour per day exposure (Nadakavukaren, 1995).

In addition, the community in which the industry is housed also may be exposed to contamination. When pipes corrode or waste products from industry are released into lakes or rivers, asbestos fibers can be released into water supplies. Effects of ingested asbestos are not as well established as those of inhaled products, but the current presumption is that there is no safe level of asbestos exposure (Nadakavukaren, 1995).

Although the morbidity and mortality experienced by the workers and their families is obvious in terms of emotional and economic loss, the impact on the community in terms of long-range detriment cannot be overlooked. Economic impacts of the exposure of large numbers of workers, who may not migrate to other communities and industries because of their morbidity, can be considerable. In addition, the industry in which the exposure occurred may be eliminated from the community as production of asbestos-containing products is deleted, thus constituting another economic impact.

At the societal level, implications also must be considered. Society's obligation to those experiencing occupational exposures to known toxic substances has both moral and legal ramifications. Societal mandates include legal and mandatory screening among groups of exposed workers, with mandated actions to be taken by the industry and subsequent compensation to those experiencing the disease consequences of asbestos exposure. Those members of the community who experience less extensive exposure may not be entitled to compensation but may be asked to participate in screening because the moral and ethical implications of not offering such remedies as can be offered are irreconcilable in the society.

RELIGION

The relation of religion and health evokes many common-knowledge examples from the media. For instance, the unwillingness of some religions to accept blood transfusions, even if death is likely, is a notorious item for the news media. Also, on a more positive outcome note, there are many religions that foster dietary or other restrictions that are known to be health promoting, such as a proscription against smoking and excessive drinking. Yet, these obvious religious-based health outcomes are not all there is to understanding the degree of influence by religion.

In a classic study, the combination of community culture, sexual practice patterns, and religion has been ascertained to influence strongly the prevalence of cervical cancer (Skegg, Corwin, Paul, & Doll, 1982). Cervical cancer had earlier been thought to be a function of female's sexual contacts, with support from the observation that prostitutes had high prevalence rates and nuns had low prevalence rates (Helman, 1994). The Skegg et al. study was generated by the observation that in highly Catholic Latin America, the cervical cancer rates were very high although there were strong sanctions against premarital and extramarital sex. There was also the expectation that women would have only one sexual partner for life. Skegg et al. hypothesized that in some communities, women's risk for cervical cancer was less related to their sexual behavior and more to that of their male partners.

Testing this hypothesis led Skegg et al. (1982) to the comparison of three postulated types of society. "Type A" were communities of people with very strong sanctions against all forms of sexual behavior outside marriage; examples were Mormons and Seventh-Day Adventists. "Type B" communities were those in which only women were strongly discouraged from extramarital sexual relations, yet men could have many partners, including prostitutes; examples were from many Latin American societies, which were similar to Europe in the last century. Finally, "Type C" communities were those in which both men and women have several sexual partners during their lives. The example was contemporary Western society, which is considered by many comparisons to be permissive.

The prevalence rates for cervical cancer were lowest in Type A communities and highest in Type B communities. Religion as a part of community culture influenced the behavior of the Type A population and the opportunities for vectoring the transmission of infectious microorganisms promoting cervical cancer. In Type B societies, in which women were strongly discouraged from have sex outside marriage, cervical cancer prevalence was high, but not because of clandestine behavior on their part. Their male partners lived in a cultural environment that allowed for sex with prostitutes, who represented a microorganism reservoir for the human papilloma virus associated with cervical cancer. Skegg et al. (1982) reported that 91% of Colombian students had premarital sex, and 92% of these men had sex with prostitutes. Type C communities had declining rates of cervical cancer because there was less use of prostitutes due to the nature of the permissive society.

In summary, this exemplar of religion and disease shows that disease prevalence from an epidemiologic perspective was closely connected to specific parts of the larger cultural system. These cultural system connections were found to be religious values, which strongly influenced not only sexual behavior but medically unsupportable beliefs about who was responsible for the cervical cancer prevalence. Without knowing these aspects of the cultural system, a biological and social epidemiologic analysis of cervical cancer would be constructed with significant errors of assumption.

SOCIOECONOMIC STATUS

Many studies of the relation of SES to health have been tests of individual SES and family-level SES (Robert, 1998). SES is statistically related to health because the items used for quantification are indirectly connected to real health behavior. Items like income and education do not have as much a direct impact on health, but they do have an indirect impact. More money and education can translate into better health. Overall, such studies have shown that there is a positive relation between SES and health (Crombie, Kenicer, Smith, & Tuntstall-Pedo, 1989; Figueroa & Breen, 1995). However, the additional question of the effects of community-level SES has received less attention. Robert, using nationally representative data, showed that community-level SES does have an effect on health indicators that is separate from the SES effects of individual and family members of the same community. For example, in a community with low overall SES, the individual and families experience lower levels of health beyond their own individual and family SES. This means that *community* must exist as a collective experience and perception of its members and is empirically sufficient to produce health effects. This is a new way of seeing the reality of the concept of community. If the SES of an aggregate of people can influence the morbidity and mortality of itself distinctly from its constituent parts, then does this mean that there is some existential component of community? Whatever the source of the effect, Robert's study further reinforces that health and disease are not simply the outcomes of biological chains of events.

Because there are huge numbers of SES studies about health effects, the issue will not be belabored here. However, caution should be taken in using such data, particularly if they are generated only from cross-sectional, statistical associations. As Robert's (1998) study of "community-level health effects" highlights, "Understanding the community context in which a person lives may also ultimately be important in improving individual and population health" (p. 31). This caveat points to the importance of understanding meaning in the lives of those comprising the community. If only statistical associations are shown, interventions for public health purposes will have no sociocultural framework on which to place the intervention design and conduct implementation. If health behavior were strictly due to SES, then it would follow that if we all had the same income and education, we would all have the same health. That would be very unlikely, because even within SES strata, there is intragroup variation.

Other components of SES, such as relative wealth and income disparity, are discussed in greater detail in relation to health in Chapter 3.

RACE, MINORITY STATUS, AND ETHNICITY

Race

Much of what passes as social differentiation in public health is described in terms of *race*, *minority*, and *ethnicity*. Unfortunately, these common terms are fraught with a multitude of limitations, including biological, political, and social definitions that cloud rather than clarify the reality of culturally diverse community life. Regarding race, James Green (1999) noted, "It is important to mention this mutable dimension of our biological heritage because Americans tend to think of race or 'a race' as something inevitable, as an unchanging part of the 'natural world,' even as something ordained by God" (p. 10). The reality of careful thought about race shows that racial constructs such as "African Americans," "Native Americans," "Mexican Americans," or actually even "white Americans" have no biologically specific boundaries. There is no way to "draw a straight line" between presumed races. Racial grouping schemes have ranged from a few color-specific brands to more highly differentiated subraces based on selected traits such as "physical type" combined with geographic location. The manifold problems of the race concept and their great magnitude of effects caused the American Anthropological Association to publish in 1998 a special issue on the concept of race in the *American Anthropologist* (Harrison, 1998).

Race is a biologically indefensible construct (Templeton, 1998). This fact is strange given the amazing longevity and seeming immortality of the concept of race in popular and professional usage. Many years ago, Frank B. Livingstone (1962) delineated the genetic specifics that show that all living humans have physical variance, but that none is exclusively limited to any one human population. This means that within one population location, the morphology of the human nose, for example, will encompass a very large range of anthropometric measurements. Moreover, nasal morphology will cross-cut populations so that broad nasal aperture width will be found in all populations, as will narrow nasal aperture width. The same is true for other physical features, such as hair type, skin color, stature, and eye color. Today, advances in molecular genetics have allowed for the confirmation of Livingstone's early article (Avise, 1994; Templeton, 1998).

It can be noted that the notion of race as a useless and biologically unjustified concept does not mean that physical variance in humans does not exist. Human variation, both genotypic (e.g., allele frequency variance) and phenotypic (e.g., blood type, bone density, hair type), can be measured easily (Beuttner-Janusch, 1966; Cartmill, 1998; Polednak, 1989; Templeton, 1998). However, most physical variation, about 94%, lies within so-called racial groups, whereas between them, the difference is only 6% of their genes (American Anthropological Association, 1998, p. 712). The issue is that variances are not useful in plotting well-defined, accurate, and analytically useful boundaries between groups. In fact, such racial boundary schemes serve more to harm than to help.

There is a way to organize thought about human physical variation in which similar traits are plotted over geographic space. This is called a map of *clines*. Clines are analogous to thermobars used by meteorologists to plot temperature variance on maps. The plots form curvilinear "bars" connecting all points of the same temperature. In a similar way, human variation, ranging from visible, surface morphology (e.g., skin color) to biochemical phenotypes (e.g., blood types), can be plotted as clines. For example, blood type O spreads from North Africa into southern Europe. However, the surface physical features of the people expressing this blood type would give the appearance of markedly different "races" that would "obviously" exist between north Africans and southern Europeans (Beuttner-Janusch, 1966). Underneath the skin, however, they are the same.

Race still is used in public health as if it were an obvious and readily understood variable. Large numbers of research and intervention projects are designed and funded that incorporate the use of race as a parameter of the effort. For example, research designs that target members of various races as participants seldom even consider such blatant issues that commonly arise from people considered part one race and part another race. Which race will they be today? Which race will they be for a certain situation? Which race will they be for the agency's intervention project? When such questions can be asked, the very concept of race is revealed as grievously flawed.

Another way in which race can be seen to obscure is in the U.S. Census Bureau's attempts to reflect some ill-defined aspect of diversity of the population by introducing "multiracial" as a category in the demographic section on race (Smedley, 1998). First, the basic problem of race is maintained and not solved. It simply is amplified by adding "multi-" to "race." Second, the interviewee self-identifies his or her "racial" category. Unless the interviewee is a molecular biologist with perfect genealogies of their family (an impossibility), they will not be able to offer even an approximation of their population genetic background, much less their own personal genetic history by which to determine race. Third, this reveals that the Census Bureau's addition of "multiracial" to the interview schedule is really asking for a socially invented, self-assigned concept of an interviewee's adopted social category, not anything related to biologic systematics. Finally, it is interesting to note that the Census Bureau has not used the same racial categories more the twice in succession (Keefe, 1992). The problem of who fits what category is not a new one.

The fact that race is still used in common research practice, demographic data collection, and in policy development is a problem. How can public health agents best defend themselves, their work, and those whom they intend to help from the fiction of race? One way is to first have an accurate understanding of the limitations of the concept. Then, as data derived from surveys using race are reported, a cautious, skeptical critique can be applied. Also, when developing interventions, the concept of race can be expunged and replaced by more meaningful categories of a community's lived experience. Such categories include "minority status" and "ethnic status."

In summary, the American Anthropological Association has developed a position on race that may be useful in conveying the most current thinking on the concept. According to the Association's position, there are no biological entities as races. Race is an ideology about human differences that was derived from ancient notions on physical differences. These differences have been irrationally mutated to serve social and political needs. Finally, the concept of race is a contemporary folktale or myth (American Anthropological Association, 1998, pp. 712-713).

Minority Status

Minority in one sense implies simply a quantitative reflection of the population numbers for a given group of people. However, there is also a political implication. Minority populations typically experience a power differential in the social and political arenas of life. This means that cultural identity can be cross-cut by minority status. For example, if minority status means the experience of being a member of a group that experiences unequal access to power, goods, and services, the cause of such treatment cannot only be racist, but it can be due to many other circumstances as well. These include being physically handicapped, homosexual, an HIV/AIDS victim, old, or even some mix of these examples. If a person is homosexual, HIV-positive, and elderly, they can be of any socially defined racial category and still be an oppressed minority receiving irrational, penalizing neglect or mistreatment. The outcome is a socially stigmatized life and separation from the life experience and opportunities afforded to others considered more favorably. Simply put, "The term 'minority' refers to social and economic disability, not to cultural differences as such" (Green, 1999, p. 15).

It is easy to imagine that communities will be comprised of many minority groups. Moreover, these minority groups will be undergoing constant change as political climates change. Also, minority groups that share affinity due to common diseases and disabilities are subject to changes resulting from medical improvements that ideally may relieve them from their debilitating symptoms. Conversely, medical research may suffer from political subterfuge at the funding level and be nearly nonexistent. This would leave certain minority groups fixed with their situation with little chance of assistance from basic and clinical research.

In summary, minority status is not equivalent to commonly used racial categories. In today's complex multicultural world, minority status has gone beyond attachment only to people of color and been extended to those who are kept from ordinary social and political power needed to maintain quality of life. Communities will have groups and subgroups that reflect the perceptions of its members and their notions of social status. Public health interventions must account for these groups, their origins, and their role in the community to increase the probability of successful programs. The key for planners, researchers, and practitioners is to assume great heterogeneity in the fabric of the social life of all communities.

Ethnicity

If heterogeneity is important in understanding minority status, it is crucially important in understanding ethnicity. Everyone can name an ethnic group, such as Irish Catholics, orthodox Jews, Asian Americans, and others. However, the problems are many in understanding these "obvious" ethnics in terms of their lived experience in the United States. Heterogeneity is seen in several factors, such as which generation they were born into after migrating to the United States, which part of a society they are from, how long they have lived in the United States, how intensively they have participated in U.S. life, what language is their most comfortable, or who they have married since being here. All these factors influence the lived daily experience of being ethnic in the United States.

The issue of ethnicity and heterogeneity is also related to the viewpoint of the observer. With regard to African Americans, one observer may think of ethnicity as a given and obvious distinction, whereas another would inquire about the African American's genetic load of genes from Africa. How many African genes are present and accounted for? What if the African American person "in question" is considered half white and half African American? What is their ethnicity then? What if an African American infant is adopted into a highly socially insulated strata of society and has a life experience of extreme wealth with a Polish American family? Is the adopted person still African American? Are they American African? Does it matter?

Like the earlier discussion of race, ethnicity as a concept must be well understood to be analytically useful. Even then, ethnicity is best considered a meager heuristic device. This means that ethnicity is so multidimensional and fluid that its reality is only based on an explicitly asserted definition of ethnicity useful in achieving a specific purpose. Consider, for example, an intervention planned for a Cuban American community. Simply put, the planners may recruit potential users of the intervention by specifying that they be Cubans. As with race, this is not a simple task. Cuba is a society with a significant history of strife, international contacts, and changing political "ownership" (Hernandez, 1992). It is not uncommon for genetic and cultural diffusion to occur as a result of such political changes. Consequently, the planners may be surprised to see plainly African-looking people speaking fluent Spanish with Chinese surnames practicing a religion based on European Catholicism and African shamanism. This mix is the result of the specific history of Cuba, which includes African contact during slavery, Chinese influx for labor via the Caribbean island chain from South America, and Spanish conquest from the natives of the island known as the Taino.

These realities of being "Cuban" still neglect the fact that many Cubans have been exposed to or have been participating in American culture for 40 or more years. Which generation of Cubans would be appropriate to label *Cuban*? The youngest generation may have English names and not speak Spanish. However, they may well participate with their grandparents in activities that are easily seen as derived from Cuban life before migration. When does a person stop "being" their ancestry?

Interventions that intend to be ethnic-specific must account for the reality of ethnicity. This reality is not easily defined. It will include a multitude of combinations of cultural experiences and current political trends. So-called ethnic people will be a synthesis of their composite life experience. However, in certain situations, some portions of their lived experience will be fully expressed and others suppressed. This phenomenon of "situational ethnicity" is a common one that is vexing to public health interventionists. In any one situation, people typically match the expectations of the immediate social environment. For example, in a clinic setting of biomedically trained practitioners, patients try to appear intelligent and understanding of the discussions related by the practitioner. The psychosocial need to fit into the biomedical model expectations are so strong that people may not truly understand what the practitioner has said but will pretend to do so (Helman, 1994; Kleinman, 1980). If patients have culture-specific beliefs about their symptoms and expected treatment, they often will suppress them, using them only at home in the familiar family and cultural environment. The practitioner only experiences one portion of the reality of the "ethnic" patient. The appearance given by the patient could cause the practitioner to conclude that there is no need to consider further the culture of the patient for optimal treatment. This is a mistake that could have significant clinical implications.

James Green (1999) summarized a critical viewpoint stated by Bennett (1975) about two types of "ethnic" concepts. First is the Categorical Model of Ethnicity. Many of the perspectives used to describe ethnicity emphasize cultural content within groups and assume high levels of cultural uniformity within ethnic groups. Both of these notions are found to be incorrect. Also, and perhaps most threatening to rational planning, is that categorical thinking about ethnicity leads to oversimplification of the reality of how ethnic people experience life. It becomes easy to solve problems when they have become contorted to fit some preexisting scheme in which artificial boundaries and definitions have been asserted. This kind of reductionism is comforting in that it gives the sense that the problems of ethnic people can be dispatched easily. Moreover, it fosters the belief that if an intervention for an ethnic group is implemented and few users appear, it is the fault of the ethnic group. The real problem is that the planning and implementation process has been conducted with false initial conditions. Actions based on wrong starting assumptions are doomed to failure.

The Transactional Model of Ethnicity is postulated in opposition to the Categorical Model of Ethnicity. This Transactional Model emphasizes heterogeneity in boundaries between putative ethnic groups, expects differential expression of surface social and behavioral features within groups, and promotes the involvement of ethnic group members in the development of intervention goals. This model is much more reality-based than the Categorical Model, particularly because it allows for the perceptions of the ethnic members themselves to be a part of the defining process for who they are and how they experience life.

Public health practitioners can expect to observe strong evidence of "ethnic culture," aspects of "ethnic group membership," and markers of "ethnic identity." Moreover, Keefe (1992) suggested that a temporal dimension exists in which members of ethnic groups who have been in the United States for a brief time will express more obvious evidence of ethnic culture in their daily lived experience. However, those who have become more established over longer periods of time in the United States will express greater evidence of ethnic group membership and identify as important parts of their lives.

Ethnic culture refers to patterns of behavior and beliefs that set them apart from others. Over time, the expression of these behaviors and beliefs may become muted or highly selectively used. *Ethnic group membership* refers to the network of people around which the person affiliates. Often, this will be those from similar cultures but can include a wide array of those with similar immigration experiences, even if they are from different cultures. *Ethnic identity* refers to the perceptions and attachments that a person has to their own group and culture. Ethnic identity can form in at least two different ways that are derived from specific ethnic experience. Keefe (1992) stated, "Ethnic identity may come about through both self-motivated allegiance and forced identity due to prejudice and discrimination" (p. 37).

Case Study: Psychogeography of Locating Community Support Group Interventions

In Tampa, Florida, a large city of nearly 1 million people, an intervention was planned to develop Alzheimer's disease (AD) support groups for ethnic caregivers (Henderson, 1997; Henderson, Gutierrez-Mayka, Garcia, & Boyd, 1993). The city had a well-established support group to which the white population responded. However, the city is largely tri-ethnic: white, African American, and Hispanic. The fact that the existing support group attracted mainly white caregivers showed an imbalance in caregiver attendance by ethnicity. The epidemiology of AD shows that no single population is totally protected from it. There was a mystery regarding what ethnic caregivers did for support in managing the long-term at-home care required for victims of AD. The disease robs its victims of memory, reasoning, and, finally, life.

Part of the plan for the intervention included finding members of the African American and Hispanic communities so that support groups could be developed for each of their communities with their help. In the African American community, an employee of the county's aging services program was asked to assist in "coaching" the project staff in learning about and becoming involved in the community. The employee agreed and also included a prominent local pastor in the African American community. As all the community public health literature on interventions in African American communities reports, the churches in the community must be incorporated into the plan.

The pastor agreed to hold support group meetings monthly at his church. To make the community aware of this new resource, the project director and the pastor went from church to church making announcements and inviting everyone interested to attend. The African American churches all had a unit of the church that was responsible for tending to the well-being of other members regarding health, transportation, or other needs. These units were generally called "Missionary Societies." Because their mission was to assist those in need, there seemed to be a perfect match between the basic purpose of the support group project and the function of the Missionary Societies.

The pastor would make arrangements for our presentation. He would be introduced by a member of that church, make a few comments about the project, and then the project director would offer some appropriate information about AD and caregiver needs. Finally, specifics about the impending support group would be noted so that everyone was fully informed should they decide to participate.

After making "the rounds" at 10 churches totaling hundreds of members, the date for the first support group arrived. No one came. So, it was tried the next month. No one came. Sensing that there may be a pattern developing, the astute project director began to make some inquiries to specific members who had been enthusiastic about the group but did not attend. These conversations were in private with the project director, and occurred in ways that were totally nonthreatening. No one else was around. There was no specific appointment made to "officially investigate a problem." There was simply (by appearance) a social call made during which the person was encouraged to jointly "think through what was needed to do better."

In multiple conversations with several people, it gradually emerged that the failure was due to an unwritten and nearly unvoiced social rule: Do not cross the loyalty boundaries to one's own pastor and church. Church members are very participatory in their church membership. There is great loyalty to pastors who are seen as pillars of the community. By leaving the "compound" of one's own church to take advantage of a resource held at another church, there was a sense of committing an act of disloyalty.

The test for this finding was to keep all project staff the same, make the same announcements, offer the same resource, but change the location. Rather than what came to be seen by the project staff as a "culturally relevant" or "culturally loaded" setting (i.e., a specific church), a "culturally neutral" site was found. The local city library operated a branch unit in a part of the city with the highest demographic proportion of African Americans. The first meeting held at this site was attended by 12 caregivers, each of whom cared for AD victims.

The culturally neutral public library branch became the meeting site through the end of the project. The invisible barrier had been broken. Even with strong efforts at prethinking possible problems and using assistance from within the community, the early efforts failed. The correction was found only after backtracking the steps that had been taken.

Planning this intervention required the discovery that even something as seemingly mundane as the bricks and mortar of a building can have powerful community symbol value. Without this examination of community cultural dynamics at a deep level of nearly subconscious experience, this project may have been abandoned. Ethnic caregivers would have continued to miss the help that is so vitally needed to weather the caregiver storm.

INTERCULTURAL INFLUENCE AND PUBLIC HEALTH

The "problem" of cultural diversity is bound up with the "problem" of ethnicity. Yet, according to Henderson (1993), without due consideration, attempting to include matters of cultural diversity in community interventions, paradoxically, can defeat well-intended plans to be culturally sensitive, that is, the use of incomplete or flawed concepts about cultural diversity in communities establishes problematic initial conditions that cannot always be overcome. The public health agents may suffer under the illusion that they are accounting for cultural dynamics very well. However, the "culturally different" recipient of an intervention always can perceive the poor fit of the interventionists' meager cultural efforts compared to their real lived experience. The effect can be counterproductive by causing the intervention recipient to feel as if they are given, perhaps again, superficial and substandard credence by interventionists.

It is not uncommon for cultural diversity in public health interventions to be included in a way like this: "We" as agents of public health intervention are confronted with a problem that "they" have, "they" being those "afflicted" with something like ethnic culture. It is as if all public health intervention must consider ethnic culture because, being defined as an affliction of some targeted group, it is a problem that needs to be stamped out or neutralized like an invading virus.

So, if "cultural diversity" is essentially a red herring, what is not? The real issue is *intercultural influence*. Intercultural influence refers to the complex interplay of cultural systems regardless of artificially demarcated group boundaries. The cultural diversity concept has implicit in it the assumption that one group (like a public health agency) must unilaterally take account of the deviant group (like an ethnic group). The reality of such a situation is that both the agency and the ethnic group are engaged in a process of mutual interaction. It is at least bidirectional.

Because there are no culturally homogeneous societies, a community is and always has been marked by dynamic processes of intragroup and intergroup interactions. It is the process of intercultural influence that is the real substantive issue for public health interventions that intend to be culturally calibrated.

Intercultural influence as a concept promotes the examination of the values, beliefs, and precepts held by all the actors of a given interaction. For example, not only is the culture of an ethnic group fully examined to facilitate program implementation, but the organizational culture of public health agencies becomes an appropriate target for culture inquiry, and even the implementers' cultural background is considered. Intercultural influence is complex. Put it into motion by examining "process" and a real kaleidoscope of culture results.

Public health specialists need first to have a good understanding of the basic concept of culture before intercultural influences make sense. There are several ways to elicit information about the culture of a group, including ethnography, key informant interviewing, focus groups, social marketing, and readily available "data sets" that portray the culture, such as newspapers, radio, TV, and activities of community organizations. However, the critical step is the process of interpretation of the elicited cultural information.

Interpretation of observed or elicited behavior requires the detection of nonobvious factors. Such factors are often subtle but significant. These factors can be very subtle because people may not be conscious of them, or they may be paradoxically counter to the actual behaviors observed, such as the workaholic who gives rhetorical blessings to the benefits of stress reduction. It is important to understand that cultural elements identified and added together do not equal the reality of that culture. Each cultural element "lives" in a matrix of interlinking values and beliefs that are situationally changeable. Understanding culture is a challenge requiring not only the formal recipe but the "chemistry" that goes on between the elements.

Finally, the culturally exotic is not. Only by being unfamiliar with cultural phenomena do they seem exotic. This persistent notion results in the significant problem that "our" culture is deemed normal and reasonable. Moreover, other cultures' "exoticness" is evidence of peculiar adaptations (i.e., not normal, or unnecessarily different). Hence, there is the need to stalk cultural diversity, wherever it exists, "out there." The point is that, no matter how often ignored, cultural phenomena exist "in here," too.

In summary, communities are richly diverse in their social and cultural nature. Community public health interventions must be based on an accurate knowledge of the culture, social systems, and symbolic values that relate to the intervention's purpose. Early public health work recognized that all populations have their own culture that is vital and adaptive. Ignoring this preexisting cultural knowledge and behavior while attempting to conduct interventions is to commit the "fallacy of the empty vessel" (Polgar, 1964). There is no society or social grouping that is an empty vessel, devoid of culturally adaptive knowledge on any topic.

The intellectual position of intercultural influence is helpful in approaching community interventions because it "levels the playing field." Adopting the perspective of intercultural influence when designing and implementing interventions assists in gaining a more reality-based balance of power. The agents of help are not implicitly superior to those in need, nor are those in need considered to be experts in public health. Both are able to codirect their destinies for the benefit of lasting community health.

CONCLUSION

There are several key concepts to improve basic understandings of complex communities for public health interventions. The full comprehension of "culture" as a writhing knot of constantly mutating values, beliefs, and perceptions that are differentially shared by members of a community will produce much more reality-based intervention plans than those based on culture as a set of traits. Also, communities and their social groups and subgroups are best considered as highly heterogeneous. Simplistic models of community culture should be avoided, and highly diverse sociocultural dynamics should be expected. Furthermore, the heterogeneity should be considered a positive attribute of adaptation and not a function of disorganization.

Intervention plans also should focus on understanding community dynamics in terms of processes of interactions. Process perspectives assume that people are always interacting and that the nature of the community is found in the interactional process. Such an analysis will show not just that one specific group relates to another, but it will show how it relates. Understanding the "how" of interaction will reveal much about the community as a dynamic entity.

Finally, the most useful concept for understanding community dynamics for public health needs is the intercultural influence model. This model requires the insight that part of the cultural dynamics involved in interventions is the culture of the public health purveyors themselves. The reality of intervention work is that of engaging the cultures of the community and intervention agencies. It also may be that the cultural experience of the agents of the intervention relate to the success of the project. The public health issues of a community can be addressed when social differentiation, cultural diversity, and intercultural influence are fully considered.

III.

Sociocultural Response to Illness

Disease, illness, disability, and death pose a threat to human populations, particularly when large numbers of people are affected or when society must respond to the needs of vulnerable groups. This section covers various forms of sociocultural response to illness, including naturally occurring processes and organized activities. Chapter 7 analyzes natural societal responses to illness from the sociological perspective of deviance and social control. Various mechanisms of control are discussed, employing concepts such as labeling, stigma, medicalization, hygienization, and collective behavior. The domain of violence is given a special focus, examining how political, community, and family violence pose threats to the well-being of social systems at all levels.

A comparative approach to medical systems, broadly defined, is taken in Chapter 8, using the anthropological concept of health cultures. The discussion lays the groundwork for understanding universal features of the complex system of beliefs, practices, and social arrangements related to the management of illness. Key concepts introduced in this discussion include cultural relativity, ethnocentrism, and emic-etic distinctions. The utility of this perspective is illustrated through case studies of Western medicine as an ethnomedical system and the professional-bureaucratic culture of public health.

Organized programs to reduce health threats are addressed in Chapters 8 and 9. The first focuses on community-based approaches to intervention, and the second overviews a more specialized approach—social marketing. Although not a comprehensive review of directed change programs in public health, these two strategies provide good examples of both established and emergent approaches to health promotion. Chapter 8 introduces the core concepts of community, community participation, and community organization and illustrates the application of basic principles of community-based approaches through a discussion of the Planned Approach to Community Health. Chapter 9 defines the four *P*s of marketing—product, price, place, and position—outlines the steps in audience segmentation and strategy planning, and shows how it all fits together in designing a social marketing public health intervention.

7

Deviance and Social Control

One of the basic functions of society is to regulate human behavior by keeping people in conformity with prevailing social norms. This is done through the social control of deviance. There is always a certain degree of variation from acceptable behavior, but too much deviance is a threat to the stability and harmony of the group. Also, some societies and historical periods are more tolerant of divergent lifestyles and conduct than are others; some are noted for rigid enforcement of correct behavior.

Medical sociologists make a distinction between normative and situational deviance (Pfuhl & Henry, 1993). *Normative deviance* occurs by choice and includes behavior we usually view as sin, immorality, or breaking established laws. Circumstances that are out of one's control, on the other hand, are considered *situational deviance*, and affected individuals are not held responsible for it. Victims of misfortune, accidents, and many illnesses are examples of the latter form of deviance.

Social control of deviance can take various forms, ranging from highly institutionalized to very subtle and informal means. Legislative bodies pass laws designed to deter activities considered harmful to individuals and groups. Law enforcement and the criminal justice system are very formal institutions with the primary purpose of controlling illegal behavior and enforcing punishment for serious crimes. Government and other bureaucratic regulation, as well as social and political policies, also serve to shape the behavior of individuals and organizations in deliberate ways. Religious institutions play an important role in upholding moral and ethical standards by condemning certain acts as sinful and by reinforcing approved values and ideals. In fact, most social institutions, such as churches, schools, and the media, play a part in the control of deviance. The less visible forms of influence include social ostracism, stigma, and everyday gossip.

Illness is viewed as a form of deviance because, in a way, it represents a threat to society. When people get sick, they are unable to function normally and may have to neglect their usual role responsibilities. They miss work and cannot take care of the personal and family duties they normally carry out. Others must fill in for them until they get well. If too may people get sick at the same time, it can cause undue strain on the system. For example, employers become concerned if workers take too many sick days and it affects productivity, and multiple ill-nesses within families can be devastating for the group. In public health, there is concern for protecting the health of communities by controlling the transmission of communicable diseases from infected persons (see the discussion of tubercu-losis control in Chapter 4, this volume). The extreme cases, of course, are epi-demic situations in which large numbers of people are debilitated or perish within single communities, sometimes leading to a breakdown in the basic func-tions of everyday life.

THE SICK ROLE

In the 1950s, sociologist Talcott Parsons developed the notion of illness as devi-ance through his delineation of the *sick role* (Parsons, 1951). Like all social roles, the sick role has attendant rights and duties that are recognized by society. The classic view of the sick role was based on American health culture during the 1950s and 1960s and had the following aspects. Becoming ill is considered out-side the person's control, therefore the sick person is blameless and deserving of sympathy and special privileges. Because of the physical debilitation of illness, the sick person is exempt from usual responsibilities, and certain indulgences are allowed. For example, we expect sick people to be more dependent, demanding, and self-centered than a well person. However, illness is thought to be undesir-able, so the sick person must want to get well and relinquish the role as quickly as possible. To do this, the sick person is expected to seek professional treatment when needed and to comply with prescribed therapy. Refusal to follow a doctor's orders can jeopardize one's claims to the privileges of the sick role.

The potential for abuse of the sick role is always there; people can use illness as an excuse for avoiding their obligations (e.g., missing work, skipping school, standing up a date). To counteract this misuse, institutions employ control mech-anisms such as requiring a note from one's doctor to miss work or, in the case of schools, a parent's written verification of illness. Likewise, someone who ap-pears to be exaggerating his or her debilitation or carrying on too long may be accused of malingering, and claims to the sick role may be questioned. In Parson's (1951) view, doctors play a gatekeeper role, exercising authority to legitimize or deny claims to the sick role. However, the changing nature of health problems and medical care management has attenuated the central role of physicians in the illness process.

There have been many criticisms of the sick role concept since its original formulation (Gallagher, 1979; Segall, 1997). To begin with, it is most applicable to acute illnesses that are time-limited and treatable with curative therapy. Chronic illnesses and disability do not fit the model very well. People with long-term conditions can control their illnesses with medication or lifestyle modifications, but they do not "get well" in the sense conveyed by a temporary sick role. In some cases, the role is lifelong, and the affected person must adapt and learn to live with the affliction. Moreover, the social construction of many chronic illnesses places blame on the individual for his or her condition. People who engage in unhealthy behaviors are held accountable for the consequences. For example, we make judgments about people who choose to smoke because of the enormous costs to society for the expense of care and lost productivity associated with smoking-related conditions. Also, we tend to attribute greater personal responsibility to illnesses with a large psychosocial component. In other words, illness has become increasingly viewed as normative deviance as opposed to its traditional conceptualization as situational deviance.

We also have come to recognize that help seeking is rarely determined exclusively by individual choice; social and economic factors such as access to care and financing arrangements play a large role in use of services. Another weakness of the model is that it does not adequately address the inherent rewards of "secondary gain," that is, in many cases people like being sick and do not want to give up the role. Finally, the Parsonian formulation of the sick role is overly "medicocentric" in that it accentuates the physician's role in treatment and ignores the broader spectrum of activities and influences in illness, such as self-care and alternative therapy at the individual level, and health care reform and corporate capitalism at the macrolevel. More recent formulations of the sick role clearly differentiate it from the "patient role" (Segall, 1997).

The transformation of the sick role in developed nations from situational to normative deviance and the complications of economic factors in help seeking have important implications for public health. With its emphasis on chronic disease prevention and concern for access to care, public health has contributed to the emergence of a new deviant role, the *at-risk role*. Unlike the sick role, individuals at risk enjoy no special privileges or support from the health care system or social environment, and they may remain in the role for an indefinite time span. People who choose to engage in unhealthy behaviors are considered at risk for various conditions, and they constitute the "target populations" of planned public health interventions. Numerous institutions of surveillance and monitoring have arisen to identify these troublesome risk groups.

Various health status and risk factor surveys, such as the Youth Risk Behavior Surveillance System discussed in Chapter 3, are periodically conducted by government agencies to keep tabs on the health and lifestyles of target groups. In addition, through the dissemination of "expert knowledge" and media representations of the "healthy body," individuals internalize ideals of body image and functioning, and, through self-monitoring, regulation, and discipline (e.g. weighing oneself daily, perpetual dieting), they strive to attain socially approved states of being (Lupton, 1995). Armstrong (1993) described a "vast network of observation and caution" (p. 407) throughout society, which sustains a level of anxiety and vigilance about the complexity of disease causation. Furthermore, environmental and technological risks have been generalized to the point that everyone, regardless of social position, is considered "at risk" (Petersen & Lupton, 1996).

Case Study: HIV/AIDS as Normative Deviance

Societal reactions to the AIDS epidemic in the United States offer an instructive example of the public health consequences of a disease viewed as normative deviance. Because the risk behaviors associated with HIV infection are perceived as basically immoral or illegal (homosexual relations, intravenous drug use, multiple sex partners, prostitution), the general public has tended to cast blame on victims of the epidemic (Rushing, 1995). Instead of being absolved of responsibility, infected individuals are viewed as social outcasts, condemned for their own bad behavior. Moreover, prevention programs have been severely hampered by society's reluctance to support education aimed at groups that engage in these risky behaviors. Promoting safe sex practices among gays and hygienic drug use is politically unacceptable because many people consider such efforts as tacit approval of immoral conduct. To allow taxpayer funds to pay for programs aimed at homosexual behavior is widely viewed as tantamount to condoning a sinful lifestyle. Consequently, despite the fact that gay men and intravenous drug users represent the largest risk groups for AIDS in the United States, federal- and state-funded prevention programs ironically target heterosexual transmission and scarcely mention those groups most in danger of infection.

Not only have prevention efforts been affected by the moral construction of AIDS, the victims themselves have suffered the consequences of stigma both within their support systems and by the medical establishment. People with AIDS experience rejection by family, friends, and community; face employment discrimination; and encounter barriers to receiving sympathetic and appropriate treatment.

LABELING THEORY

Another way in which society controls deviance is by assigning labels to certain categories of individuals and behavior (Waxler, 1981). The labels, in turn, may lead to special privileges, stigmatizing reactions, marginalization, or other controlling measures. Labeling signals the need for some kind of special or different treatment by society. Terms such as *homeless, disabled, problem patient*, and *indigent* set apart those so labeled as different and in need of special attention. Thus, the social consequences of labeling can be positive or negative.

According to labeling theory, once a label is assigned to a person, others tend to perceive him or her through a lens colored by the stereotype associated with the deviant characteristic. For example, the behavior of someone labeled as *mentally ill* is likely to be perceived differently than a *normal* person, even if there are no actual differences in the behavior itself. Likewise, a *problem child* often gets treated differently than other children. It is not uncommon for labels to have a lifelong impact, with the person's social identity becoming closely meshed with the original category. People "become the label," and society treats the person accordingly. Physical disabilities are particularly powerful influences on identity in this way.

The social consequences of verbal labeling parallel older physical practices of "marking" deviant individuals to indicate their stigmatized or privileged status. In colonial America, thieves and other criminals were branded on the right palms to identify them with their transgressions permanently. To reveal repeat offenders, the accused were asked to raise their right hands in court, which is the origin of the "swearing in" practiced today. African slaves were branded to signify their status as owned property and were denied basic human rights. In the 20th century, European Jews under Nazi rule were required to wear the Star of David on their chests and later in the concentration camps were tattooed with serial numbers to signify an inferior status.

Sometimes, labeling can lead to *secondary deviance* when the individual's self-concept or a group's identity subsequently becomes altered after being labeled. Often the labeled person's life and self-image become organized around the fact of their "differentness" (Lemert, 1967). Examples of this phenomenon include the recovering alcoholic whose life is focused around the principles of Alcoholics Anonymous, the physically challenged person whose handicap becomes the focal point of interaction with others, the mentally ill person whose diagnosis tends to dominate his or her identity, and gay, lesbian, bisexual, or transgender persons whose sexual orientation assumes central importance in how others relate to them and how they view themselves.

In a number of cases, labels originally intended to benefit a deviant group have, in reality, had a mixed impact. For example, the federal legislation mandating public education for "handicapped" children ("special needs" is the more current label) was enacted to ensure special education in public schools for children with disabilities. Some observers have argued that such programs also have led to stigmatization within the school system and have questioned whether the benefits outweigh the downside. Other examples of well-intentioned labels with negative repercussions include posttraumatic stress syndrome, attention deficit disorder, addiction, and premenstrual syndrome (PMS). In the latter case, for instance, the recognition of PMS as a legitimate medical condition with psychological features was initially welcomed by feminists, only to backfire in some respects when it was subsequently used to reinforce negative stereotypes of women as emotionally unstable.

MEDICALIZATION

Medicalization is the process by which nonmedical problems become defined and treated as medical conditions (Conrad, 1992). Issues that formerly were considered social problems, family concerns, or even normal life experiences have become viewed increasingly as illness diagnoses, subject to labeling and management by health professionals. For example, compulsive behaviors, childbirth, homosexuality, developmental changes, eating disorders, and even death itself have moved into the realm of medical pathology with associated treatment protocols. First noted and criticized in the psychiatric field, the scope of medicalization appears to have no bounds, and concerned observers worry about the negative consequences of what social critic Ivan Illich (1976) calls the "medicalization of life."

Like other processes of labeling, medicalization is a form of social control that casts the experience or behavior in question within the framework of deviance from some idealized "normal" state. We need look no further than the vast field of addictions therapy to see how many behavior patterns have come under the rubric of compulsive disorders: gambling, drinking, overspending, promiscuity, child abuse, excessive cleanliness, all of which used to be viewed as criminal behavior or moral failings, matters best handled by the legal system or one's spiritual adviser. The line between social problems and medical conditions has become progressively blurred. So pervasive is this transformation that some observers make the claim that medicine has replaced religion as the dominant moral ideology and social control institution of contemporary society.

Critics argue that the appropriation of life problems represents yet another aspect of medical imperialism, part of the insidious process of dominance, monopolization, and surveillance that places everyone under the watchful eye of the medical system. And this gaze includes public health institutions as well, such as the redefinition of "bad habits" such as smoking, speeding, and unprotected sex as threats to the health of the nation. Medicalization individualizes problems, that is, it transforms socially rooted conditions into personal pathologies. Moreover, it decontextualizes social problems from their multifaceted background, reducing a complex systemic process to a clinical diagnosis. On the other hand, some aspects of medicalization have been hailed as welcome progress from archaic notions of sin and depravity. Certainly, the more humane treatment of the mentally ill represents an improvement over earlier centuries' confinement of the "insane" in deplorable "lunatic asylums." Also, in many cases, medicalization has led to destigmatization, as we have seen with physical disability, infertility, and learning disorders.

Within public health, a parallel process of medicalization has taken place, with more and more issues and situations being defined as *public health problems*. Our concerns now reach far beyond the traditional bounds of sanitation and hygiene, disease control, and protecting the health of vulnerable populations. Now, public health encompasses a myriad array of interests, from injury prevention, noise pollution, and disaster management, to domestic violence, chronic sleep deprivation, and genital mutilation. To a large extent, social problems generally have been conflated with public health issues, and a process analogous to medicalization is taking place that we might call *hygienization* (from the Greek term for health practices). Through hygienization, any phenomena concerned with the well-being of large groups of people can be labeled as conditions with public health significance or, often enough, as public health "emergencies" or "crises" that are "reaching epidemic proportions."

One of the consequences of hygienization is that public health has taken on an agenda that has become unwieldy and controversial, with effective solutions difficult to attain, as seen in an essay that argues that public health has become its own worst enemy:

> We have claimed as "public health problems" violence, drug abuse, teen pregnancy, and homelessness, all of which are deeply rooted in societal determinants. Yes, we can and should research these problems. Yes, they impact on health. But no, we do not as yet have the technical understanding and tools, or the political support, to do much about them. (Somers, 1995, p. 658)

In certain arenas, we find *incomplete medicalization*, in which competing definitions of a phenomenon vie for legitimation. For example, within the field of family violence, competing views of *spouse abuse* define it variously as a sociomedical problem, a criminal issue, and a feminist cause rooted in patriarchy. These different constructions have important implications for treatment and control, that is, whether the proper authority for management should be social workers, medical professionals, law enforcement and the courts, or structural change within the gender order. The women's movement has worked consistently against the tendency to medicalize women's lives and the problems with which they deal, particularly in the areas of reproduction. Likewise, mental health professionals have lobbied vigorously against the narrow definition of *psychopathology* as chemical imbalance to be treated exclusively with drugs.

Finally, *demedicalization* also occurs with conditions formerly considered pathological but now redefined otherwise. For example, masturbation and homosexuality used to be considered psychiatric conditions, complete with official diagnoses in standard reference books. Both have been eliminated as recognized conditions and are no longer listed in psychiatric handbooks. To a lesser extent, pregnancy and childbirth also have been demedicalized in response to consumer demands that natural life events such as birth and death be humanized and recontexualized in the larger scheme of existence. However, it should be noted that demedicalization does not necessarily imply normalization. Homosexuality may no longer be considered a psychiatric disorder, but large segments of society continue to view the behavior as immoral.

DEVIANCE AND PUBLIC HEALTH

In Chapter 8, we discuss some of the features of the culture of public health, such as its values relating to serving the poor and disadvantaged, which contribute to prestige and salaries that are somewhat lower when compared to the private medical sector. There are other factors related to social deviance that influence the image of public health. This has to do with the fact that the kinds of problems, groups, and behaviors that dominate the public health agenda are heavily weighted toward stigmatized issues and marginalized groups. The field addresses some of the most disreputable behavior (e.g., smoking during pregnancy, drug abuse, violence, drunk driving, environmental pollution) and low-status people around (e.g., indigent patients, child molesters, homeless families, pregnant teenagers, senile elderly). These associations naturally affect the position of public health in the social hierarchy.

Public health is also very involved with the collective response of society to medical problems perceived as threats to the well-being of the community. We previously mentioned, for example, the exaggerated societal response to adolescent childbearing over the ages, including the social construction of teen pregnancy as a grave menace warranting vigorous attack. Similarly, we can mention the problematizing of single-parent families, the aging of the population, and other issues that provide interesting perspectives on societal response to perceived deviance. The magnitude and severity of the societal response to deviance reflects the degree of perceived danger posed by the problem. For example, the large number of "cocaine babies" born to crack-addicted mothers in recent years triggered stringent public health and legal measures to curb the problem in the United States. This issue conjoined several forms of social deviance and medicalized problems, compounded by adverse effects on innocent victims. It involves addiction, itself a large arena of stigmatized behavior and multi-sectoral societal control. It involves women's reproductive health, a generally medicalized domain, because women at risk for drug use can be screened during prenatal care. Finally, it involves adverse infant outcomes with long-term demands on social services, hence its public health implications.

Sometimes, efforts to control public health problems through legal measures can have repercussions that conflict with therapeutic goals. For example, women may be reluctant to report spouse abuse because such disclosure within the legal system may place them at risk of having their children taken away from an unsafe environment (see the next section on violence). Similarly, drug-using pregnant women may avoid seeking prenatal care in areas in which drug screening may lead to incarceration or losing one's infant to state care. For example, Whiteford (1996) reported on the repercussions of such a situation in Florida. In 1987, Florida was the first state to pass a statute that allowed authorities to incarcerate pregnant women who test positive for illegal drugs and to take custody of their infants after birth. Although the rationale for jailing the pregnant women was to protect the health of the fetus, few incarceration facilities provide prenatal care or addiction treatment. Moreover, jailed women were separated from their other children, putting the welfare of the latter in jeopardy. Consequently, the statute had the undesirable consequence of keeping needy women out of prenatal care. Although drug use among pregnant women cuts across all social classes, it is primarily poor, minority women who seek care at public clinics who are most likely to be "caught." Private providers of obstetrical care rarely screen their patients for drug use. Applying a political economic analysis to the problem, Whiteford concluded that "laws that jail pregnant women for their addictions are less about protecting the unborn than they are about punishing women for being poor, pregnant and addicted in a society that denigrates each of those conditions" (p. 249).

An extreme example of collective response to disease threat are societal reactions to serious epidemics. *Collective behavior* refers to evolving, noninstitutionalized responses as opposed to institutionalized, day-to-day behavior (e.g., riots and mobs are forms of collective behavior). In such situations, irrational behavior is not uncommon because people respond to social definitions of the problem that may have little basis in reality. The usual, everyday instututionalized means of coping often prove inadequate, so people turn to desperate means. During the global pandemics of the Middle Ages, for example, all of the extreme forms of collective behavior were evident: massive migration, desertion, persecution, punitive quarantines, ostracism of the sick, scapegoating, and conspiracy theories.

During epidemics, society tends to respond by constructing a moral interpretive framework for the crisis and by placing blame on the victims for their misfortune. Very commonly, the source of the problem is attributed to foreigners and stigmatized groups. Members of any group against which the dominant population holds suspicion and hostility are frequent targets for blame. Issues of class and racial conflict often surface in the design of measures to control contagion. Indeed, it is the fear of contagion that propels much of the action geared to protect upright citizens from the unsavory sources of infection. The following case study of the Black Death illustrates these points.

Case Study: The Black Death

Also known as the Great Plague, the Black Death epidemic during the 14th century was one of the worst disasters in human history. About one third of the world' population perished from this highly contagious bacterial infection. Although we know now that the plague was spread by fleas, at the time its cause and transmission were a mystery; none of the learned people of the time could offer a plausible explanation. Consequently, doomsday interpretations abounded, and most people believed the disaster signaled the end of the world. The dominant theory about the cause of the epidemic was that God had sent his wrath upon the world to punish people for their sinful ways. Because of the massive toll on mortality, the breakdown in social order was extreme, with almost complete chaos and anarchy in many places.

Avoidance and desertion of sufferers was common. There was mass exodus from communities, and riots and lawlessness prevailed. People engaged in self-flagellation as a means of expiation for sins believed to be causing this calamity. Most significantly for this discussion, certain groups were singled out as scapegoats for the epidemic. Noblemen, deformed people, suspected witches, and even physicians were accused of spreading the disease, but Jews received the largest share of the blame. During a reign of terror, they were lynched and burned by the thousands across Europe (Rushing, 1995). The fact that Jews became the primary targets is not surprising given their long-standing status as the enemy of flourishing Christianity. Strict rules prevented contact between gentiles and Jews in the form of marriage, commerce, and domestic service. The scapegoating of Jewish people during the Black Death reflects the social divisions preexisting in Europe.

VIOLENCE

Violence is part of the human condition, but it generally is viewed as socially disruptive and undesirable. All societies, even the most technologically simple ones, have had to deal with various forms of violence, and most societies maintain official institutions to control and deter violence. Violence can take many forms: suicide, homicide, rape, spouse abuse, war, political oppression, terrorism, and ethnic conflict. In recent decades, all forms of violence have been increasingly recognized as public health problems that warrant attention from diverse disciplines and sectors of society, not just the criminal justice system or the medical profession. Indeed, the discourse on violence has expanded to include complex processes of *structural violence,* the abusive impact of poverty and discrimination on disadvantaged segments of society (Farmer, 1999). In the following section, we discuss different types of violence from a public health perspective, highlighting current issues in domestic violence.

In the United States, violence has been called a leading national health problem for decades. There is a widespread perception that the country is becoming increasingly violent. The significance of this problem for public health lies in the fact that violence affects large numbers of people both directly and indirectly by contributing to a social climate that is insecure, unsafe, and disruptive of healthy functioning for individuals, families, and communities. Violence destabilizes social systems, creating shock waves that affect multiple levels of human ecosystems. For the purposes of this discussion, we group the various forms of violence into three categories: *political violence, community violence,* and *family or domestic violence.*

Political Violence

Political violence encompasses a wide range of actions involving organized efforts to subordinate, control, coerce, or exterminate a target group. In recent years, the world has witnessed horrendous acts of political violence, including genocide and "ethnic cleansing," human rights abuses, and terrorism, as well as many forms of war and civil disorder. The 20th century has been described as the most politically violent era to date in human history. In addition to the millions of lives lost from political violence, the impact of such destructive forces on individual societies and the world community has been enormous. Severe political turmoil incapacitates the basic functioning of governments and social service systems. The ability of citizens to secure fundamental survival resources, such as food, water, and shelter, is often curtailed for extended periods. Essential public health activities frequently are devastated in such situations, including the provision of health care and preventive services for vulnerable populations, such as the delivery of vaccinations for infants and children.

In war situations, immense resources are appropriated for the support of military forces, weapons, and logistical operations, diverting resources from social welfare programs. Even in times of peace, many countries invest huge proportions of national budgets in defense in response to the possibility of aggression. In developing countries, for example, it is common to see defense budgets several times larger than appropriations for health and welfare. A common sequela of war is the dislocation of large populations, who become refugees in other nations or internally displaced persons, vulnerable and dependent on international assistance efforts. Long-term effects include increased immigration from conflict areas to more stable countries, with attendant demands on the host governments to provide for health and welfare needs of immigrant populations. Recognition of the far-reaching social impact of political violence has led the public health community to embrace human rights advocacy and antiwar efforts within its agenda, including raising awareness of the role of profit-motivated military industries in perpetuating world conflict.

Terrorism represents a special form of violence that became increasingly prevalent in the late 20th century as politically motivated collectives turned to extreme means such as assassination, hijacking, bombing, and kidnapping to exert pressure on opposition groups. One particular form of terrorism that directly affects public health concerns is abortion clinic violence. In the United States, attacks on abortion clinics increased markedly during the 1980s and 1990s. The types of violence perpetrated on abortion clinics include murder, arson, bombing, kidnapping, death threats, vandalism, harassment, and intimidation. Since 1977, there have been more than 2,000 reported acts of violence, more than 28,000 reported acts of disruption, 7 murders, and 16 attempted murders directed against abortion services, providers, and clients (National Abortion Federation, 1998). Public awareness and concern about the issue heightened markedly following the murder of physician David Gunn in March, 1993, at a clinic in Pensacola, Florida. In response to the escalating violence, local law enforcement agencies stepped up surveillance and protection of clinics, and, in 1994, Congress passed the Freedom of Access to Clinic Entrances Act (FACE) (1994). FACE places legal restrictions on the types of interference that citizens may engage in on the premises of abortion clinics.

Legislation and policy aimed at curbing abortion clinic violence led to a reduction in incidents since 1995; however, levels of violence remain significantly higher than those prior to 1984 (U.S. Bureau of Alcohol, Tobacco, and Firearms, 1999). The goal of these organized efforts is to curtail women's access to abortion services systematically through the intimidation of staff and clients and ultimately the closing of clinics. The agenda is political, but it has complex underpinnings related to religious ethics, moral principles, human rights, and access to health care. The abortion question represents a good example of a controversial issue in which there are strong, competing norms and ideologies surrounding a behavior, with no consensus regarding what is acceptable or deviant. Abortion clinic violence represents an extreme manifestation of the conflict between prolife and prochoice factions. However, most activists on both sides denounce violence as a strategy and favor legitimate, legal means of social change.

Community Violence

Like political violence, community violence encompasses a wide range of antisocial acts, including suicide, homicide, rape, gang violence, assault, and battery. High rates of community violence are associated with increased urbanization and poverty, particularly in inner-city neighborhoods. In the United States, availability of firearms has been linked to the elevated rate of violent crime involving guns. Homicide is of particular interest not only because of its severity but also because it is a fairly reliable indicator of violent crime in general. Between 1960 and 1990, the homicide rate for the entire country increased dramatically, doubling from about 5 to roughly 10 per 100,000 population. However, rate increases were even greater in the largest American cities, peaking at 35.5 in 1991 (Fox & Zawitz, 1999). However, a noteworthy trend has been the marked decline in homicide victimization rates in large metropolitan areas since 1991. Both the rise and fall of homicide in recent years are largely attributable to changes in gun violence by adolescents and young adults. By 1997, national homicide rates had declined to levels last observed in the 1960s. The decline in youth homicide is paralleled by a corresponding decline in violence-related behaviors among high school students, such as fighting, possession of weapons, and feeling unsafe (Brener, Simm, Krug, & Lowry, 1999).

Sociological studies of violent crime have identified constellations of factors associated with this type of deviant behavior (Reiss & Roth, 1993). At a very broad level, community violence has been linked with social and economic inequality, ethnic heterogeneity, and residential mobility. In particular, it is the concentration of poor families in urban areas—characterized by rapid population turnover, high housing/population density, and illegal markets for drugs and firearms—that contributes to violent crime. In these settings, legitimate routes to social status, income, and power are severely limited, so youth turn to illegal activities, with their attendant risk of violence, for a livelihood.

The structural impact of racism is evident in differential homicide trends for African Americans. Blacks are seven times more likely than whites to be murdered and eight times more likely than whites to commit homicide. However, these differences occur only in poor populations; homicide rates are similar for the two ethnic groups at middle and higher levels of socioeconomic status (SES). Nevertheless, because of the higher prevalence of poverty among African Americans, violent crime is a serious problem, particular for young males. Homicide is the leading cause of death among African American males aged 15 to 24 (CDC, 1999). The situation is further complicated by social context. Research has shown that community characteristics affect violence independent of income or ethnicity, and a much larger proportion of poor blacks than poor whites live in high-risk neighborhoods conducive to violence (Reiss & Roth, 1993).

Consider the fact that at this point in time, a teenage male in the United States is more likely to die of a gunshot wound than from all natural causes combined. The alarming increase in youth violence that occurred in the late 1980s and early 1990s in the United States, coupled with the occurrence of several mass shootings in schools during the late 1990s, has focused national attention on this problem and potential strategies for addressing it. As with homicide generally, the bulk of juvenile crime is committed by boys. Youth are most often victimized by their peers. Risk factors associated with violence include early childbearing, low school achievement, rigid parental discipline, parental conflict, poverty, and disorganized neighborhoods. Various programs to curb youth violence have been implemented at the level of families, youth groups, and communities: "In general, interventions applied between the prenatal period and age 6 appear to be more effective than interventions initiated in later childhood or adolescence. Community-based programs that target certain high-risk behaviors may be beneficial as well" (Kellerman, Fuqua-Whitley, Rivara, & Mercy, 1998, p. 271).

Family Violence

One public health problem that spans all stages of family development is family violence. It includes spouse abuse, child maltreatment, and elderly abuse. This is a fairly recent field to develop, with national attention emerging only in the 1970s for child maltreatment and in the 1980s for spouse abuse. Before that, a veil of silence and ignorance shrouded domestic violence; signs of abuse went unnoticed, and families kept such matters secret, seldom seeking outside help. The field of family violence has been influenced by many disciplines: medicine, nursing, psychology, women's studies, and criminology. Each discipline takes a different perspective and uses distinctive terminology. In public health, the emphasis has been on documenting the prevalence of different kinds of abuse, identifying risk factors for its occurrence, understanding the effects of abuse on families, and developing appropriate policies and intervention programs to reduce the negative consequences of family violence.

One of the early milestones in the professional recognition of child abuse occurred in 1946 when radiologist John Caffey identified the link between a distinctive series of long bone fractures in children and a history of child battery. In 1962, Henry Kempe and his colleagues published "The Battered Child Syndrome" in the *Journal of the American Medical Association* (Kempe, Silverman, Steele, Droegemueller, & Silver, 1962). However, it was not until the 1970s that the field of child abuse studies began to take shape. An important impetus for the development of public awareness and legislation was the notion that society is responsible for the protection of the health and well-being of children. This line of thinking has led to important control measures, such as laws requiring mandatory reporting of child abuse by professionals and the development of screening protocols for identification of children at risk. Studies show that the prevalence of severe battering on children is about 4%, with about 70% experiencing physical acts such as spanking and slapping, although reporting problems lead many to believe that these are conservative estimates. Attention to sexual abuse in children came later than attention to physical abuse; there has been a notable increase in reported sexual abuse, but it is not clear whether this reflects an increase in incidence or in reporting.

Research on child abuse has focused on aspects of the child victim, pathology in the parents, precipitating events, and the larger social and cultural environment that engenders and tolerates certain kinds of physical acts toward children. Culturally, there is a traditional acceptance of physical discipline for children, and what is defined as excessive force varies significantly from one ethnic and social group to another. Such variable norms have created complicated legal challenges for the prosecution of parents from backgrounds where community standards are at odds with the dominant majority. Studies also have implicated the social environment in child abuse in terms of degree of family integration in a community, SES, and other contextual factors. Family history of domestic violence is a key risk factor; having witnessed abuse as a child is an important determinant of later involvement in an abusive relationship. Other dysfunctional elements, including substance abuse and mental illness, often play a role. The long-term effects of child abuse can include low self-esteem, aggressive behavior, depression, and passivity.

Spouse or partner abuse most often takes the form of a man battering his female partner, although female-to-male and same-sex abuse also occur. Actual rates of spousal battery are unknown, but studies report between 15% and 25% of couples experience violent conflict of some form (Schafer, Caetano, & Clark, 1998). About three fourths of victims are divorced or separated from their partners, and about one third of all female murders are committed by spouses and lovers. Theoretical understandings of spouse abuse have been multiple, drawing from an early concentration on feminist theory to newer contributions from other perspectives, including early learning theory (Koss et al., 1994). Deeper understanding of the dynamics of spouse abuse has revealed that it usually occurs in a cyclical fashion involving periods of relative peacefulness, conflict escalation, and explosive battery, although overall conflict tends to escalate over time. Also, the core elements of the syndrome appear to be attempts by the perpetrator to exercise power and control over the victim. Recent research has focused on the need for the recognition that not all batterers are alike and that intervention programs for the most seriously violent batterers may require additional development. Most attention has focused on victims, including attempts to identify risk factors and programs to assist abused individuals. Yet research has been more successful in identifying risk factors for perpetrators, such as experiencing violence as a child, drug and alcohol use, low assertiveness, low SES, and sexual aggressivity toward spouse. Also, only recently have programs offering services for perpetrators become widely available. In contrast, a great deal of attention and resources have been directed to promoting public awareness of female abuse and improving access to community shelters and other services.

In the case of elder abuse, it is estimated that about 32 out of 1,000 older people in the United States have experienced some form of physical violence. Research suggests that elderly abuse is primarily a white, middle-class phenomenon, but underreporting may exist in some ethnic groups that value respect for the aged. We know that the more dependent an older person is on others for daily living, the greater the likelihood that abuse will occur. Related to this is the fact that older males are more at risk because they are more likely to be living with someone. Also, there is a high rate of psychopathology among female abusers. Although one's spouse is the most frequent perpetrator, sometimes it is the victim's adult child that inflicts harm. Elder abuse is believed to be one of the most underreported events in the domestic violence domain.

In addition to the dependency explanation, other theories of elderly abuse point to the role of the stressed caretaker, a history of family violence, and the notion of the pathologic abuser. The consequences of caretaker stress have become a central focus of gerontology. Researchers refer to *generational inversion* in describing the common phenomenon in which aged parents take on childlike dependencies as their health declines and they lose functional capacity. However, empirical support for the caretaker stress theory has been limited, and there appears to be no relation between an older person's level of impairment and the risk of being abused. The evidence does suggest a link between the degree of dependency of the caregiver on the elder, such as financially or through housing or living arrangements, and the prevalence of abuse. Some analysts have attempted to explain elder abuse in terms of *social exchange theory,* which posits a principle of reciprocal giving in social relations. Because of their dependency, it is argued, aged individuals cannot fulfill societal expectations for balanced exchange, leading to aggressive retribution on the part of caregivers. This explanation, however, is refuted by Groger's (1992) notion of *delayed reciprocity,* which holds that parents earn their care in late life by accumulating years of investments in the well-being of their children.

Professionals working in the field of family violence have taken strong positions regarding the need for improved services of all types. First, better screening is needed, they argue, for identifying cases of maltreatment at all ages. This would involve a broad range of health and educational professionals and would entail integrating screening measures as part of routine work. The extra time and effort required to do this makes some service providers reluctant to take on the added responsibility; in addition, they sometimes feel frustration in finding services for identified cases. Second, improvements are needed in reporting systems. Often, reports fall between the cracks of overburdened bureaucracies, and reporting practices are inconsistent from one state to another. Although all states require reporting of child abuse, only five require reporting of woman or partner abuse, and those that do are not certain of its usefulness. Fewer than half the states have any legislation on elderly abuse, and, of these, only one half enforce mandatory reporting of incidents. Third, the response system in place to handle reported cases of abuse is shamefully inadequate, fraught by underpaid workers assigned too many cases and given too little support to do their jobs adequately. Job turnover in child protective services is amazingly high, and although the public regularly becomes outraged by newsworthy cases of abuse, few voices are raised to protest the current situation. Although shelters for battered women have expanded in recent years, the demand for shelters and other community resources exceeds the supply. Victims in shelters increasingly exhibit needs for both substance abuse and mental health services, and a shift is identifiable in the field away from the informal "woman-to-woman" nature of services and toward more clinical services. The future role of shelters remains to be seen as many agencies move toward outreach, community-based services, and walk-in centers.

Overall, the public health system has not been very responsive to the problem of family violence. For example, for years studies have documented the fact that some women have an elevated risk of physical abuse during pregnancy (although overall elevated risk is questionable), yet little attention has been given until recently to involving the health care system in screening high-risk women and detecting battery during this especially vulnerable period. Of all the types of family violence that occur, child abuse is taken most seriously, and most investigatory efforts are directed there; yet, much more could be done to prevent child abuse and to address the other problems from many angles. A well-developed system of prevention, early detection, and management would require a more organized approach that integrates the health and social welfare systems.

CONCLUSION

This chapter examined various forms of societal reaction to health problems from the perspective of the sociology of deviance. Within the book's overarching framework, social control of illness can be viewed as part of the macrolevel response component of the Health Impact Model. As we saw, the more extreme forms of collective behavior in response to threatening situations include irrational behavior, as in the case of deadly epidemics, along with moral sanctions against "sinful" transgressions. Intertwined with such responses are the social processes of labeling, stigmatization, medicalization, and hygienization.

Although the classic Parsonian delineation of the sick role has limited utility for contemporary chronic diseases linked to normative deviance, it nevertheless has enduring relevance in the general sense that we can identify consistent ways that society sets limits on acceptable behavior for sick persons.

Society also must control other threats to group well-being, such as the deleterious effects of violence in all its forms. Whether the violence is based in political, community, or domestic contexts, various social institutions are engaged in the prevention and management of the problem. Competing definitions of the problem are advanced by law enforcement, the medical profession, and social service agencies. Political and community violence can impede public health efforts directly, and family violence increasingly has been recognized as a serious public health problem.

8

Comparative Health Cultures

The *comparative study of health cultures* can be defined as the cross-cultural study of preventive and therapeutic traditions, both past and present. Anthropologists use the term *health culture* (Weidman, 1988) to describe the complex system of beliefs, practices, and social arrangements related to the management of illness. The goal of this field of inquiry is to better understand how human populations anticipate and respond to illness. Thus, the focus is on prevention as well as the process of evaluating signs and symptoms of sickness and the actions that people take once illness is recognized. The theoretical perspective underlying the approach taken in this chapter is *social constructionism,* which assumes that people interpret or assign meaning to their experiences based on a worldview shared with the social milieus in which they live. Like other life experiences, illness is socially constructed by individuals and their reference groups through processes such as symptom recognition, illness labeling, and patterned help-seeking responses.

Key concepts in the study of health cultures include the contrasting notions of *cultural relativity* versus *ethnocentrism* and *emic* versus *etic* perspectives. In a sense, the concept of *cultural relativity* implies a value principle—the assumption that aspects of one cultural system can be judged or evaluated only within the context of its own parameters. In contrast, *ethnocentrism* applies the ideology and standards of one culture to assess another. A good example of ethnocentrism in the health arena is the strong tendency within industrial societies to apply the standards of Western medicine in studying illness and healing in other cultures. For example, what is considered the "real" cause of an illness might be defined quite differently in Western medicine compared to a traditional medical system in which supernatural etiology is recognized. In a similar way, an emic view takes the "insider" perspective, whereas the etic approach attempts to adopt a more universal and culturally relative stance. The terms are derived from the linguistic terms *phonemic* and *phonetic*, the former referring to speech sounds having meaning within a particular language and the latter including all sounds found in human speech. Later in this chapter, we discuss universals in healing systems, such as a culturally recognized role of "healer." The generic healer role exemplifies the etic category, whereas a specific type of healer, such as a *curandero*, would be one of many possible emic examples of the role.

Four central questions frame the scope of inquiry into health cultures. First, we ask, "What are the universal and particularistic features of healing systems?" or, to use the terminology set out previously, we seek to differentiate between etic and emic components of medical systems. Second, we ask, "What is the range of beliefs and practices related to sickness and healing found across human societies?" Related to this, we want to know what is most common and what is rarely observed. In the past, researchers have been particularly attracted to the rare and exotic, but more pragmatic attention to common practices has gained increasing emphasis. Third, we have a utilitarian interest in knowing "What works in different situations and why?" Finally, related to the latter question, we ask, "What lessons can we apply to our own health system to improve the quality of life?"

Largely drawing from the field of medical anthropology, a broad range of topics has been covered in the cross-cultural study of health cultures. An important part of the literature can be described as the study of *ethnomedicine*, that domain of cultural systems dealing with knowledge, beliefs, treatment practices, and values related to illness. Another segment focuses on the organization and structure of health care systems, including not only the various practitioner roles but the complexity of social and political structures that connect providers and receivers of care. The systems in question may range from very simple to extremely complex in scope and degree of differentiation. Efforts to encompass the range of complexity have included the development of various frameworks for classifying health systems. For example, some of the basic typologies found in the literature include Western and non-Western systems, local/regional/cosmopolitan distinctions, modern and traditional, orthodox and unorthodox, and mainstream versus alternative practices. One problem with classification systems, however, is that they can never sort out the diversity into neat categories. This is because the real world rarely fits our neat conceptual schemes, and because there is ongoing change both within and across health systems. Like all natural systems, health systems are constantly in flux, responding to internal and external forces and adapting to evolving circumstances. Consequently, change processes in health systems represent another area of focused study.

The ethnomedical literature applies various typologies for categorizing different kinds of illness, along with their etiology, prevention, progression, and treatment. For example, Murdock's (1980) fivefold typology differentiates among *natural* causes of ill health, including infection, stress, organic deterioration, accident, and human aggression. Others have identified various *supernatural* forces behind ill health, such as sorcery, witchcraft, divine punishment, evil eye, magical fright, and breach of taboo. Combining both natural and supernatural causes in a simple typology, Foster (1976) proposed a dichotomy between what he calls *naturalistic* and *personalistic* etiology, the latter including willful intent on the part of human or spiritual agents. Still others have chosen to differentiate between *ultimate* and *proximate* causes of disease, similar to the Causality Continuum we presented in Chapter 3. Ultimate causes include abstract teleological concepts such as God's will or natural selection, as well as sociological constructs such as the political, economic, or gender order of society. Proximate causes typically encompass specific medical diagnoses, biological processes, or pathogenic agents.

UNIVERSALS IN HEALTH CULTURES

As a way of framing the study of health cultures, it is helpful to outline some basic features that are found in all societies, no matter how simple or complex, that can be considered "cultural universals in health beliefs and practices." Although our list of 12 features may not be exhaustive, it covers the major components of interest to comparative ethnomedical research.

1. Illness and Care

Disease, disability, and general health problems are part of the human condition; there is no evidence of a time or place in which people lived completely healthy lives free from disease. All societies face multiple health problems, and all groups differentiate among specific illness conditions. Furthermore, organized systems for caring for the sick are a cultural universal; no records exist of human groups that simply allow illness to take its course without attempting to alleviate the pain and suffering associated with sickness.

2. Prevention and Treatment

Not only do all human groups respond in an organized way when someone becomes ill, but they also take deliberate actions to maintain health and prevent the onset of disease (Colson, 1971). In preindustrial societies, preventive efforts

might include eating healthy foods, ingesting fortifying teas and herbal preparations, avoiding exposure to extremes of temperature, practicing ritual activities,
and observing behavioral taboos. Indeed, some folk preventive measures were
quite sophisticated and disease-specific, such as variolation, the ancient practice
of inoculating individuals with infectious material from infected persons, which
evolved into modern immunization practices.

In recent years, there has been growing interest in indigenous therapies of
various forms, but most notably in the area of herbal remedies as a source of new
drugs for diseases that affect large numbers of people. About one quarter of
pharmaceutical drugs currently on the market are derived from plants, including many used as traditional herbal remedies for centuries. For example, the
common aspirin, made from a compound extracted from the bark of willow
trees, is a remedy shared with many Native American groups. For centuries, the
common plant foxglove has been used to combat circulatory conditions, including its derivative digitalis, a drug used to treat heart failure. Some of the newer
cancer-fighting drugs also derive from plant sources, such as vincristine and
vinblastine, used to treat leukemia and Hodgkin's disease, are extracted from the
common rosy periwinkle, a plant native to Madagascar and part of the local
pharmacopeia. One of the most widely used antimalarial drugs, quinine, derived from tree bark, in this case the cinchona tree of South America, and was first
introduced to the developed world by the Jivaro in the early 17th century. A more
recent herbal remedy from China, wormwood, has spurred interest for its ability
to control some forms of drug-resistant malaria (see Chapter 12, this volume).

3. Role Specialization

Contrary to popular myth, the oldest profession was not prostitution, but
healing. Even in the most simple societies in which division of labor was based
largely on age and gender, role specialization was found in the activities of healing the sick. The earliest healers were magico-religious practitioners called *sha-
mans*, respected community leaders who specialized in the management of all
kinds of human misfortune, both spiritual and natural. The healing arts were
tightly integrated with religious practices. As societies became more complex,
other specialized secular healer roles emerged, such as the *traditional birth attendant*, *herbalist*, and *bonesetter*. For centuries, *physicians* were the primary medical
professionals providing general care for all kinds of illness, and since the 19th
century, *nurses* have become increasingly important in staffing health institutions. Over time, highly bureaucratic medical systems have evolved, along with
many different occupational categories to handle the increasingly specialized
management of illness. Today, we have literally hundreds of distinct practitioner

categories in the health field, from highly specialized medical fields, to a plethora of nursing specialties, to a diverse array of allied health practitioners. Also part of this array is a complex spectrum of mental health, social welfare, and public health professionals. Clearly, the trend is toward ever-increasing role specialization, a phenomenon related to the growing fragmentation of health care.

4. Explanatory Models of Disease

Everywhere, when someone becomes ill, there are patterned and organized responses to the event based on assessment of the particular episode. The response is very focused and tailored to the particular kind of illness the sick individual is suspected to have. In other words, there is rarely an all-purpose sick-care response. The concerned caretaking group attempts to determine the nature of the illness, what caused it, what sequella are likely to occur, what treatments and help-seeking actions are warranted, and what the likely outcome will be for the patient and significant others. Taken as a whole, this series of actions produces an *explanatory model* (Kleinman, 1980) for the illness. Explanatory models of illness are socially constructed for specific episodes, but they share many aspects with more general cultural models of illness categories. For example, if someone develops a runny nose and watery eyes, he or she may decide the symptoms are caused by a simple cold and act according to a personal explanatory model of the common cold. On the other hand, sudden loss of consciousness in some societies is immediately suspected to indicate supernatural etiology, setting into motion appropriate care for spiritual disorders.

5. Metamodels of Disease Causation

Comparisons of divergent cultural models of illness reveal the ubiquity of several metamodels of disease etiology that appear to constitute ideological universals. Although similar to the notion of general typologies such as Murdock's (1980) categories of naturalistic causes, the concept of metamodels differs from these formulations in that it is based on emic theories of causation. For example, the concept of *equilibrium* (or disequilibrium) is found in most if not all theories of disease (Cassidy, 1996). Equilibrium models may be expressed in terms of a balance of hot and cold humors, as found widely in Latin American, Arabic, and Chinese folk medicine, or they may be embedded in highly technological measurements in Western medicine, such as hypertension, hypothermia, hypoglycemia, and hyperthyroidism. Another metamodel of disease causation is the *hydraulic system,* the notion that the healthy flow and movement of various body fluids or energy is disrupted, leading to pathology. Examples of this model include African folk theories of blood rising or concentrating in certain parts of the body, Eastern notions of blocked breath or wind, and Western explanations for lymphedema. Our final example of metamodels is *contamination*, the invasion or pollution of the body by impure, foreign, or pathogenic matter. This broad category covers many things, ranging from poisoning, breach of taboo, and exposure to noxious agents to the germ theory of disease and mutagenic processes underlying cancer. Other metamodels of disease causation probably could be identified; we offer the three to illustrate commonalities across seemingly disparate ideological systems.

6. Ritual and Faith

When we talk about the role of ritual and faith in healing, what comes to mind are exotic folk traditions involving mystical ceremonies and trust in the powers of a spiritual healer to intercede with cosmic forces. For example, Native American healing rituals have been widely described, such as the many ceremonies performed by Navajo "singers" to remove the source of different ailments (Kunitz & Levy, 1981). Less salient, but certainly no less real, is the presence of metaphysical elements in all forms of medical care, including even the most sophisticated technological procedures of Western medicine. Researchers have described the elaborate rites that shroud the practice of surgery, such as rules for hand washing and delineation of sterile and nonsterile fields. Even mundane activities such as a trip to the doctor's office are imbued with ritual aspects, and the entire hospitalization experience is loaded with ceremonial features from the moment of admittance through discharge. Faith, too, has come to be recognized as an essential component of healing. A large body of research on the placebo effect documents the power of belief in people's response to treatment; indeed, in clinical trials, participants' response to a placebo is often larger in magnitude than the effects observed in the experimental group (Moerman, 1982). In recent years, there has been growing interest in the spiritual dimensions of all therapy, including the use of prayer and meditation in conjunction with high-tech procedures. This body of research and practice has dispelled the notion that scientific medicine is strictly rational and empirical and highlights another universal in therapy.

7. Core Cultural Values

Medical systems, like other domains of culture, express core values within the larger cultural system. For example, Western biomedicine embodies the core values of Western culture, which traditionally have been identified as individualism, mastery over nature, future time orientation, "doing" activity orientation, and internal locus of control (Stein, 1990). These values underlie aspects of Western medicine, such as the focus on the individual patient, the conquest mentality toward disease, and faith in the healing power of applied technology; these are but a few examples. In Chapter 7, we discussed the sick role in Western society, which prescribes that appropriate steps be taken to treat illness; this can be linked to the action orientation of the larger culture. Moreover, patients are expected to behave in a manner that shows concern and planning for the future, such as in keeping appointments, getting regular check-ups, and living healthy lives to prevent illness. And we expect all this because people also are supposed to be in control of their lives and responsible for their own health, not acquiescent to some external forces, sometimes to the point of "blaming the victim." Other aspects of biomedicine shaped by cultural values are further elaborated in the discussion of Western medicine as an ethnomedical system. Values also are touched on in the section on the culture of public health.

8. Structure: The Sectors of Health Care

Although Western medicine has become the dominant cosmopolitan system of care throughout the world, a great deal of medical pluralism remains, and this is not likely to change. One way of conceptualizing the heterogeneity that characterizes the medical arena across cultures is to apply the tripartite structure of *popular, folk,* and *professional sectors* (Kleinman, 1980). According to this scheme, the popular sector of medicine is the largest and most frequently used resource. It consists of self-care, over-the-counter medication, family care, advice from friends and neighbors, peer support groups, and other sources of help from lay persons. The professional sector, on the other hand, includes organized systems of bureaucratic medicine practiced by individuals who have undergone formal training and who are bound by government regulation (e.g., licensure). Professionals differ from folk healers in that they learn a codified body of knowledge and must conform to established, peer-controlled standards of practice. In contrast, individuals who fall within the folk sector of medical care learn their trade informally, usually through an apprenticeship; they operate independently of bureaucratic regulation and are not expected to conform to any set standards. Examples of folk sector practitioners in European and North American countries include traditional midwives, energy channelers, root doctors, and spiritualist healers.

Yet another way of differentiating among diverse therapeutic practices in pluralistic systems is the dual sectors referred to as mainstream or *orthodox medicine* and *alternative medicine* (Wardwell, 1994). The distinction here is primarily political-economic—what is defined as orthodox has more to do with legitimation and control of the medical marketplace and less to do with normative use or even professionalism. For example, a 1993 study of alternative medicine use in the United States included chiropractors in its scope of inquiry (Eisenberg et al., 1993), despite the widespread public acceptance of chiropractic as a valued professional form of care that is typically covered by health insurance. In most instances, insurance coverage can serve as an indicator of what is considered orthodox care, but in this case chiropractors remain marginalized politically from the powerful and monopolistic medical profession. Other forms of alternative medicine, such as massage and relaxation therapy, are treated as orthodox and covered by insurance only if they are prescribed by a physician, again reflecting the political-economic nature of the legitimation process.

9. The Sick Role

As described in Chapter 7, the sick role postulates that society controls illness, a form of social deviance, by enforcing strict rules for appropriate sick behavior, including certain rights and responsibilities bestowed on ill persons. In Western society, the sick role exempts the sick from normal role obligations, such as going to work and cleaning the house, but requires that professional advice be sought and followed correctly. Although originally developed to describe expectations in Western countries, the notion of a sick role can be identified in any health culture. It appears that the universal aspects of the sick role include some combination of rights (exemptions) and duties (responsibilities), like all social roles, but the specific content of the expectations varies across cultures. For example, the expectation to consult a physician and follow medical advice is not found everywhere; in some settings, the family is expected to take a major role in managing the illness episode. In other words, it is a universal expectation that sick people should follow prescribed behavior to maintain their good standing in society.

10. Social and Moral Control

Like the sick role, the idea of social and moral control through illness was described in greater depth in Chapter 7. Suffice it to say here that it is a universal feature of health cultures to treat illness in such a way that underscores the prevailing moral precepts of the times. In addition, part of the response is aimed at controlling deviance per se, a threat to the social order. The key point is that societal response to illness goes beyond the needs of the individual; illness is used by society to enforce morals and reduce nonconformity. Sometimes, control is exercised through a process of labeling, such as defining alcoholism as a "disease" and thereby centering its treatment within the medical system. Another control mechanism is stigmatization, the pejorative treatment of classes of people and categories of behavior deemed dangerous, unacceptable, unworthy, or a threat to the public good. For example, in Haiti, families sometimes deliberately seek out orthodox medical care to forestall possible public accusations of involvement with voodoo, and they avoid as long as possible a diagnosis of supernatural illness because of the unsavory moral implications (Brodwin, 1996). In the United States, certain illnesses such as sexually transmitted diseases and smoking-related conditions are socially stigmatized because they are associated with what is considered immoral behavior. Other examples of moralistic dimensions of illness discussed in various chapters of this book include HIV/AIDS, tuberculosis, and the Great Plague.

11. Therapy Managing Group

Very rarely do individuals go through an entire illness episode without getting help or advice about it from someone they know. For routine, minor illnesses limited to self-care, this may be more the case, but when the services of medical specialists are brought into the picture, the illness usually comes under the supervision of a *therapy managing group*. There is almost always one or more significant others whose views are taken into consideration for decision making about a patient's treatment. In some cases, the group might involve only one or two close family members, whereas other instances might involve a large network of kin, friends, and professional case managers. One of the authors once served as a member of a complex network of friends, family members, church members, social workers, and medical professionals involved in the management of a middle-aged woman's psychiatric illness. The group communicated regularly by electronic mail, and major decisions were made by ad hoc subgroups composed of the patient plus at least one family member, one friend, and one professional. In the former Zaire, Janzen (1978), who coined the term, described elaborate *kin-based therapy managing groups*, which supervised multiple stages of therapy-seeking from various specialists. Some patient advocates explicitly lobby for greater involvement of natural therapy managing groups in medical care.

12. Therapeutic Networks

Also referred to as *lay referral systems* or *hierarchy of resort*, the concept of *therapeutic networks* encompasses the process of seeking help from different sources and the patterned sequence and regularity of the various components involved (Helman, 1994). People do not respond to illness in an ad hoc, trial-and-error approach. They use past experience, accumulated knowledge, contemporary advice, and referral to develop a strategy for obtaining the best results for the means available. Therapeutic networks become patterned within health cultures, and their basic outlines can be discerned through research. For example, in the vast majority of illnesses, people do not immediately seek professional care following the first symptom; they watch and evaluate what happens and seek informal advice from family and friends. The decision to consult a medical specialist may be based on recommendations from someone they know and trust who has experienced a similar problem. Once in the system, a patient may "shop around" among providers until he or she is satisfied with the diagnosis and/or care received. Often, the therapeutic network will be profoundly influenced by the perceived nature of the illness. For example, if supernatural etiology is suspected, this may dictate involvement of a magico-religious healer right away. In another instance, an illness may at first appear to be caused by natural forces and a Western practitioner will be consulted, and then only after repeated failures to effect a cure will a traditional healer be consulted.

WESTERN MEDICINE AS AN ETHNOMEDICAL SYSTEM

Early comparative studies of health cultures tended to describe non-Western medical systems in terms of how they differed from "modern, scientific medicine," the latter implicitly assumed to represent the standard against which to evaluate other health beliefs and practices. This somewhat ethnocentric approach has been replaced by a more critical perspective that views Western medicine as just one among many equally legitimate ethnomedical systems, though acknowledging its global political and geographic dominance (Rhodes, 1996). In keeping with this critical stance, anthropologists and others have offered fairly consistent ethnographic descriptions of the "culture of medicine" as practiced in Europe and North America, including some of the following components. First and foremost, Western medicine is founded on the principles of modern science and, like other scientific traditions, gives primacy to the rational and empirical study of physical phenomena. Only that which can be objectively observed and measured is considered real. Thus, patients' subjective reports of experience and perceptions are accorded much less significance than the physical and chemical data derived from physical examination, laboratory tests, and electronic machines. If something cannot be seen or measured, it does not exist, because the primary language of science is mathematics.

Like Western thought generally, scientific medicine divides the world into two distinct realms, the physical and the mental. Often referred to as *mind-body dualism*, this separation of phenomena into thought and matter has profoundly shaped our theories of illness and the organization of medical practice. Because of this dichotomous thinking, a separate specialty, psychiatry, has developed to deal with mental illness, and even within this discipline, chemical therapy through medication has dominated treatment patterns. Traditional constructions of illness view what goes on in the mind as independent of bodily processes. Diseases generally tend to be viewed as "entities" within a mechanical body, analogous to foreign enemies invading a physical terrain. The germ theory of disease dominated most of the 20th century, complete with military metaphors of war and defense (e.g., germ-fighting drugs, the war on cancer, one's battle with illness, and campaigns to eliminate threats to health). Furthermore, the locus of treatment in Western medicine is the individual person, with clinical practice organized around patient-centered care. Environmental factors have been given much less attention than what goes on inside the bodies of sick persons. Thus, the war is seen as a series of individual battles with the goal of warding off disease.

Research and practice in Western medicine relies heavily on technological developments such as those associated with surgery, chemotherapy, radiology, and advanced life-support systems (Hahn, 1995). Sometimes called the *cult of technology*, this bias toward the use of sophisticated equipment and machines parallels the weaponry of modern warfare. It also underlies the prestige and status associated with those medical specialties that rely heavily on advanced technology. The "high-tech" orientation of Western medicine, and particularly the American version of it (see subsequent discussion), has become a point of much debate and criticism in recent years. Critics point out the dehumanizing effects of a system that worships technology at the expense of emotional sensitivity and respect for people (Davis-Floyd, 1994).

Another distinctive feature of modern medicine is the *cult of efficiency*, the organization of care so as to maximize the economic use of time, personnel, and other resources. Nowhere is this value more evident than in hospital settings, where patients are treated like vessels for sick organs, tightly regimented, managed, and controlled through round-the-clock procedures and routines. The importance of efficiency is also manifested in doctors' offices, where activities are organized to maximize the most productive use of staff time, particularly that of the physician. Across diverse studies of patient experiences in medical settings, recurrent complaints point to deep-seated patient dissatisfaction with what they perceive as being insensitively treated like commodities in a production factory. Not only are patients treated as "goods," but the entire health care system has been transformed into a vast industrial complex. Health and health care have become "big business," leading to increasing commodification and marketing like other products for sale in the marketplace (although more so in the United States than in Europe and Canada).

Finally, as we saw in Chapter 7, Western medicine has demonstrated a tendency to take over more and more areas of life under its purview, a process sometimes described as the *medicalization of life*. Vast areas of human welfare formerly considered social, moral, family, or behavioral problems and issues have been labeled *illnesses* or *disorders* of some sort, with medical views on proper management replacing traditional wisdom. Bad habits, personal failings, disorderly conduct, and moral transgressions have been given diagnostic medical labels. Furthermore, many natural bodily processes and changes previously viewed as part of the normal process of human development likewise have been medicalized and brought under the oversight of medical treatment. For example, a range of events related to women's reproductive lives, adolescence, and old age in general have been reconstructed as medical problems to be addressed by professionals.

Within these broad outlines of Western medicine, differences can be observed across national boundaries and sometimes by regions in a single country. For example, medicine as practiced in the United States has been contrasted with other industrialized countries on several points. U.S. medicine has been described as "aggressive" and invasive, quick to intervene with the "biggest guns" technology has to offer. For example, rates for most types of surgery are by far the highest in the United States, and end-stage life-prolonging treatment is used much more vigorously than in other places. Most antibiotics and other medications are used more extensively, and there is far heavier reliance on high-tech apparatus and tests. Payer (1988) summed up American medicine as aggressively attacking "the virus in the machine," highlighting its approach to the body as a set of parts to be tuned, repaired, or replaced, much like the way we view an automobile.

However, the picture of Western medicine drawn previously represents an ideal type and does not take into account the vast heterogeneity of an increasingly complex system. There are many areas of medicine that depart from this stereotypical view. It is partly an issue of semantics, because we use the term *medicine* to include all activities within the health care system, and there are many different professions involved. For example, the field of nursing is widely recognized as oriented to holistic patient care that does not reduce a patient to a diseased organ. Other allied health professions, and certain medical specialties as well, likewise take a more psychosocial view of illness, so it is misleading to think of medicine as a monolithic entity. Even within mainstream, "hard-core" medical practice, noteworthy changes have taken place in recent years. There is increasing recognition of the psychogenic origins and social embeddedness of illness and of the need to approach treatment from a holistic perspective that goes beyond the boundary of physical bodies. The walls separating mind and body are eroding as researchers and practitioners demonstrate the integration of thoughts, feelings, and physiology. Alternative and complementary healing are rapidly gaining legitimacy within orthodox medicine, and greater attention is being accorded the therapeutic environment.

Social scientists have devoted considerable attention to studying the profession of medicine, including its systems for training and socialization of practitioners. Such studies have identified ways that the core values of medicine are inculcated among its acolytes, such as devotion to "doing something" and achieving real "cures." The following case study illustrates some of these ideas.

Case Study: Doctor Do Much and Doctor Frustration

> I like to do a lot of OB (obstetrics). There's an end point, and you know, you're done. The woman is pregnant, I deliver her baby, and that's a cure. You can see the results of your work, a finished product. I know they say now that pregnancy isn't a disease, but you know what I mean. I get the same feeling doing surgery, and I know that's the reasons people go into surgery and OB. They want results. They want something to show for it when they're done. Surgeons like to cut it (the disease organ or tissue) and be finished. They go in, take out the appendix, and there's no question they've made a cure. A generation ago the patient would have died because they didn't have surgery and they couldn't do a cure. It's so different treating chronic illnesses. You do your goal setting, but end up feeling like a failure because the patient isn't cured. (Stein, 1990, p. 30, quoting a family physician)

As Howard Stein (1990) noted, "For healers, intervention often seems less an opportunity to help than a compulsion to change others. It is as though they must prove to themselves through their patients that they are able to heal" (p. 30). Socialization into a culture, society, family, or other way of being also applies to professional occupations. In the health sciences, there has been an enormous interest in understanding the process by which physicians are trained. However, the scientific curriculum is only one level of medical socialization. Moreover, there are also the personality factors that relate to occupational selection.

One common value theme in medical training and practice is to do as much as possible in the time available. The ability to master technology and biology promotes the *physician-as-technician* and the perspective of *people-as-machine* model, an approach considered one of the "highest aspirations" of physicians (Stein 1990, p. 30). Although there is a wish to "take charge" over a situation, person, or procedure, there is also the frustration of being at the mercy of another, unable to do anything in the face of death.

Frustrations also accrue to the physician from the patient's sense of what to expect of the practitioner:

> Some patients *dare* you to try to take their disease away. They really drive you crazy if you try to cure them. Take away one symptom, they come back at you with another one, as if they're trying to beat you at some game. I like the kind of patient who wants to get better. They're good compliers, and you don't have to worry about what tricks you've got left up your sleeve to outsmart them. Why can't we dissect every medical problem like we did in anatomy? (Stein, 1990, p. 31, quoting a family medicine resident)

Physicians as healers are willing to engage in a complex contest of fate. Even if acute problems can be seemingly healed, there is always some other imperfection that needs attention. Ultimately, death occurs; it is just the time of death that is elusive.

THE CULTURE OF PUBLIC HEALTH

As with all cultures, public health professionals working in the prevailing U.S. system share certain implicit assumptions—its practitioners take them for granted until someone from outside the group challenges them. Many of these cultural orientations are incorporated into this textbook and taught in schools of public health as part of students' enculturation into the profession. Examples of these basic assumptions include the conceptualization of health as a state of complete well-being rather than the mere absence of disease; the belief that disease states are influenced by multiple factors, as presented in the Social Ecology of Health Model; and the value placed on primary prevention.

Some of the most implicit assumptions that guide public health professionals mirror the dominant value orientations shared by the broader society. Public health professionals, like most North Americans, believe it is possible to uncover the causes of disease (*rationalism*) and search for a better understanding of the factors that placed people at risk for premature death, disease, and disability. They believe the world acts according to laws that can be understood, and although change is inevitable, laws can be discovered to predict and direct its course (*positivism*). They are also optimists—they believe it is both desirable and possible to improve society. Government is expected to work toward greater equity, and public health professionals typically view themselves as part of a systematic effort to make society a better place to live. Like other health care providers, public health professionals are guided by a strong value placed on "doing" and the expectation that humans can master nature. These orientations are manifest in large-scale efforts to eradicate problems; public health has officially waged "War on Poverty" and "War on Cancer" and mounted a multimillion-dollar campaign—"America Responds to AIDS." Even when their efforts prove to be ineffective, public health professionals continue their fight, believing increased funding or new tactics will yield the desired results. The view that disease and poverty are intrinsic to life and can never be eradicated is inconceivable.

The prevailing culture of public health also guides the way its practitioners are organized and how its services delivered. In the following section, we describe the culture of public health's impact on how maternal and child health services are delivered. Our description is based on research conducted primarily in the southeastern and south central portions of the United States, with special attention to maternal and child health services such as the Food and Nutrition Supplemental Program for Women, Infants and Children (WIC); prenatal care; and immunization programs delivered at the local or county level.

Almost everywhere, state and local county and city health departments are structured as nonprofit governmental agencies and administered by health professionals and staff who are trained to follow strict ethical codes. Guided by a shared commitment to serve, administrators and staff try to help everyone possible within resource limitations. Of special concern are disenfranchised populations and those at increased risk of disease, death, and disability. Even when efforts to help these "hard to reach" populations fail, public health professionals find it distasteful to shift their efforts to other less-deserving segments of the population who may be more responsive to their efforts. Not only is it unimaginable to give up trying to reach resistant populations, but because these groups are usually the poorest or neediest, public health professionals feel obliged to allocate the greatest amount of time and other resources in an effort to do something to help them.

Public health professionals' almost religious zeal to "make a difference" is such a dominant value that it may supersede efficiency, cost effectiveness, and accountability. As in many service cultures, public health administrators may tolerate misdirection and inefficiency in the short run as long as the programs are fulfilling their self-generated mission in the long run (Kotler & Andreasen, 1991, p. 76). Some health departments have hired program managers trained in corporate culture with the expectation they will more closely evaluate program cost effectiveness and eliminate waste. But, when these administrators try to eliminate programs that have failed to demonstrate their effectiveness, they often encounter widespread resistance and resentment by staff members who view programs intended to "do good" as the ends rather than just one means for fulfilling their mission.

Public health employees' commitment to the ultimate goal of the programs they work in is also evident in job satisfaction studies. In surveys of employees working for the WIC program, for example, the most frequent reason given for working in the program is the desire to "make a difference." Even when higher-paying positions become available elsewhere, many employees continue to work for WIC because it gives them an opportunity to help families in need. In fact, the sacrifices employees make in terms of lost wages, longer hours, and stressful work settings makes some feel superior to those who opt for easier, less meaningful work (Bryant, Davis, Unterberger, & Lindenberger, 1993).

> The deepest satisfaction I have is the knowledge that women, infants, and children get the necessary food and education, and a feeling of family. And I also enjoy being a help to the nutritionists and clerks because they are MY family.

> I think one of the things that I feel good about is the fact with all the research that we have to prove that WIC makes a difference, that we know that it's really making a difference in pregnancy outcomes, and in the health of mothers and babies.

> I think [WIC] is an important program because it helps women, infants, and children. It gives them a healthy start and that is why I think it's important. It's kind of like working for our future, building America's future.

> I was in a restaurant talking with somebody and I said "I work for this program called WIC" and this total stranger across the table said, "I just want you to know I love WIC; it helped me so much," and you could see that she was quite successful now, but she said, "There was a time when I needed WIC and it made all the difference." Those are the kind of success stories that helps us think why we're doing this job . . . because we do make a difference.

The desire to make an impact can also be a source of frustration for public health professionals. Clients are expected to be needy, humble, and grateful for the assistance provided them and, when they do not meet these expectations, employees are frustrated. When WIC employees were asked what they disliked about their jobs, many responded with distasteful stories about WIC participants who are ostentatious, own expensive goods they cannot afford, or fail to appreciate help offered.

> What's the most difficult part? Dealing with participants that act like the world owes them everything.

> What gets me is when [clients] come in and say, "I pay my taxes, I want my milk."

They come in with new clothes, fancy jewelry, and $300 purses. Then they tell you they don't have any income. They get pregnant every nine months.

At the local level, the culture of public health is also reflected in the physical setting in which its practitioners work. The saying that "poverty rubs off on those who work within its midst" has visible support in the U.S. public health system. Employees typically are required to work in small work spaces separated by partitions rather than private offices with doors. Waiting areas are usually crowded and noisy. Many health departments are located in economically disadvantaged neighborhoods where needy families can access their services easily. A proposal to house public health services in expensive, spacious buildings with lavishly furnished private offices would probably be rejected by both taxpayers and many public health professionals as incongruous with the organization's self-image.

Camaraderie flourishes among employees in most public health departments. Teamwork is highly valued, and knowledge is shared freely. It is rare for individuals to be concerned with getting credit for an innovative idea; when a new program is successful, everyone involved shares a sense of satisfaction. Salaries in public health are typically lower than in the private medical sector. However, many nurses and nutritionists enjoy greater autonomy than their counterparts working in physician-dominated hospitals and private medical practices. Employee attributes valued highly include compassion, kindness, thoughtfulness, humility, and dedication, as well as the more typical employee characteristics, such as competence and dependability.

Recent changes in the health care market have highlighted the cultural boundaries that separate the public health and private medical sectors. Most public health professionals mistrust profit-motivated organizations, including the managed care companies with whom they now compete for Medicaid patients. Public health professionals expect the profit motive to override the service mission. They claim medical providers working for private, for-profit organizations do not understand the special needs of the poor and worry that the emphasis on efficiency and profit will limit the resources allocated to education and ancillary services (health education, WIC, social services) needed by economically disadvantaged clients. Some public health workers claim that private providers are poorly prepared to work across ethnic and class lines, and many resent the private sector's sudden interest in caring for a population overlooked when government reimbursement levels were not profitable. They are concerned that, if and when managed care services cease being profitable, poor patients will be pushed back into a public health system no longer prepared to serve them. These attitudes reflect the implicit values that unite public health workers as members of a professional culture focused on caretaking of the poor and distinguish them from other health-related organizational cultures.

Case Study: "Folk Flu," "Viral Syndrome," and Influenza

We have said that people construct explanatory models for specific illnesses. Why is it important to understand people's explanatory models for specific illnesses? A comparison of explanatory models of the flu by lay people, medical providers, and epidemiologists illustrates the impact that divergent perspectives can have on infectious disease control and surveillance. McCombie (1999) made such a comparison while she was working as a communicable disease officer for a county health department. She relied on participant observation in a wide variety of public and medical settings; formal and informal interviews with clinicians, patients, and coworkers; and medical chart reviews to document each group's explanatory models of the flu or influenza. These data and the results of formal investigations were used to examine the impact that the divergent explanatory models had on medical treatment, infectious disease control, and surveillance activities.

Epidemiologists use influenza or "flu" to refer to a respiratory tract infection caused by a single-stranded virus of the Orthomyxoviridae family. Symptoms include fever, headache, sore throat, runny nose, and myalgia. Only rarely does influenza cause diarrhea or vomiting. Public health professionals monitor flu outbreaks to assess the efficacy of influenza vaccines and identify changes in viral strains. In contrast to the epidemiologists' explanatory model, most lay people use the word *flu* to refer to a much broader set of symptoms affecting both the respiratory and gastrointestinal tracts. Some people distinguish between a type of flu that affects only the respiratory tract and the "stomach flu" that causes gastrointestinal disturbances. For others, diarrhea and vomiting are defining symptoms of the flu—a clear deviation from the scientific definition or explanatory model—whereas a respiratory tract infection accompanied by fever, myalgia, and other symptoms characteristic of influenza is considered a bad cold.

As with all explanatory models, the folk or lay model of the flu has important functions. It gives people a way to explain their illness, thereby reducing uncertainty, and it directs them to seek appropriate treatment. In the case of "folk flu," however, some people mistakenly think they have a stomach flu when they actually may be suffering from a foodborne illness such as *Salmonella* or other gastrointestinal bacterial infection, such as shigellosis, requiring antibiotic treatment. For example, in a large outbreak of shigellosis that occurred in a county where McCombie (1999) worked, 44% of the people affected did not seek medical care because they thought they had the flu.

Physicians and other medical providers also construct explanatory models for diseases like influenza. In addition to adopting lay terms, such as the flu, to communicate more effectively with patients, medical providers often blend elements of the folk explanatory model with aspects of the scientific explanation. In McCombie's (1999) study, many clinicians used the term "viral syndrome" or, when talking with patients, "the flu" in initial diagnoses of illnesses presenting with a broad range of symptoms, including diarrhea, vomiting, and nausea when accompanied by fever. Misdiagnosing gastrointestinal diseases such as the flu is not always problematic because both diseases are usually self-limiting and the patient can recover without medical treatment. However, McCombie's medical chart review revealed that viral syndrome had been used as the initial diagnosis for many serious bacterial infections, such as typhoid fever, shigellosis, and *campylobacter*. As a result, several patients failed to receive life-saving antibiotic treatment and died.

McCombie's (1999) case study illustrates how divergent explanatory models create barriers for infectious disease control. People who think they have the flu but actually have a contagious gastrointestinal disease or viral hepatitis may not follow the hygienic measures needed to prevent the disease's spread. Day care centers are common sites for infectious gastrointestinal diseases because of young children's fecal incontinence. McCombie described one instance in which an investigation and subsequent control of giardia were stymied because the director misdiagnosed the disease as the flu and failed to adopt practices needed to stop the disease from being transmitted to attendants and other children. Another example comes from Tampa, where a recent outbreak of hepatitis was traced to a food handler who believed he "just had the flu" and returned to work.

Infectious disease surveillance is also hindered when communicable diseases are misdiagnosed. McCombie (1999) documented numerous false leads in which reported influenza outbreaks were actually caused by foodborne illnesses. Because people were convinced they were suffering from the flu, few were willing to complete 3-day diet records needed to investigate and document the problem. The opposite situation also occurs. For example, a principal sought help from McCombie's health department to investigate a disease believed to have been caused by pigeon droppings in the school ventilation system. When McCombie suggested the children were suffering from influenza, a teacher became angry and responded, "We have a lot more than just the flu here!" (1999, p. 33).

It is important to note that folk explanatory models of disease vary between lay people; not everyone holds the same beliefs about diagnosis or treatment of an illness, making it necessary for clinicians to elicit each patient's views. Medical providers also differ in their explanatory models, so public health professionals need to understand the explanatory model of the clinicians they work with as well as the public they serve.

In addition to highlighting the public health implications of divergent explanatory models, McCombie's (1999) case study illustrates how the culture of public health influences its practitioners. Public health professionals' explanatory models are socially constructed and, as a result, may differ from those held by clinicians socialized in the culture of medicine. Failure to recognize these differences can have serious consequences for public health practitioners and their efforts to protect the public's health.

CONCLUSION

Cultural dimensions of illness, medical care, and public health are important in all societies, both simple and complex. Perspectives in comparative health cultures have changed radically from the early days when Western scientific medicine was used as the standard for evaluating other healing traditions. A more relativistic view characterizes current frameworks that recognize the constructed nature of all emic therapeutic concepts, including those of scientific medicine. Nevertheless, we can identify universal features of health cultures that, treated as general etic categories, highlight the core components and functions of therapeutic systems. In reviewing some of these universals, we highlighted dimensions that have relevance for public health practice.

Although most of the early ethnomedical research by anthropologists focused on non-Western healing traditions, which reinforced the more general societal view that "cultural difference" was something "others" had, in this chapter we emphasize the cultural dimensions of mainstream health institutions. We overview the culture of medicine as described in the scholarly literature, including the distinctively American brand of practice, drawing on the sizable body of published work in this area. Curiously, almost nothing has been written to date about the culture of public health per se, although some researchers have addressed the issue indirectly through more narrowly defined questions such as the case study on folk flu presented in this chapter. Thus, we offer some formative ideas on the culture of public health, with particular emphasis on the worldview of local public health departments.

9

Community-Based Approaches
to Health Promotion

During the past two decades, public health professionals have come to recognize the importance of community in the formation of an individual's health status. An ecological perspective of health makes it clear that changes must occur in the social and physical environments as well as at the level of individual behavior to decrease disease and disability. Recognition of the importance of an ecological perspective has been accompanied by an increased reliance on community-based interventions in which public health professionals work with community members to modify the social and physical environments as well as individual behavior in an effort to improve community health.

This chapter begins with an examination of the concept of community and then discusses the distinguishing features of community-based approaches to health promotion and disease prevention. After a description of various community-based intervention models, the chapter ends with a brief discussion of the challenges of evaluating community-based interventions and the benefits of involving community partners in the evaluation process.

COMMUNITY

Community refers to a group of people who share a sense of social identity, common norms, values, goals, and institutions (Israel, Schulz, Parker, & Becker, 1998). A community may be based on geographical boundaries (a neighborhood, city, or other place), social identity and/or interests (the lesbian community, an ethnic group), or shared political responsibilities (an advocacy group for the homeless) (Eng & Parker, 1994; Patrick & Wickizer, 1995). Not all neighborhoods, interest groups, or political groups are communities. To be considered a community, a group must be characterized by the following elements:

> 1) membership—a sense of identify and belonging; 2) common symbol systems—similar language, rituals, and ceremonies; 3) shared values and norms; 4) mutual influence—community members have influence and are influenced by each other; 5) shared needs and commitment to meeting them; and 6) shared emotional connection—members share common history, experiences, and mutual support. (Israel, Checkoway, Schulz, & Zimmermann, 1994, p. 151)

This shared identity and sense of belonging develops when people come together to share their experience and act to transform it.

It is important to keep in mind that groups do not always fit neatly into our definitions of community or respond to our efforts based on these definitions. Calling a group a community does not make it so. For example, initial efforts to target the "gay community" in addressing HIV/AIDS did not reach all gay men because not all gay men are at risk for contracting the virus associated with AIDS or consider themselves a member of the gay community. Many gay men do not share a sense of identify with other gay men and do not come together to share their experiences or act together to transform their experience.

Even when individuals do share an identity and work together as a community, the group may be very heterogeneous. Societal trends toward greater geographic mobility and the use of communication technologies now make it possible for communities to be broader based and more heterogeneous than was once possible (Patrick & Wickizer, 1995). Communities are less likely to develop around geographical units today because people change residences more frequently, have weaker extended family networks, and lack social ties with their neighbors (Pilisuk, McCallister, & Rothman, 1996). At the same time, many people are sharing their experiences and joining together to improve their lives by communicating through the Internet. Because communities are more flexible and may fluctuate more drastically in their membership, our ability to conceptualize community in terms of distinct categories is limited, to say the very least. Although this limitation does not preclude the grouping of individuals into communities, it does demand attention to the diversity within them in terms of values, norms, needs, commitment, emotional connection, and acculturation that affect the success of public health programs aimed at the community level.

DISTINGUISHING FEATURES OF COMMUNITY-BASED INTERVENTIONS

Community-based interventions not only take place in the community but, more important, they are guided by a philosophy that can be characterized by three principles (Brownson, Baker, & Novick, 1999).

First, community-based interventions are guided by an ecological framework. Because individual, interpersonal, community, organizational, and governmental factors are believed to affect individual health status, community-based programs attempt to address multiple factors, either simultaneously or sequentially (Brownson et al., 1999). A community-based approach to breast-feeding promotion, for example, might address individual factors by offering classes or individual counseling to increase knowledge and build skills. At the same time, peer counselors or lay health advisers might be trained to act as local advisers and referral sources as a way to build social ties. And community members might advocate for changes in hospital policies to make lactation management and support more readily available and to encourage employers to allow mothers to pump their breasts or breastfeed during their breaks. Finally, a community coalition might lobby for changes in federal policies that affect the role WIC program or prenatal care services play in promoting breast-feeding or create new lactation management and support services.

Second, community-based interventions are designed to meet the felt needs and wants of the community and its members. The notion of "starting where the people are" is a fundamental principal of health promotion. Community-based interventions typically begin with a needs assessment and the development of ties with community leaders who understand the community's strengths and problems. If a group's "sense of community"—their shared identity and ability to work together—is poorly developed, then work must begin with the development of trust, mutual support, and leadership needed to work together to solve common problems (Brownson et al., 1999). In some community-based intervention models, the community selects the issue or issues to be addressed.

The third characteristic of community-based interventions is community participation. Community participation refers to the process by which individuals and families take an active part in discussions and activities to improve community life, services, or resources (Bracht & Tsouros, 1990). In contrast to public health interventions planned and implemented by public health professionals for communities where they neither work nor live, community organization strategies place public health professionals in a collaborative partnership with community members. Community members may include community professionals, lay leaders and activists, representatives of local businesses, churches, voluntary organizations, and citizens. This partnership brings people together who share common goals, resources, and problems (McWilliam, Desai, & Greig, 1997). Working together, these partners define and critically analyze community problems, set goals, and, ultimately, design, implement, and evaluate interventions aimed at achieving these goals.

In Florida, for example, the state program designed to reduce teen smoking has enlisted support from teenagers in many aspects of program planning and implementation. High school students have formed SWAT teams—Students Working Against Tobacco. These teens have developed and implemented numerous strategies for dissuading others from smoking. Their participation is believed to improve program design and enhance program effectiveness in several ways. First, the teenagers who participate in program activities acquire new information about the problems associated with smoking, acquire drug refusal skills, and acquire methods for persuading others not to smoke. Second, these skills and commitment are also reinforced and maintained by their participation in the program and the public commitments they make to not smoke. Third, participation gives program designers valuable information about teen views and

TABLE 9.1   Guiding Principles for Health Promotion Organizing

---

Planning must be based on a historical understanding of the community. Conditions that inhibit or facilitate interventions must be assessed.

- Because the issue or problem is usually one of multiple (rather than single) causality, a comprehensive effort using multiple interventions is required.

- It is important to focus on community context and work primarily through existing structures and values.

- Active community participation, not mere token representation, is desired.

- For the project to be effective, intersectoral components of the community must work together to address the problem in a comprehensive effort.

- The focus must be on both long-term and short-term problem solving if the longevity of the change is to endure beyond the project's demonstration period.

- Finally, and most important, the community must share responsibility for the problem and for its solution.

---

the factors that influence their decisions about smoking. Bracht and Kingsbury (1990, p. 72) summarized other guiding principles of community-based approaches to health promotion (see Table 9.1).

TYPES OF COMMUNITY-BASED APPROACHES

Community-based health promotion programs use a wide variety of strategies, including grassroots organizing, professionally driven community organization, coalition development, use of lay health advisers, development of community identity, and legislative advocacy (Minkler & Wallerstein, 1998). Although there is no widely accepted taxonomy of community-based intervention models, most practitioners distinguish between true *community organizing* directed by community members and other community-based interventions directed by professionals from outside the community.

Community Organization

When community groups identify common problems, set goals, mobilize resources, and implement strategies for reaching those goals, we call the change process *community organization* (Minkler & Wallerstein, 1998). Community organization attempts to improve public health by empowering communities to manage and control the change process to influence the human, economic, social, and physical environment. Community organization is distinguished from other community-based approaches by the degree of control and ownership the community has over the change process and the emphasis placed on enhancing community competence as opposed to solving a community problem.

The first distinguishing feature—community control and ownership—refers to the community's role in setting the agenda—selecting the issue to be addressed, goal setting, and determining the strategies used to achieve those goals. Public health educators have long known the importance of starting with an individual or group's felt needs rather than problems identified by outside professionals or organizations. Projects that address the issues a community considers important are more likely to be accepted and, therefore, more effective than projects imposed by outside experts. For this reason, many community organizers believe it is essential for the community to define the problem or problems it wants to address and assume control and ownership of the change process. The community's control over the change process in community organizing differs from other community-based approaches in which the health professional defines and names the problem and then seeks input and consultation from community members in developing strategies for remedying the problem.

Although these principles of community relevance and self-determination are central tenets of community organizing, they are often difficult to implement. Funding sources are one source of constraint on how issues are selected. Most public health projects are funded by national, state, or other agencies that have allocated resources for specific issues they have decided to target (Altman, 1995). Even when funding is not tied to a specific problem or health category (e.g., HIV prevention), health departments or other lead community organizations, who are used to categorical funding, may be unable to make the transition from a strict problem-solving focus to a broader community development project (El-Askari et al., 1998). The time constraints placed on funding also significantly affect a program's potential for success and comprehensiveness, with longer funding periods making it possible to develop a realistic timeline and objectives (Israel et al., 1994).

Another distinguishing feature of community organization is the emphasis placed on community empowerment as a desired outcome of the change process. *Empowerment* refers to a "social action process by which individuals, communities, and organizations gain mastery over their lives in the context of changing their social and political environment to improve equity and quality of life" (Minkler & Wallerstein, 1998, p. 40). Unlike community-based interventions that are focused primarily on solving a specific health problem, a primary objective of community organization activities is to build the community's capacity to work together to achieve consensus about their problems and ways to solve them. Professionals who live outside the community may help citizens learn new skills or provide important resources needed to implement change strategies. However, community members are actively involved in prioritizing health problems in their communities, selecting the health condition or conditions to be addressed, and designing interventions to achieve the goals they have set. Community members also have primary responsibility for program implementation, including community education and grassroots organizing. During the process, indigenous leaders are developed who can stimulate critical problem-solving activities and direct sustainable change activities (Bracht, 1990; Minkler & Wallerstein, 1998). As community members work together to solve their problems, they gain a stronger sense of collective efficacy and learn how to engage in effective problem solving. Participation increases community members' sense of mastery and their realization that they can improve their lives and those of others. Through participation and increased competence, citizen groups gain more power over resources—social and tangible assets. As citizens support each other, address problems within the community, and develop the ability to work together to influence decisions in the larger social system, they learn to use their collective skills and power to obtain a more equitable share of resources (Israel et al., 1994; Robertson & Minkler, 1994).

STAGES IN THE PROCESS

Community organization typically unfolds in five basic stages (Bracht, Kingsbury, & Rissel, 1999). The first stage, *community analysis,* consists of data collection and analysis to gain a better understanding of the community's problems and to set priorities. Community organizers also assess the community's strengths, its readiness to change, its barriers, and other factors that may influence the change process.

In the second stage, *design and initiation,* a community planning body—a coalition, committee, or board—is established to plan and coordinate the change process. Other tasks include recruitment of members, establishment of bylaws or procedures to guide the planning process, and identification of goals and objectives. The makeup of community planning consortia is a critical element of this phase. Ideally, members are selected who truly represent the entire community, and the group is structured with clear roles and responsibilities.

Once a problem has been targeted and objectives set, the group then develops strategies for resolving the issue. Key tasks to be accomplished in this *implementation* phase include the generation of broad citizen participation; development of a sequential work plan; use of comprehensive, integrated tactics; and the integration of community values and norms into programs, materials, and messages used to bring about change. In some community organizing approaches, research is conducted among representative samples of potential audience segments to enable program planners to benefit from feedback from people whose time and interest preclude more active participation in planning consortia.

During the fourth phase, *maintenance and consolidation,* the program is implemented and successful elements are more fully incorporated into community structures. A key element in this phase is the development of a positive organizational culture, with cooperation, trust, and recruitment of new volunteers or staff.

Finally, the program moves into the *dissemination and reassessment* phase. Program activities are evaluated and revised and the results disseminated. Community groups may update their community analysis, review changes in community resources, and assess the program's effectiveness in changing norms or behaviors. Some groups may search for new sponsors of successful activities or find other ways to institutionalize the change so it is sustained while they turn their attention to new issues. As they begin planning new directions for the future, the five-stage process begins again.

HIGHLIGHT ON PARTICIPATORY RESEARCH

Many community-based intervention models rely on data to assess community needs and assets and gain an understanding of the factors that affect the conditions the program is attempting to change. Research, like other aspects of the planning and implementation process, often involves community members. *Participatory research* or *community-based research* refers to the active involvement of community members in all phases of the research process. Community members work with researchers to define the research problem and set research objectives, design the methodology and data collection instruments, collect and interpret the data, and use the results to guide program planning and evaluation (Schulz et al., 1999). Community members' involvement in creating new knowledge and in determining how that information is used in the community change processes addresses underlying social and political inequities and empowers the community. Participatory research also democratizes program planning and evaluation by putting community members in control of the types of questions that are asked and issues that are investigated (Coombe, 1998). Barbara Israel and her associates (Israel et al., 1998) developed key principles for conducting community-based or participatory research, which are summarized in Table 9.2.

A community organization approach that relies heavily on participatory research is the Community Organization and Development (COD) model. COD attempts to decrease excess deaths by empowering economically disadvantaged communities of color (Braithwaite, Bianchi, & Taylor, 1994). COD actively involves disenfranchised persons in data collection and analysis and applies results to program decision making.

The most prominent guiding concepts of COD are self-determination, bottom-up planning, community problem solving, shared decision making, and cultural relevance:

> The philosophy underlying this approach is that health promotion is likely to be more successful in those populations when the community at risk identifies its own health concerns, develops its own prevention and intervention programs, forms a decision-making board to make policy decisions, and identifies resources for program implementation. (Braithwaite et al., 1994, p. 408)

Participatory research plays a key role in the COD process. Working with outside health educators, community members use rapid ethnographic assessment

TABLE 9.2   Principles for Conducting Community-Based or Participatory
Research

Key Factors	Description
Focus on community	The concept of community as a unit of social identity is central to community-based research. Community-based research attempts to identify and work with communities and to strengthen a sense of community through collective engagement.
Community assets	Community-based research attempts to identify and build on community assets—skills, resources, and social relationships—as a way to address communal health concerns.
Equal participation	Community members are equal partners in all phases of the research process. Individuals from outside the community who can assist the community in improving the health and well-being of its members also may participate in research activities.
Beneficial knowledge	Community-based research generates knowledge that is mutually beneficial to all partners by informing the social change process and contributing to a broad understanding of the factors related to health and well-being.
Empowerment	Community-based research encourages colearning and empowerment. Community members acquire new skills, and academic researchers learn from community members' knowledge, experience, and unique perspectives of local problems. By acknowledging inequalities between themselves and community members and sharing power, researchers help empower the community.
Cyclical and iterative research	Community-based research is cyclical and iterative. Steps include "partnership development and maintenance, community assessment, problem definition, development of research methodology, data collection and analysis, interpretation of data, determination of action and policy implications, dissemination of results, action taking (as appropriate), specification of learnings, and establishment of mechanisms for sustainability" (Israel et al., 1998, p. 180).
Ecological perspective	Community-based research uses an ecological model of health and addresses the concept of health from a positive model, emphasizing physical, mental, and social well-being.
Broad dissemination	All partners have access to research findings. Results are disseminated to community members and other partners in a format and language that is easy to understand and use. Community participants all have a voice in how the results are published, and their contributions/ownership of the information is acknowledged.

methods to build a detailed profile of the community. They conduct in-depth interviews, focus groups, and surveys and use existing demographic information to provide locally relevant baseline data from which to design program interventions and measure change. These ethnographic techniques also help to clarify existing bonds and relationships between community members (Braithwaite et al., 1994).

The COD model follows a formalized and coherent step-by-step approach:

1. Identify community leaders.
2. Conduct a demographic profile of the intended community.
3. Develop a community resource inventory.
4. Organize a coalition board that will serve as the governing body.
5. Obtain coalition board incorporation.
6. Apply for Section 501(c)(3) status (a nonprofit designation under the U.S. Internal Revenue Code).
7. Conduct needs assessments.
8. Conduct community forums.
9. Plan and implement health interventions.
10. Provide ongoing board training and technical assistance.
11. Conduct intervention evaluation.

The COD process has been used in Atlanta, Georgia, where it involved two local health departments, a medical and public health school, two suburban communities, and one inner-city community. The overriding goal of the project was to empower the community by developing a community-controlled coalition board. Formal bylaws, articles of incorporation, and other contractual relationships were important in establishing the coalition's power and authority.

Participatory ethnography played a key role in the project. Community researchers and health educators used participant observation, in-depth interviews, focus groups, surveys, and existing data to build rich community profiles that captured the social and cultural context, interpersonal dynamics, and needs of the community. Research results were used to educate community residents about health conditions, equip them with sufficient information to support and protect their interests with agency policymakers, and serve as a basis for mobilizing community-wide interest and action.

INTERVENTION MODELS

Even within community organization, there are numerous intervention types or approaches. The most widely recognized typology (Rothman & Tropman, 1987) categorizes these into three models of practice: *locality development, social planning,* and *social action.* Locality or community development emphasizes community participation and consensus building with the goal of increasing community competence. This approach is heavily process-oriented, drawing on a broad cross-section of people to determine and solve their own problems. Although an outside facilitator or catalyst may coordinate the process and teach problem-solving or other needed skills, the goal is to build community consensus and a sense of community through community action.

Social planning is a more carefully controlled approach to solving substantive community problems, such as crime, AIDS, or drug use. This approach is heavily task-oriented and based on empirical problem-solving methods. The process is often directed by expert planners who, "through the exercise of technical abilities, including the ability to manipulate large bureaucratic organizations, can skillfully guide complex change processes" (Rothman & Tropman, 1987, p. 27). Social planners often rely on research and the manipulation of formal organizations or power structures to achieve specific program goals to solve specific community problems. This model is the most similar to other community-based approaches and no longer is considered community organization if the external expert assumes control of the planning process and/or focuses more heavily on solving the problem than empowerment as the central goal.

The third model, social action, focuses on a disadvantaged segment of the population that needs to be organized to achieve equity and justice. Conflict and dissatisfaction with the status quo are often used as means to create pressure for change and place demands on the larger community for increased resources or more just treatment. The ultimate goal of social action is to enable communities to change major institutions or community practices to redistribute power, resources, and decision making (Minkler & Wallerstein, 1998; Rothman & Tropman, 1987).

Many public health professionals combine elements from each of Rothman's three intervention models, relying on technical experts, for example, to guide the change process but focusing primarily on the goals of increasing community participation and empowerment. One hybrid model that has gained widespread popularity among public health professionals is the Planned Approach to Community Health (PATCH).

PLANNED APPROACH TO COMMUNITY HEALTH

PATCH is a planning model that provides communities with a structured process for identifying and prioritizing health problems and then implementing and evaluating programs to resolve them (USDHHS, 1995a). The PATCH process is usually directed by a local or state health department; however, other organizations, including hospitals, military institutions, universities, and other voluntary groups or agencies, have used PATCH to address a variety of health concerns (USDHHS, 1995a). Community participation is a central feature of the PATCH model—community members form health promotion committees/groups; collect and utilize data; establish health priorities; and design, implement, and evaluate activities that are geared to modifying established behavioral risk factors (USDHHS, 1995a).

As a community-organizing model, PATCH represents a combination of locality development and social planning models (Rothman & Tropman, 1987). Because PATCH uses data in a systematic approach to solving substantive health problems, it can be classified as a social planning model for community organizing. However, PATCH is similar to locality development models in its "use of broad participation of a wide spectrum of people at the local community level in goal determination and action" (Rothman & Tropman, 1987, p. 26).

PATCH is predicated on the belief that improving the health of individuals and communities must involve a process of empowering individuals to increase the control they have over their health (USDHHS, 1995a). Building on this desire to increase individual control over one's health and the knowledge that communities have a tremendous influence on individual health behavior, the primary goal of PATCH is to increase communities' capacity to address local health priorities effectively (Kreuter, 1992; USDHHS, 1995a). Through participation in the PATCH process, communities learn the skills necessary to analyze health problems critically; set goals; and plan, implement, and evaluate programs aimed at increasing the health of the community. According to Kreuter (1992), a secondary goal of PATCH is to provide a practice guide that state and local health education leaders can use to work with community members to address local health priorities. The Centers for Disease Control and Prevention (CDC) encourages PATCH coordinators to use the model to work toward the Year 2000 and 2010 national health objectives. PATCH is used to compare community rates of the leading causes of disease, death, disability, and injury to state and national rates and to create programs to reduce behavioral risk factors prevalent in their community (USDHHS, 1995a).

The emphasis on individual and, ultimately, community control of the PATCH process encourages increased participation, investment, and institutionalization of the process; thus, communities who use the PATCH process successfully are more likely to sustain healthy behavior changes over the long run than are communities who have been targeted by an outside, expert-driven health education program (Kreuter, 1992; USDHHS, 1995a). PATCH encourages collaboration between academic-based researchers, local public health professionals, state representatives, lay leaders and activists, representatives of local business, churches, voluntary organizations, and residents. This collaboration brings together people who share a common goal, who offer a variety of resources and expertise, and who share a vested interest in solving the problem (McWilliam et al., 1997). The PATCH process also encourages the development of local expertise and empowers community leaders and representatives to access the information and resources necessary to improve the health of the community. The end result of the PATCH process should be greater collaboration between state and local public health agencies and increased communication between local agencies and organizations and between state and federal agencies. This collaboration, or developing infrastructure, also results in a decreased risk of overlap of services targeted to the same health priority (Kreuter, 1992). Most important, individuals and communities are empowered to work together in addressing behavioral risk factors that are present in the community, and they have developed the skills necessary to obtain knowledge, funding, and other resources that can help them help themselves (Bogan, Omar, Knobloch, Liburd, & O'Rourke, 1992; Kreuter, 1992; USDHHS, 1995a).

History and Theory

PATCH was created through a collaborative effort between state and local health departments and community groups in the mid-1980s (USDHHS, 1995a). It was designed to be a user-friendly, community-based process that incorporated information from health education, health promotion, and COD theories within the context of the Precede Model. According to the CDC (USDHHS, 1995a),

> Patch was built on the same philosophy as the World Health Organization's Health for All and the Ottawa Charter for Health Promotion, which specifies that health promotion is the process of enabling people to increase control over their health and to improve their health. (p. CG1-2)

Elements considered critical to the success of the PATCH include the following (USDHHS, 1995a):

- A wide range of *community members participate* in the process and are actively involved in the processes of analyzing community data, setting priorities, planning interventions, and making decisions about the health needs of their communities. This participation should result in a greater sense of community ownership of the program.

- *Data guide the process* from planning to implementation and evaluation. Community members use many types of data in an effort to gain a comprehensive view of the health status of the community.

- Based on the analyses of the community data, *participants develop and implement a comprehensive promotion strategy.* Community members are encouraged to relate the goals and objectives of their health promotion strategy to relevant year 2000 national health objectives.

- *Evaluation activities emphasize feedback and improvement* to make timely changes if needed. Both process and impact evaluations are crucial.

- The *community's capacity* for health education and health promotion is *strengthened.* Once the community's capacity to address local health priorities is strengthened through learning and initiating the PATCH process, the community is then more capable of repeating the process to address other health priorities.

Phases in the Process

There are five phases in the PATCH process that are standard across health problems and communities; in other words, although PATCH may be modified to meet the specific requirements of each individual community and health priority, the phases remain the same. The phases of the PATCH process are

- Phase I: Community Mobilization
- Phase II: Data Collection and Organization
- Phase III: Selection of Health Priorities
- Phase IV: Intervention Plan Development
- Phase V: Evaluation

Mobilization of the community is considered to be the initial phase of the PATCH process; however, attempts to recruit new partners and retain current partners should continue throughout the process. Mobilization efforts begin with defining the community and attempts to gain commitment to and support of the PATCH process, which can take several months to 1 year (USDHHS, 1995a). An important part of this phase is the creation of an organizational structure that will guide the PATCH process. This structure consists of the community group, steering committee, and a local coordinator (USDHHS, 1995a). Evaluations of PATCH in several communities reveal that some local coordinators need training in volunteer recruitment and retention to have a diverse range of people involved in PATCH committees and activities (Orenstein, Nelson, Speers, Brownstein, & Ramsey, 1992).

Once the community is mobilized, *community members collect and analyze data* on mortality, morbidity, and factors related to health risk behaviors, such as opinions, beliefs, knowledge, and motivating, enabling, and rewarding factors (USDHHS, 1995a). The use of the Behavioral Risk Factor Surveillance System (CDC, 2000) is no longer required by the CDC; instead, communities are encouraged to use preexisting sources of data and to collect data via focus groups, face-to-face interview, surveys, and other mixtures of qualitative and quantitative methods (Kreuter, 1992; USDHHS, 1995a). PATCH participants also consider means of sharing their results with the broader community during this phase. Data collection activities are key to the success of PATCH programs, and communities may differ in how much time is needed for this critical phase of the process. However, community members may grow impatient if large amounts of time and effort are spent on data collection, especially if insufficient attention is devoted to the development and implementation of interventions (Bogan et al., 1992; Orenstein, Atkinson, Mason, & Bernier, 1990).

The *selection of health priorities* to be addressed by the intervention begins once the community data have been analyzed. The community group also must consider micro- and macrolevel factors that influence health risk behaviors, including social, cultural, economic, political, economic, and environmental factors. The community's capacity to address the particular health priorities also must be assessed during this stage, along with the presence of existing programs and policies that already may address the health priority under consideration. Guided by the Precede model, PATCH calls for consideration of the "importance" and "changeability" of the behavioral risk factors when selecting a health priority (USDHHS, 1995a). In other words, is the behavior prevalent in the community and is there a strong association between the behavior and the health priority (importance)? And is there evidence that the behavior can be changed (changeability)? Finally, community objectives related to the selected health priorities are established during this phase to provide an initial framework for the next phase in the process.

The next phase focuses on *developing a comprehensive intervention* plan based on the information obtained in Phases II and III. The identification of existing programs and resources that seek to address the same health priority the community has chosen is vital during this stage to prevent "duplication of services" and to include leaders who may be threatened by another program addressing the same issue (USDHHS, 1995a). The community group creates a health promotion strategy, establishes objectives, and develops a plan during this stage. The CDC (USDHHS, 1995a) recommends that community members attempt to include education, policy, and environmental strategies as part of their intervention plan and components that motivate, enable, and reward the target audience to change relevant health risk behaviors.

Evaluation is labeled "Phase V"; however, monitoring and assessment activities should occur throughout all phases of the PATCH process. The community establishes evaluation criteria to measure the success of the program based on relevant and shared goals and objectives. Process and impact evaluations are crucial to the PATCH process. Process evaluations are based on community objectives and work plans and allow the community to compare actual implementation to ideal implementation. Process and impact evaluation data are particularly important for planners to use for program improvement purposes.

PATCH in Sarasota County, Florida: A Case Study

In 1984, Sarasota County was selected by the CDC and the State of Florida's Chronic Disease Program to become the first county in Florida to initiate a PATCH program. Sarasota County is located in southwest Florida and is home to approximately 320,000 individuals. Demographic information indicates that the population of Sarasota County is predominantly white (95% white, 4% black), older (45% of population is 55 years of age or older), and divided approximately evenly between male and female residents (53% female, 47% male). Approximately 13% of the population have less than a high school education, and 7% fall below the poverty level. Although Sarasota County is not necessarily representative of the state of Florida, due to its lower number of minority residents (7% vs. 29%) and lower percentage of people falling below the poverty level (7% vs. 13%), it provided an opportunity to test a relatively new planning model in an environment that was both able to initiate the process without intensive community development efforts and capable of supporting the process once initiated. The following sections provide a brief overview of the initial phases of the PATCH process in Sarasota County.

The Phases of PATCH in Sarasota County. PATCH in Sarasota County provides a good example of the need to include community mobilization efforts throughout every phase of the process. Public health leaders from the Sarasota County Public Health Department initiated the process by contacting representatives of local community organizations, including hospitals, local foundations, national foundations (e.g., the American Cancer Society), schools, senior centers, fire departments, and mental health centers, and inviting them to participate in a partnership between the community of Sarasota County, the state of Florida, and the

CDC that would allow the community to address local health problems in a unique way. Leaders of PATCH in Sarasota County mobilized the community through traditional methods, such as word-of-mouth, meetings, newsletters, and personal letters that emphasized the importance of individual community members in the success of the program. For example, one newsletter described the role of individual community members in the following way:

> YOU. Your involvement makes PATCH our program. You may participate in several different ways—
>
> ... come to workshops to make decisions about the direction of the program and learn about community health promotion: Volunteer to play an active role in carrying out PATCH activities.
>
> ... help the state and local coordinators manage PATCH activities.
>
> ... take responsibility for completing a specific activity such as conducting a survey, carrying out public relations, or exploring the resources in the community.

Efforts to mobilize the community were present throughout the initiation of PATCH in Sarasota County and continue to be central to the success of the program. A community outreach subcommittee was responsible for generating a comprehensive list of agencies and organizations in the local area that would serve as resources for a wide variety of community activities. The use of local representatives and health leaders was also an important component of mobilization efforts.

After the initial structure of PATCH in Sarasota County was developed, a workshop titled "Diagnosing the Community" was held to discuss ways in which the current health status of community residents could be assessed. The participants in the workshop determined the sources of information to use and designed an opinion survey that would be used to interview community members regarding the major health problems in the area. Ultimately, data on the health status and presence of risk factors in the community were collected through the use of the Behavioral Risk Factor Surveillance System; a CDC-recommended community opinion survey; and analyses of state and county mortality and morbidity data. The community survey was conducted with health, religious, civic, and business leaders, and a booth was set up at a local mall to interview local community members. Community members' opinions were solicited through the use of the following questions: "What are the major health problems in Sarasota County?" "What do you think are the causes?" and "How should these problems be reduced?"

A second workshop was conducted to organize the material gained from data collection efforts and to establish objectives for the community. Participants in this workshop interpreted the results of the opinion survey and the results of the other data collection efforts, ranked the major health problems in the community, set objectives to reduce the major health problems, and planned dissemination of the results to the community.

Community representatives, based on the information gained in Phase II of the PATCH process, determined that there were 22 concerns identified through the community health assessment process. PATCH representatives decided initially to select the top six areas that were of concern to Sarasota County: HIV/AIDS, community wellness education, lack of access to affordable health care, geriatric problems, substance abuse, and teen problems. Six countywide working committees were then formed to address these areas. Ultimately, the "Teen Problems" committee moved from PATCH to a committee of the Sarasota County Youth Related Services Associate, and four additional committees were formed: "Mental Health Issues," "Environmental Health Issues," "Perinatal Resource Network," and "Healthy Sarasota 2000." Each committee then developed objectives for their specific health priority area and developed *interventions* based on these objectives. Table 9.3 provides an early representation of PATCH in Sarasota County.

Specific evaluation activities and outcomes are beyond the scope of this discussion due to the number of committees involved in PATCH in Sarasota County; however, overall results of the program suggest PATCH has been successful in mobilizing the community to address priority health concerns and in enabling community members to develop skills that can be generalized to a variety of health issues in a variety of settings. The membership of PATCH in Sarasota County remains active and continues to generate new interests. Currently, 120 agencies are involved and more than 250 community members regularly participate in quarterly PATCH meetings, committees, and activities. The success of PATCH in Sarasota County also resulted in the selection of the Sarasota County Public Health Unit as a CDC demonstration site for evaluating other planning models and contributed to the development of numerous community-wide initiatives that continue to the present day.

ADVANTAGES OF COMMUNITY-BASED INTERVENTIONS

Community-based interventions offer public health program planners many benefits. First, as we have already noted, community-based approaches recog-

TABLE 9.3 Early Representation of Planned Approach to Community Health (PATCH) in Sarasota County, Florida

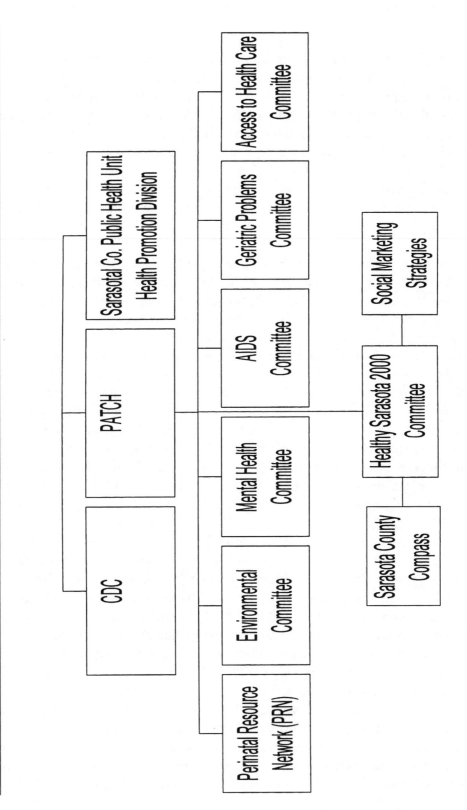

nize that health problems have multiple causes, requiring multiple interventions to affect individual behavior and simultaneously modify the social, political, and economic environment in which health conditions are based (Butterfoss, Goodman, & Wandersman, 1993). By modifying the social and physical environment, community organization augments individual members' ability to change: The introduction of supportive norms, values, and policies makes it easier for individuals to adopt healthier lifestyles.

Second, community participation has an indirect effect on health by strengthening the social networks of community members who come together to define and solve problems. In this way, community participation enhances participants' sense of social connectedness, perceived control, individual coping capacity, and health status (Minkler & Wallerstein, 1998). Thus, community participation increases the social cohesiveness of the broader community. Evidence for the positive health benefits of social cohesion comes from the small town of Roseto, Pennsylvania. Roseto captured researchers' interest because its residents had dramatically lower myocardial infarction mortality rates than did neighboring communities with similar demographic characteristics. Studies conducted in the late 1950s and early 1960s found an important association between mortality rates and social cohesion. In addition to lower mortality rates than neighboring communities, Roseto's citizens enjoyed closer family ties, more ethnic and social homogeneity, and more social support. Even the poorest citizens shared a sense of connectedness and benefited from social ties to other community members. Additional support for the link between social cohesiveness and health came from a longitudinal study of myocardial infarction rates in Roseto over the next 30 years. As the community's stability, family cohesion, and supportiveness declined, myocardial infarction rates climbed (Patrick & Wickizer, 1995). Other studies have focused on the flip side of social cohesion, documenting increased rates of suicide and other health problems among socially isolated individuals. As we have seen already, people who are socially isolated have far greater rates of death from many causes than do those with one or more close social ties.

A third benefit of community-based interventions comes from community participation and a shared a sense of ownership that citizens develop together. In addition to the impact this sense of ownership has on participants' own health, local control also ensures the longevity of change. Members are more likely to sustain efforts they have had a role in designing and implementing.

Fourth, the community's participation in all phases of the process facilitates the development of interventions that are integrated into existing community structures. Programs, services, and other activities are compatible with community norms, values, and beliefs, and the endorsement of local leaders or opinion makers can foster acceptance by other community members (Bracht, 1990, p. 21).

Fifth, community-based approaches can be very cost-effective. Even small successes can reap important economic benefits because of the large number of people reached. Compare the impact of a community-wide program that assists just 5% of its 50,000 members to exercise regularly with a 75% success rate among 500 participants in an exercise class or other intervention targeting small groups of individuals. Economic benefits are especially impressive when community-based interventions bring about permanent changes in community norms or environmental structures that reinforce and thus facilitate long-term change (Bracht, 1990; Frankish & Green, 1994).

Finally, by focusing the public health professional's attention on multiple environmental and interpersonal factors, community organization avoids an overreliance on education, communications, and other strategies criticized for "blaming the victim" (Ling, Franklin, Lindsteadt, & Gearon, 1992; Rothschild, 1997).

The health benefits to be gained when community members participate in an effort to solve their own problems are succinctly summarized by Minkler and Wallerstein (1997):

> As individuals engage in community-organizing efforts, community empowerment outcomes can include increased sense of community; greater participatory processes and community competence; and outcomes in the form of actual changes in policies, transformed conditions, or increased resources that may reduce inequities. As communities become empowered and better able to engage in collective problem solving, key health and social indicators may reflect this, with rates of alcoholism, divorce, suicide, and the social problems beginning to decline. Moreover, the empowered community that works effectively for change can bring about changes in some of the very problems that contributed to its ill health in the first place. (p. 252)

CHALLENGES ASSOCIATED WITH COMMUNITY-BASED INTERVENTIONS

Although community-based interventions offer public health program planners many benefits, there are challenges that must be addressed when working with communities to affect change. Because community direction of the change process is a defining theme in community-based intervention models, success requires the formation of an effective working relationship between public health professionals and community members. Many factors have been reported to affect these partnerships and the effectiveness of their work. These factors are summarized here.

- Community-based programs are affected by their ability to incorporate the values, norms, and language of community members. Cultural values of a specific population that affect health issues may not be understood or adequately expressed by someone not embedded in the cultural belief system (Bailey, 1992). Views from those in a community may differ drastically from the views of those outside the community, including advisory board members and researchers (Chalmers & Bramadat, 1996).

- Community planning consortia or work groups vary in terms of how well their members represent the larger community. Community leaders may not understand issues of importance beyond their individual concerns. A community's capacity will not improve if activities are driven solely by a small group of powerful people. For this reason, many community-based interventions rely on research among representative samples of potential audience segments to give program planners an understanding of the views of community members whose time and interest preclude more active participation in community affairs. By obtaining information from a broad sample of community members, research allows a community planning group to meet its responsibility to serve all its constituents (Eisen, 1994).

- Stereotyping of communities also may affect program performance adversely. Outside experts often underestimate the strengths of communities and lack an "appreciation of the expertise of potential participants" (McWilliam et al., 1997, p. 32). For this reason, many community organizers now assess communities' assets as well as needs.

- Many disenfranchised populations or communities have considerable mistrust of public health efforts, including public health professionals and experts (Alter & Hage, 1993). This barrier must be addressed through open dialogue about varying perspectives, professionals' acquiescence of power, and the allowance for additional time needed for community participation.

- Power differentials between public health professionals and community members may hinder the building of an equal, collaborative relationship (Brownson, Riley, & Bruce, 1998; Plough & Olafson, 1994). Community members and representatives must feel like equals in the planning process. To build trust, public health professionals must be willing to be guided by the needs and desires of community representatives and ultimately the community itself (Flynn, Ray, & Rider, 1994).

- Confusion over lines of authority and/or the roles individual members play in the collaborative process can inhibit seriously the achievement of program goals. Problems may arise due to differences in socialization of community organizations and academic members. Community organizations tend to be more democratic and focus on shared decision making and responsibility, whereas public health organizations (e.g., health departments and schools of public health) are accustomed to hierarchical leadership with a "clear chain of command" (Buchanan, 1996, p. 265). This difference in structure has the potential to paralyze the collaborative process unless an explicit delineation of roles and responsibilities and leadership responsibilities is made at the onset of the program (Brownson et al., 1998).

- The development of community-based interventions is a complex, time-consuming process. If the intervention is begun before the community is ready or if the evaluation is done before adequate time is allowed for the intervention to have an impact, the program may falsely appear to have been inadequate. Public health professionals must be prepared to allocate sufficient time for community members to feel comfortable participating in the program and for the actual intervention and evaluation of the program (Brownson et al., 1998).

CONCLUSION

Many public health professionals now believe that change strategies directed by community members are far more likely to succeed than those planned and executed exclusively by outsiders (Green & Kreuter, 1991; Minkler & Wallerstein, 1998). This approach reflects the social ecological perspective of health and the belief that social and physical environments can be modified to augment individual behavior change. Community-based efforts use multifaceted strategies to address the environmental, social, behavioral, and political factors that affect health. Some community-based programs address multiple factors simultaneously, whereas others use a sequential approach, addressing one set of factors at a time. In addition to the ecological approach adopted by community-based interventions, these programs are tailored to the needs of the target community—"starting where the people are at"—and involve community members in the planning and implementation phases.

Community organization differs from other community-based approaches in its emphasis on community empowerment and the level of control the community exerts in defining the issues it will address and planning, implementing, and evaluating strategies designed to meet the goals they set. Community organizing models, such as PATCH, attempt to empower communities by helping them work together to set goals, develop strategies for achieving those goals, and gaining mastery over the social and political environmental factors that influence the health and well-being of their members.

Community-based interventions are challenging because of the additional time and skill needed to build effective partnerships with community members. Many public health practitioners are used to controlling planning activities and find it difficult to allow the community to be in the driver's seat. When successful, however, community-based interventions can be more effective in addressing the multiple factors that influence health and in bringing about changes that are sustained longer than efforts directed from agencies outside the community.

10

Social Marketing

S *ocial marketing* is a widely accepted approach to solving public health problems (Ling et al., 1992). It has been used to reduce AIDS risk behaviors (Fishbein et al., 1997; Smith, Helquist, Jimerson, Carovano, & Middlestadt, 1993); to prevent youth from smoking (Hastings, MacFadyen, MacKintosh, & Lowry, 1998); to fight child abuse; to increase utilization of public health services (Siegel & Donner, 1998); to combat many chronic diseases (Andreasen, 1995); and to promote breast-feeding (Bryant, Coreil, D'Angelo, Bailey, & Lazarov, 1992), good nutrition (Lefebvre et. al., 1995), physical exercise, contraceptive use (Rangun & Karim, 1991), infant weaning foods (Manoff, 1984), childhood immunizations (Cabanero-Verzosa et al., 1989), and oral rehydration therapy (Zimicki, 1993). Although social marketing's foundation was laid in 1971, its application to public health problems in the United States has emerged primarily within the past 20 years. Today, social marketing is used by a wide range of public health and social service organizations in the United States, including the Centers for Disease Control and Prevention, the National Cancer Institute, and the American Association of Retired Persons (Andreasen, 1995).

Social marketing is "the application of commercial marketing technologies to the analysis, planning, execution, and evaluation of programs designed to influence voluntary behavior of target audiences to improve their personal welfare and that of their society" (Andreasen, 1995, p. 7). Although social marketers rely on marketing's philosophy and techniques, their objectives are different from those of their commercial counterparts: Social marketers promote "socially beneficial" behavior change rather than commercial products and services.

In this chapter, we examine the distinguishing features of the social marketing approach and the steps used to design multifaceted behavior change interventions. A case study is used to illustrate how social marketing can be applied to improve public health service design and delivery.

DISTINGUISHING FEATURES OF THE SOCIAL MARKETING APPROACH

Social marketing is distinguished from other behavior change models used in public health by six principles: (a) the use of marketing's conceptual framework-exchange theory and the "4 Ps"; (b) a consumer orientation; (c) reliance on formative research to understand consumers' desires and needs; (d) segmentation of populations and careful selection of target audiences; (e) continuous monitoring and revision of program tactics; and (f) the desire to promote socially beneficial change.

The Conceptual Framework

Marketing provides the conceptual framework that guides program development. This conceptual framework views the consumer at the center of an exchange process in which she or he is acting primarily out of self-interest—attempting to maximize their ability to satisfy wants and needs and minimize what they must sacrifice to obtain them (Kotler & Armstrong, 1996). This framework includes five key concepts involved in the exchange process: the *product* (the health behavior being promoted) and its *competition* (the risk behavior currently practiced); the *price* (social, emotional, and monetary costs exchange for the product's benefits); *place* (where the exchange takes place and/or where the target behavior is practiced); and *promotion* (activities used to facilitate the exchange).

The product refers to the behavior being promoted. Social marketing may be used to get people to adopt new protective behaviors (e.g., start a regular exercise regimen), or stop practicing risky behaviors (e.g., eating too much fat). Product also may refer to a public health service, with the behavioral objective of increasing people's utilization of a program or changing how they use program services, such as increasing older people's consumption of the meals offered at congregate feeding sites. Finally, the product may refer to a tangible commodity, such as a condom, but, again, social marketers keep their eye focused on the behavior—the proper use of the product.

To be marketed successfully, social marketers believe the product must provide a solution to problems that consumers consider important and/or offer them a benefit they truly want. For this reason, they are very interested in people's aspirations, preferences, and other desires as well as their health needs. Most teenagers, for example, want to be between 1 and 5 years older, and, therefore, marketers often use older teenagers as spokespersons or role models when trying to reach them (Brightman, 1994).

Social marketing also reminds public health professionals to consider the competition. For many behaviors of interest to public health practitioners, the consumer must make a choice between the protective or healthy behavior and a risky alternative—the competition. In these cases, the product's benefits must be more highly valued than the benefits provided by the competition. Social marketers ask, "What products [behaviors] compete with those we are promoting? How do consumers compare the product's benefits with those offered by the competing product?" Answers to these questions enable social marketers to emphasize the product's benefits that best distinguish it from the competition, thereby maximizing its attractiveness to consumers.

Breast-feeding offers a good example of the difference between a social marketing and a traditional view of a public health product and its benefits. For more than a decade, public health professionals at the federal, state, and local level have promoted breast-feeding actively. Public health officials have been motivated to promote breast-feeding largely because of the protection it offers infants against gastrointestinal, respiratory, and middle ear infections, allergies, and other chronic diseases. They also have been impressed with breast-feeding's potential to decrease expenditures on infant formula supplements given to WIC participants and to decrease Medicaid expenditures for hospital and outpatient medical care. Despite widespread efforts to promote breast-feeding as a health behavior that offers important medical benefits and cost savings, breast-feeding rates remained low, especially among economically disadvantaged populations. In the late 1980s, some public health professionals turned to social marketing for a different approach (Bryant et al., 1992). Their marketing research revealed that public health professionals' view of the product and its benefits did not correspond with how the audience viewed breast-feeding and bottle-feeding. In fact, pregnant women are far more attracted to the emotional benefits breast-feeding offers than to its clinical or economic advantages. Women's aspirations as mothers center around the love they hope to give and receive, not the clinical aspects of infant care. Also, although mothers clearly want their babies to be healthy, the medical risks associated with bottle-feeding are not visible enough to convince them that breast-feeding is truly superior to formula. In marketing terms, the medical benefits were not sufficient to distinguish breast-feeding from bottle-feeding. The emotional benefits—a closer bond with the baby, the opportunity to relax and establish a special relationship with the baby—were distinctively better. In keeping with these findings, the Best Start social marketing project has promoted breast-feeding by emphasizing the close, loving bond and special joy that breast-feeding mothers share with their babies (Bryant et al., 1992). Health and other benefits are discussed in promotional materials, but campaign materials frame all of breast-feeding's benefits within the emotional benefits that its competition, infant formula, does not provide.

It is also important to view marketing's second *P*—price—from the consumer's perspective. What does the consumer have to exchange for the product's benefits? Some public health behaviors require consumers to exchange money for the product, such as the cost of an exercise or weight loss program, or low-fat foods. Other public health products may appear to be free, but closer examination reveals indirect monetary costs, such as lost wages or child care fees while being served at a health clinic. Most common, however, are nonmonetary costs—time, effort, embarrassment, loss of pride and dignity, and the psychological discomfort associated with change, especially lifelong habits. With respect to breast-feeding, research among pregnant women revealed many women were attracted to the products' benefits but were not willing to pay the costs. They worried breast-feeding would create many embarrassing moments, especially when they were required to nurse in front of others. Breast-feeding would open them to criticism from friends or relatives who see breast-feeding in a sexual light. Some women were unwilling to invest the additional time it takes to nurse a baby and worried about how breast-feeding would affect their ability to return to work, school, or an active social life. Other costs associated with breast-feeding were the pain associated with nursing, changes women mistakenly thought they must make in dietary and health practices, and anxiety about their ability to produce the quality and quantity of breast milk needed to meet their child's nutritional needs. Finally, some women were unwilling to alienate spouses, boyfriends, or their own mothers and other kin who might feel left out of the special relationship breast-feeding creates between a mother and child.

To make the exchange more attractive to consumers, social marketers work to lower costs and enhance benefits. The Best Start campaign used a variety of means to lower the price of breast-feeding. A three-step counseling strategy was designed to enable health providers to quickly identify the perceived costs and help mothers develop their own ways to overcome the problems they anticipated. Public information and consumer education materials were used to change the public's attitudes about breast-feeding in public and to counter misperceptions about the time required to breastfeed. These materials also informed people of how they could learn how to breastfeed after returning to work. The overall theme of the program—"Loving Support Makes Breastfeeding Work"—and mass media materials were designed to elicit support from family, friends, and the public at large for women who breastfeed. Finally, media advocacy and policy development were used to change regulations restricting breast-feeding in public and to promote policies supportive of breast-feeding in hospitals and workplaces (Best Start, 1997).

Unfortunately, the price of many social marketing products is difficult to control. In fact, many protective health behaviors come with a high price that is difficult to lower. Safe sex practices are not as pleasurable as the riskier competition. Most people have a hard time sacrificing the special taste, texture, and satiety that accompany a high-fat diet.

In setting "the right price," it also is important to know if consumers prefer to pay more to obtain certain "value-added" benefits and if they consider products inferior when they are given away or priced too low. A good example of how important is an understanding of consumers' perceptions of price comes from a condom promotion program coordinated by Population Services International (PSI). Consumer research designed to discover why teens did not use condoms given away by health programs found that teens assumed condoms that were free must be of inferior quality and unreliable. Research also revealed that many teens could not pay the high price of condoms in retail outlets but could easily afford to pay 25 cents for them. This price was determined as sufficient to reassure consumers that the product was reliable but not so high as to make them unaffordable.

Place, the third *P*, refers to the location where services are provided, where tangible products are distributed, and where consumers receive information about new products or behaviors. Research is conducted to identify the "life path points" where people visit routinely, so that products and information can be placed there. Social marketers also want to know when and where the target audience will be in the most receptive mood to listen and respond to our messages. Breast-feeding promotion pamphlets, for example, will be far more effective if placed in prenatal care clinics than at large shopping malls, emergency rooms, or sporting events.

Place also refers to channels for distribution of tangible commodities. Again, it is important to determine where consumers will be when they are ready to purchase the product. In their safe sex marketing campaign, PSI placed condom machines in bathrooms at fast-food stores where teenagers took their dates just before going home for the evening.

The fourth *P* is promotion. Many people expect social marketing to rely exclusively on mass media to communicate with target audiences. However, health communications is but one small part of a carefully designed set of activities designed to bring about change. In fact, an effective promotional strategy usually includes several communication elements: specific communication objectives for each target audience; guidelines for designing attention-getting and effective messages; designation of appropriate communication channels; and credible, trustworthy spokespersons. Specific health communications activities vary: Some large-scale, multifaceted projects rely on mass communications, public information, public relations, consumer education, lotteries, direct mail, and/or other means. Projects with more limited communications components may rely solely on personal counseling and print materials.

The promotional strategy also includes many activities besides health communications, such as service delivery improvements, policy changes, community-based activities, the use of coupons, and many other means for attracting potential consumers. We have seen the mix of health communication, policy changes, personal counseling strategies, consumer education, and other activities used in the Best Start breast-feeding promotion campaign. The Texas WIC case described subsequently gives another example of a multifaceted marketing plan used to increase program use.

Finally, to be effective, promotional strategies must be coordinated carefully with other components of the marketing mix (Lefebvre & Flora, 1988, p. 308). Social marketers know promotional efforts must be carefully integrated into the marketing mix; promotional efforts cannot succeed if the product's benefits, price, and placement are not also in line with consumers' wants and needs. To develop a well-coordinated marketing plan, as opposed to a communications program, intervention strategies are based on a careful analysis of an audience's perception of each of the four Ps and how these variables interact. To this end, social marketers rely on consumer research—the next distinguishing feature of the social marketing approach.

A summary of the components of the social marketing mix and a description of key questions that must be answered in determining the "right mix" are provided in Table 10.1.

Consumer Orientation

Inherent to the marketing mind-set is a steadfast commitment to understand the consumer. Social marketers want to know everything they can about the people whose behavior they want to change—their aspirations, values, beliefs, attitudes, and current behavioral patterns. They also study the broader social and cultural factors that influence consumer behavior, recognizing that behavior change is influenced by a combination of external and internal factors.

Social marketing's consumer orientation distinguishes it from traditional top-down approaches to program planning and implementation. Many traditional program planning models rely on experts and "best practice models" for guidance on how to design service delivery programs or health education cam-

TABLE 10.1   Conceptual Framework: Key Concepts in the Exchange Process

Product   The behavior, good, service, or program being promoted

- What are the *benefits* of the product from the consumers' perspective—what needs or wants do they have that the product can fulfill?
- How can we enhance the product's benefits to make it more attractive to consumers?

Price   The cost to the consumer—what he or she must exchange for the product's benefits

- What are the monetary (direct and indirect) costs of the product?
- What are the nonmonetary costs? Does the consumer have to exchange time, effort, or psychological discomfort in order to get the product?
- How can we lower the product's costs?
- How can we make them more acceptable to consumers?

Competition   Products (services, behaviors, or commodities) that compete with the product

- What are people doing now that puts them at increased risk for premature death, disability, or disease?
- What services or commodities do they use now?
- How can the benefits of the competing product(s) be diminished?
- **How can the price of the competing product(s) be raised?**

Place   The locations where services are provided, tangible products are distributed, and consumers receive information about new products or behaviors

- What are the "life path points" people routinely visit where they make decisions about the product?
- Where do consumers practice the behavior, utilize the service, or purchase the commodity?
- When and where are consumers in the most receptive mood to listen and respond to our message?
- How can the product be made more accessible? Where should it be offered? Displayed?
- Where should information be placed about the product?

Promotion   A combination of activities designed to bring about behavior change

- What activities are needed to promote the product, for example, service delivery improvements, policy changes, community-based activities, incentives, or public relations?
- What messages will promote behavior change?
- What media are appropriate—for example, mass media or print materials—for disseminating information?

paigns. When people do not use public health services, discard educational materials, or ignore professionals' advice, they are labeled "hard to reach." Conversely, the marketing mind-set requires us to look to the consumer, not the expert, for guidance in program planning. When services are underutilized or professional recommendations are rejected, social marke'ers search for what is wrong with the product rather than for what is wrong with the customers.

Also inherent in marketing's consumer orientation is a willingness to change the product or "offer" to fit consumers' wants and needs. This willingness to modify the product is a central feature of social marketing and distinguishes it from health communication that uses persuasion or an educational approach to elicit change. Unfortunately, many public health professionals mistakenly turn to social marketing hoping that they can use it to sell their services by hitting consumers' motivational buttons the right way. They do not realize that promotional campaigns cannot convince consumers to use programs that do not offer them something they truly want or need.

Consumer Research

Consumer research serves as the bedrock upon which program strategy is developed. Qualitative and quantitative research is conducted to understand the consumers' perception of product benefits, product price, the competition's benefits and costs, and other factors that influence consumer behavior. Information channels, community resources, and the social and physical environment in which change will occur also are studied (Ogden, Shepherd, & Smith, 1996).

Marketing of protective health behaviors (e.g., exercise or seat belt) relies on the social and behavioral sciences to guide formative research and subsequent program design (Middlestadt, Schecter, Peyton, & Tjugum, 1997). Formative research is used to identify and prioritize behaviors that are both protective (i.e., that significantly affect disease outcomes) and feasible to promote among members of the community (compatible with cultural values, likely to be adopted). Program objectives are then defined in behavioral terms: what the program will help people to do to protect their health and prevent disease. A program designed to facilitate healthy aging could focus on promoting a variety of healthy behaviors—low-fat and low-caloric dietary intake, regular exercise, smoking cessation, and moderate alcohol consumption. Research would be used to identify the specific behavioral recommendations most compatible with the consumers' norms, beliefs, and values and set behavioral objectives for the intended audience (Middlestadt et al., 1997).

In social marketing, consumer research is guided by many of the behavior theories set out in this text. These theories are used to identify potential behavioral determinants—perceived susceptibility and severity; self-efficacy; social norms, beliefs, and values; previous behavior and intentions with regard to the target behavior; and many others. Research is then conducted to identify the mix of individual and environmental factors that have the greatest impact on people's health behavior (Fishbein et al., 1997; Middlestadt et al., 1997; Smith et al., 1993). This behavioral orientation enables program planners to design strategies that address the critical factors that determine a specific audience segment's adoption of the targeted behavior (Middlestadt et al., 1997).

Audience Segmentation

Another distinguishing feature of social marketing is its reliance on audience segmentation in selecting target audiences. Audience segmentation refers to the process of dividing a population into distinct segments based on characteristics that influence their responsiveness to marketing interventions, such as the price they are willing to pay for a product or the spokespersons they would trust the most. Social marketers segment a potential target population for several reasons. First, segmentation allows them to identify the subgroups they can realistically reach with the resources they have available to them. When allocating time or funds, many public health professionals look first to the neediest members of the population or those at greatest risk. Unfortunately, these groups are often the least likely to respond to public health activities designed to change their behavior. Although social marketers realize that the neediest groups could benefit the most, they also know they do not have the resources needed to reach them. They also know many people who resist outsiders' attempts to change them will adopt new practices or products after most of their friends, relatives, and neighbors—people they know personally and/or admire—have done so already (Rogers, 1995). For this reason, social marketers look for *targets of greatest opportunity*—segments that are likely to respond to their efforts as well as benefit from the change. In this way, they are reaching opinion makers, who encourage others to follow their lead, thereby influencing the behavior of the hard-to-reach segment via the diffusion process.

Another reason to segment a population is to determine the best way to reach each group. Segments may differ in terms of the benefits they find most attractive, the price they are willing to pay, the best place to communicate with them or locate services, or their differential responsiveness to promotional tactics. Many social marketers use the stages of change (Prochaska & DiClementi, 1992) as a *basis variable* when dividing a potential audience. They can then select one or more segments that are sufficiently large to warrant attention and design strategies most appropriate for reaching each target group. In designing a program to promote annual mammography screening among economically disadvantaged women, very different interventions would be designed to reach women in each stage of change. A program designed to enhance perceived benefits of mammography use would be appropriate for reaching women in precontemplation, but it probably would be useless for those who know the benefits but have decided not to have mammograms because of the pain and embarrassment they experienced when screened the first time. The latter group would best be reached with information about how they can obtain mammograms in special facilities designed to minimize pain and embarrassment.

Continuous Monitoring and Revision

As program interventions are implemented, each is monitored to assess its effectiveness in bringing about the desired changes. Monitoring is used to identify activities that are effective and worthy of being sustained and to identify activities that require midcourse revision. Although many public health programs rely on process and impact evaluations to identify the components that are working and those that should be discontinued, social marketing devotes considerable resources to this activity. Social marketers are constantly checking with target audiences to gauge their responses to all aspects of an intervention, from the broad marketing strategy to specific messages and materials.

Socially Beneficial Change

Social marketing differs from its commercial counterpart in terms of its mission. Commercial marketers design and sell products to create profits. Social marketers do not benefit financially from their efforts but rather use the marketing approach to promote socially beneficial behavior change.

Social marketing is also more difficult than commercial marketing because of the nature of products being promoted. These difficulties include negative demand for products/services (e.g., taking medications), lack of flexibility in modifying products to meet consumer demands (e.g., breast-feeding), and targeting nonliterate audiences that have limited resources. Public health professionals who use social marketing also must overcome challenges associated with the types of change they hope to bring about. Healthy lifestyle behaviors are often less appealing than the risk behaviors with which they compete. Long-term change in habitual behaviors is far more difficult than promoting single purchases of a commodity. Many public health products are controversial or "sensitive" social products, making it difficult to collect valid information from consumers and to communicate effectively about them (e.g., condom use to prevent sexually transmitted diseases) (Andreasen, 1995; Bloom & Novelli, 1981). Also, public health professionals must have their work scrutinized by the funding agency and general public (Andreasen, 1995) that may hinder research activities and restrict the types of communications and other interventions used.

Focus: Marketing, Education, and Law as Behavior Management Tools

Social marketing's distinctive approach also can be understood by comparing it with other tools used to manage behavior change. Michael Rothschild (1999) developed a valuable conceptual framework that contrasts marketing with education and law or policy development.

Education informs and persuades people to adopt healthy behaviors voluntarily by creating awareness of the benefits of changing and by modifying their attitudes and beliefs about the behavioral choice. When health professionals educate people about the benefits of adopting healthy lifestyle behaviors, citizens have free choice in how they respond, and the society accepts the costs when some continue to practice undesirable behaviors. Education is most effective when the goals of society are consistent with those of the target audience (e.g., poison prevention); the benefits of behavior change are inherently attractive, immediate, and observable; the risk or costs of changing are low; and the skills and other resources needed to change are readily available.

Law uses coercion or the threat of punishment to achieve behavior change. Law is the most effective tool when society's goals are not consistent with citizen's self-interest—people do not benefit immediately or directly from adopting the recommended behavior and they must pay a high price. Public health professionals may need to enact laws when society is not willing to pay the costs associated with continued practice of an unhealthy or risky behavior (e.g., driving while intoxicated) and citizens are unlikely to find it in their immediate self-interest to change.

In contrast, marketing manages behavior by creating alternative choices (offering incentives and/or consequences) that invite voluntary exchange. Marketing alters the environment to make the recommended health behavior more advantageous than the unhealthy behavior it is designed to replace and then communicates the more favorable cost-benefit relations to the target audience. Marketing is the most effective strategy when societal goals are not directly and immediately consistent with people's self-interest but can be modified to elicit behavior change by maximizing benefits and minimizing costs (e.g., regular physical activity and weight control). Like education, marketing offers people freedom of choice, but, unlike education, it alters the behavioral consequences rather than relies on individuals to make a sacrifice on behalf of society (for an insightful discussion of other conditions that affect the relative effectiveness of education, marketing, and law in managing behavior, see Rothschild, 1999).

STEPS IN THE SOCIAL MARKETING PROCESS

The social marketing process is a continuous, iterative process that can be conceived as consisting of six major steps or tasks:

- Initial planning
- Formative research
- Strategy development
- Campaign development (material and nonmaterial interventions)
- Implementation
- Tracking and evaluation

Initial Planning

The overall goal of this stage is to identify preliminary behavioral objectives, audience segments, and a list of potential behavioral determinants. A group of program planners is assembled to discuss potential target audiences, health behaviors to be promoted, and the factors believed to influence each target group's adoption of the recommended health behaviors. During the discussion, a list is made of the subgroups affected by the problem and of basis variables (demographic, ttitudes, wants, needs, stages of change, etc.) that could be used to segment the population at risk. A list of environmental and individual factors believed to influence people's adoption of the proposed health behaviors is also generated. These lists guide the development of research objectives, selection of sampling frames, and development of data collection instruments in the next phase.

Formative Research

Because social marketing demands a thorough understanding of consumers and the people who influence their decisions, the formative research phase requires a far more in-depth analysis of consumers' beliefs, values, and behavior than is typically accomplished in program needs assessments. As noted previously, research is used to investigate the factors identified during the initial planning phase to determine those that must be addressed to bring about behavior change. Researchers attempt to answer questions such as, What factors motivate people to adopt the recommended behavior? What deters them from changing? Which external and individual factors have the greatest impact on behavior change? What benefits will they find most attractive in adopting the recommended behavior? What prices are they unwilling to pay and how can this be made more acceptable? Where will they be in the right frame of mind to attend to information about the product, remember it, and act on it? Where should tangible products or program services be located? What types of spokespersons are most credible and persuasive in recommending change? What types of promotional activities will be effective in encouraging them to adopt a healthier lifestyle? How can programs be changed to fit the beliefs, customs, norms, and values of the people they hope to influence? Which groups within the population are most likely to adopt specific behavioral recommendations?

Strategy Development

The purpose of this phase is to prepare a realistic marketing plan comprised of specific, measurable objectives and a step-by-step work plan that will guide the development, implementation, and tracking of the demonstration project. This plan contains a clear statement of the overall goals or mission of the project, a description of the audience segments being targeted, the specific behaviors that will be promoted with each audience segment, and strategies for addressing the critical factors associated with the health behaviors being promoted.

The marketing plan is organized around marketing's conceptual framework of the four *P*s and product competition. The product strategy delineates the benefits target audience members find most attractive about the recommended health behavior (or product) and determines how the product should be distinguished from its competition. The product strategy also determines the product's image; for example, exercise can be something fun and easy to do anywhere or a way to stay healthy.

The pricing strategy focuses on the costs consumers associate with adopting the recommended behavior. This part of the marketing mix specifies the costs the audience is unwilling to pay to practice the behavior and recommends ways to lower them or make them more acceptable. Other barriers that impede adoption and recommendations for overcoming them and recommendations for maintaining regular practice of the recommended behavior are also delineated.

The placement strategy is developed for distributing information and any tangible products related to the proposed behavior. This portion of the plan outlines the support materials or activities needed (e.g., signs, display racks, audiovisual equipment, reorganization of waiting room) and methods used to ensure a steady supply of the product to distribution outlets. It also identifies methods to properly train and to motivate the people who will work directly with consumers, for example, health providers or business personnel involved in promotional activities.

The promotional strategy describes the tactics and activities to facilitate change. Such change can include legislative change, policy development and organizational change, professional training, peer counselor programs, curriculum development, consumer education, public relations, direct marketing, advertising, face-to-face communication, media advocacy, and grassroots advocacy.

A step-by-step work plan summarizing the product, price, place, and promotional strategies, timetable, and budget for each campaign component is also prepared. An evaluation and monitoring plan is also developed. Health and behavioral outcome measures are identified and methods for monitoring these are specified.

Campaign Development

This phase involves the development of all campaign materials and strategies. Often, an advertising agency or other creative team is hired to design messages and prepare materials. Instructional designers, professional trainers, and public relations firms are hired to develop new products, curricula, campaign messages and materials, and public relations activities. Program strategies, campaign messages and materials, and other products are pretested and revised.

Program Implementation

Many social marketing projects do not reach the implementation phase for a year or longer. Although coordination is important for any program, social marketing projects typically require managers to balance an unusually large number of staff, consultants, or subcontractors and manage multiple activities, each of which requires careful timing. Proper sequencing of legislative advocacy, organizational policy and procedural changes, professional training, materials distribution, public relations, and public policy formation is essential to the success of a project.

Tracking and Evaluation

Tracking and evaluation activities begin before the program is launched to give program planners a baseline against which to measure changes. As the program is implemented, a process evaluation or monitoring is used to document the progress of individual program components (when, where, and what has been done, and who has been reached). Evaluation of overall program performance (media exposure, product/service usage patterns, number of staff trained, adoption rates) allows managers to decide what to continue to do, what to refine, and what to abandon (Balch & Sutton, 1997; Siegel & Donner, 1998).

After the program has been implemented for sufficient time to bring about the desired changes, an evaluation of program outcomes can be conducted. Results are used to identify objectives, target audiences or activities that should be refined, and identify new problems that require additional planning and improvement. Ideally, this step leads back to the first phase and the selection of new program goals.

PUBLIC HEALTH SERVICES MARKETING: A CASE STUDY

Although we have focused on using social marketing to promote healthy behaviors, this approach also offers public health professionals a powerful mind-set for organizing and promoting public health services. Social marketing can be used to increase utilization of public health programs, improve consumer satisfaction with those services, increase employees' job satisfaction and productivity, and make service delivery more consumer-friendly. One example of how public health administrators have applied social marketing to increase program utilization comes from the Texas Special Supplemental Nutrition Program for Women, Infants and Children (WIC). Their success demonstrates how management in public health care can effectively use the social marketing process to understand the needs and expectations of social groups and use this information to develop marketing strategies to encourage target groups to use specific health services voluntarily.

The Texas WIC program provides target populations of women, infants, and young children with nutrition education, supplementary nutritious foods, and referrals to appropriate health and social services. Numerous studies have documented WIC's positive impact on the nutritional status of pregnant women, nursing mothers, and young children (Rush, Alvir, Kenney, Johnson, & Horvitz, 1988) as well as reductions in low birth weight, preterm delivery, and fetal death (Rush, Leighton, et al., 1988).

Despite the program's proven efficacy, many families who could benefit from WIC do not participate in the program. To meet the challenge of offering the Texas WIC program to more families in need of its services, public health administrators contracted with a social marketing firm, Best Start, to develop marketing strategies to increase enrollment among the state's diverse, rapidly growing population.

Steps in the Texas WIC Marketing Project

During the initial planning phase, Texas public health administrators and Best Start staff identified pregnant women who had never enrolled in the WIC program as the primary target audience. A large proportion of women who were receiving Medicaid benefits and who were therefore income-eligible for the WIC program were not enrolled in the program. A comparison of census data and WIC program participant data (pregnant women enrolled in the program) suggested that program participation was higher among women whose incomes fell below 150% of the poverty guidelines than among those whose incomes fell between 150% and 185%—the upper limit for eligibility in WIC. The behavioral objective set for this target audience was to motivate them to enroll in the program.

Relatively little was known about the reasons for this particular group's reluctance to use the program. Extensive formative research was used to identify the program benefits they desired and the perceived costs and other factors that influenced their decisions to participate in WIC. A computer match of pregnant women enrolled in the Texas Medicaid program and the Texas WIC program generated a list of 36,743 Medicaid recipients who were not currently participating in WIC yet who were automatically income-eligible for the program. A random sample of 15,000 pregnant Texas Medicaid recipients was selected and sent a 28-item mailed survey. Twenty percent returned the survey in time to be included in the study sample. Five focus groups and 81 telephone interviews also were conducted with women who indicated on the survey that they would be willing to talk further with researchers.

Research results identified several important attitudes and perceptions that could be changed. With respect to program benefits, most women had a positive impression of the program but did not know its full service offerings. Focus group discussions, for example, revealed that most women were familiar with portions of WIC's food package, especially the infant formula and dairy products. Yet, few were aware that WIC also offers many other nutritious foods, individualized nutritional risk assessment and counseling, education classes, and immunizations—services that greatly enhanced the program's attractiveness.

Research also indicated several costs or barriers women associated with program participation. One of the most formidable costs to enrollment was the embarrassment some women would feel if identified as a recipient of free food. This attitude was especially prevalent among white women of European descent and Asian Americans.

A number of women also did not want to enroll in WIC because they felt that it would "rob" them of their sense of self-sufficiency, and they did not want to rely on yet another government program.

A third reason women were reluctant to accept WIC benefits was because they mistakenly believed WIC benefits were in short supply and should be accepted only by those with the greatest need. These women felt strongly that government programs are designed to help only those who cannot provide for themselves. Although they did not think it was shameful for people to accept help when it was truly justified, they believed others should feel embarrassed to accept help if they could work and be self-sufficient. A related concern expressed by women was the fear that their enrollment would displace other women and children whose needs were far greater than their own.

Another major barrier was created by confusion about WIC's eligibility criteria. Despite being automatically income-eligible, almost half of the survey respondents who were not enrolled in WIC did not recognize that they were automatically income-eligible for WIC. Focus group discussions provided insight into why these women did not realize they qualified for WIC. Some women mistakenly believed their family income was too high to qualify. Some did not think women would qualify if they or their husbands worked. Some believed they were ineligible because they lived with relatives whose incomes were too high. And some believed they were ineligible because they had been denied food stamps (the food stamp program has stricter income guidelines than WIC).

Finally, some women were also apprehensive about participating in a program about which their friends and relatives complained. The difficulties mentioned most frequently were long waits at WIC clinics to obtain food cards and listen to educational videotapes, rude treatment by WIC staff, lack of Spanish-speaking staff, and rude treatment while redeeming WIC food vouchers at the grocery store.

Formative research was also helpful in identifying characteristics of women who never had enrolled in the Texas WIC program. Audience segmentation made it possible to identify subgroups of never-enrolled women who would benefit from intensive outreach efforts and the specific issues that should be addressed to recruit them. For example, women who were employed, who had completed high school, and whose incomes were 135% to 185% of the federal poverty level were the least likely to be enrolled and the least likely to know they were income-eligible for WIC. This segment was selected as an important target for outreach efforts designed to clarify eligibility requirements.

Research findings were then used to develop a comprehensive social marketing plan for reaching the audience segments with the highest proportions of women who had never enrolled in the WIC program. First, the plan addressed women's misperceptions of the program's benefits. Outreach materials were designed to emphasize the nutrition education, health checkups, immunizations, and referrals WIC provided. These materials featured the variety of nutritious foods WIC offers in an attempt to reframe WIC as a program parents can be proud to use because it helps them raise healthy children.

The plan also included recommendations for lowering the price of participating in WIC. To make participation less embarrassing, the program's image was redefined from a "free food" or government assistance program to a health and nutrition program. In light of women's concerns about self-sufficiency, WIC's image was also reframed as a temporary assistance program, "Helping Families Help Themselves." The "new" WIC program was depicted as one in which families can maintain their pride and self-esteem as they earn their WIC benefits and learn about nutrition and other ways to help their families.

Because many women did not know they were eligible for the program, the marketing plan also emphasized ways to help families understand eligibility guidelines, streamline the certification process, and make it easier for health and social service professionals to refer eligible women. One television ad addressed the most common misperceptions about WIC eligibility, featuring a working father and his two daughters, a pregnant teen who lives with relatives, and a married woman as participants who are qualified for program benefits. During the ad, the narrators inform people that many families do not realize they qualify for this valuable program, including those who do not qualify for food stamps, working families, and those living with relatives, and the narrators encourage viewers to call a toll-free line to find out if they are eligible.

Placement and promotional strategies also were designed for the Texas WIC program. Message design guidelines were developed to guide the creative team in preparing television, radio, and print messages consistent with the plan's overall goals. Audience segmentation results were used to determine the regions in the state and specific stations to air radio and television spots and purchase billboards. Audience segmentation data showing that whites or Anglos were the most likely to believe it is embarrassing to accept government assistance were used to select a family with these characteristics to appear in the second television spot. This spot was designed to reposition or redefine the WIC program as a health and nutrition program that "brings lots to the table."

Finally, service delivery improvements were planned to make the program more consumer-friendly, making it possible to retain women who enrolled and minimize the number of complaints participants made to other eligible families. A training program was designed to teach grocery store cashiers how to handle difficult WIC transactions while treating WIC participants respectfully. And a permanent data collection procedure was designed for tracking program enroll-ment and program satisfaction. A summary of the Texas WIC Marketing Plan is displayed in Table 10.2.

Using the social marketing plan as a guide, Best Start social marketers, health department personnel, and an advertising agency then developed the messages, outreach materials, training programs, data collection instruments, and other re-sources needed to implement and evaluate the program. A key element in this phase was ensuring that each component was consistent with the overall mar-keting strategy. Marketing messages and mass media materials were rigorously pretested and redesigned until they proved to be effective. These materials in-cluded a new WIC logo, two television spots and three radio spots (each of which are in English and Spanish), billboards, a set of outreach brochures and posters, a community organizer's kit to facilitate coalition building at the local agency level, several training modules, and data collection instruments for tracking and evaluating the program.

The Texas WIC program was launched in fall 1995. Approximately $250,000 was used to purchase television and radio air time and billboard space. Mass me-dia and consumer education was augmented with other outreach efforts, service improvements, and other activities. To help women learn about WIC through other social service programs and prenatal care providers, materials clarifying WIC services and eligibility guidelines and offering helpful suggestions were distributed to health providers and social service workers who refer clients to WIC. To create a positive introduction to WIC, user-friendly certification proce-dures were designed to help each new enrollee feel as if she is a very important person. Also, the program was made more consumer-friendly by offering child-safe play areas, a peer-buddy system, decreased waiting times, new educa-tional materials, and customer relations training for clinic staff and grocery store cashiers.

Finally, the permanent data collection system was used to collect baseline data from new participants, regular participants, and program employees. These satisfaction surveys were used to identify problems that affect satisfaction among these three groups and make midcourse revisions. The survey results also were used to further clarify eligibility messages and improve enrollment procedures, thus creating an effective feedback system. Unfortunately, the Texas WIC Program has not continued to collect these data, and funds were not re-leased for a formal evaluation of the program's impact. Program data, however, point to significant increases in the number of families who called the toll-free number for more information after the program was launched and, more impor-tant, in the number of people participating in Texas WIC. The program's case-load grew from 542,000 in 1993 to almost 700,000 in 1998.

TABLE 10.2   The Texas WIC Social Marketing Plan

Major Components	*Examples of Specific Strategies*
Policy recommendations	1. Recognition for staff performance, including customer service awards. 2. Career growth opportunities for staff, with a clear career ladder structure. 3. Use of computers to communicate policy changes more effectively between state and local staff. 4. Revised appointment scheduling policies to improve clinic efficiency and create more "user-friendly" certification and food card issuance procedures (e.g., online, computerized policy manuals for staff).
Service delivery	1. Increased accessibility by offering WIC services at day care centers, employers, grocery stores, migrant camps, and more flexible clinic hours (night, lunch time, and one Saturday per month). 2. Child-friendly clinics where children can play, eat nutritious snacks, and learn about nutrition in child-proofed areas supervised by staff, paraprofessionals, and volunteers. 3. Peer buddy system—paraprofessionals act as advocates/guides for participants waiting for clinic services, ensure that participants have required documentation, answer questions about certification and food cards, and give "smart shopping" tips. 4. Improvements in grocery store experiences with a new food card redemption system (fewer cards to be signed at register) and a "products brochure" to depict allowable WIC foods for participants and serve as a reference for cashiers.
Training	1. Staff training and continuing education. 2. Grocery store cashier training program, videotape about customer service and the WIC transaction.
Nutrition education	1. Nutrition education facilitator training in interactive teaching skills to discuss nutrition and new, nontraditional WIC subjects (e.g., parenting, child development) with participants. 2. "Food and Family" educational magazine for WIC participants.
Tracking system	1. Monitoring system to track participant satisfaction with the food package, nutrition education, food redemption, clinic service, and clinic environment and staff satisfaction with supervision, clinic environment, ability to provide WIC services, and participant contact. 2. Training for local agency directors in interpreting results and identifying and overcoming service delivery problems.
Health communication plan	1. Messages to reposition WIC's image—to a comprehensive health and education program offering nutritious foods, screening, social support, and referral to other services, for example, through 30-second "Nutrition Tips" radio spots. 2. Messages to increase awareness of income eligibility criteria.
Community outreach	1. Community organizers' kit to assist local agency directors in working with program partners in increasing referrals of eligible families to WIC. 2. Kit includes outreach materials targeted to health professionals and eligible families.

NOTE: This table includes examples of the many strategies that have been developed for each component of the social marketing plan. The first five components are designed to increase participant and staff satisfaction; the last two are intended to increase participant enrollment (Bryant et al., 1994).

CONCLUSION

Social marketing offers public health professionals an effective approach for developing programs to promote healthy behaviors. Social marketing is distinguished from other program planning models by its use of marketing' conceptual framework (exchange theory and the four *P*s), a consumer orientation; reliance on formative research to understand consumers' desires and needs, segmentation of populations and careful selection of target audiences, and continuous monitoring and revision of program tactics.

Although social marketing often uses mass media to communicate with its target audiences, it should not be confused with health communication, social advertising, or educational approaches that simply create awareness of a behavior's health benefits or attempt to persuade people to change through motivational messages. Social marketers use data to identify the product benefits most attractive to target audience segments, determine what costs will be acceptable and those that must be lowered, identify the best places to offer products, and communicate with consumers and design the best mix of promotional tactics to elicit behavior change.

Social marketing also offers public health a new institutional mind-set, one in which solutions to problems are solicited from consumers. An organization that adopts the social marketing mind-set continually evaluates and remakes itself so as to increase the likelihood that it is meeting the needs of its ever-changing constituency. This mind-set makes it an effective tool for increasing enrollment in public health programs and enables them to ensure continued satisfaction and program participation.

IV.
Special Topics

The areas of specialization within public health are remarkably diverse, spanning all age groups, subpopulations, geographic areas, types of services, health problems, and domains of human activity. Thus, it is impossible to cover all of them in a volume of this scope. However, we feel the selection of four special topics for inclusion in this section provides at least a sample of the range of issues for which social and behavioral foundations are important.

Chapter 11 overviews the social context of health problems and health behavior in developing countries. Trends in the application of methods and models in international health research are discussed. Finally, a life span framework is used to examine current health issues in poor areas of the world. In Chapter 12, "Food and Society," the life cycle reappears as an organizing concept for understanding the interaction of biological, psychological, cultural, and social dimensions of diet and nutrition. Symbolic and religious aspects of food also are discussed, along with particular conditions such as geophagia, in this broad overview.

The final two chapters address areas of growing importance in public health, particularly in regard to the relevance of social and behavioral science perspectives. These areas are mental health and aging. Following closely the introductory section of this book, Chapter 13 discusses public mental health from a historical, epidemiologic, and theoretical perspective and systematically applies the organizing frameworks of Social Ecology, Health Impact, and Causality Continuum. Competing explanations of mental illness based on social selection and social causation theories are discussed. The final chapter advocates attention to gerontological health as a new imperative for public health. Like Chapter 2, it draws heavily on demography as a foundation for understanding changing population patterns and associated health repercussions. Whereas clinical perspectives on treating older patients have dominated this field in the past, the future lies in prevention-focused public health initiatives.

11

Health Behavior
in Developing Countries

T he distinction between developed and developing countries has become increasingly blurred as many less developed countries make important strides in social conditions as well as economic development. Although it long has been recognized that the nations of the world do not fall neatly into two categories of "more" and "less" developed, but instead extend across a wide continuum of socioeconomic diversity, only recently have observers noted that health and quality of life indicators can be quite variable within countries traditionally considered underdeveloped (Pillai & Shannon, 1995). Some very poor countries have made remarkable improvements in the health of their populations, whereas comparatively wealthier nations have not fared so well (Caldwell, 1990). It is common to find a fourfold typology used to classify nations into least developed, less developed, newly industrialized, and developed countries.

The criteria used to define development have included economic, demographic, social, and political indicators. According to World Bank (1993) definitions, the term *developing economies* refers to those falling within the low to middle range of gross national product (GNP) per capita. *Low-income economies* are those with a GNP of $635 (U.S.) or less, and *middle-income economies* include those with a GNP of more than $635 but less than $7,911. Low- and middle-income countries are also defined as demographically developing, in the sense that their age distributions, owing to their high fertility rate, are young compared with industrialized nations. Composite social/health indicators have been devised to measure quality of life conditions, such as the Physical Quality of Life Index and the Index of Suffering (Pillai & Shannon, 1995). In recent decades, the term *Third*

World often has been used synonymously with developing countries in the economic sense; however, the original use of the term was primarily political in meaning, growing out of the Cold War era when three worlds of development corresponded to democratic, communist, and nonaligned nations (Horowitz, 1966). This review uses the labels *developing countries* and *Third World countries* interchangeably.

In discussions related to health, it is helpful to consider the social and health-related indicators that often are cited in discussions of the health conditions of developing countries. These include urban/rural population distribution, literacy rate, access to clean water, infant and under-5 mortality, maternal mortality, fertility rate, and life expectancy. Table 11.1 contrasts typical norms for these indexes for developing and developed countries, bearing in mind that many countries fall somewhere between these two ideal types. Although developed countries are highly urbanized and industrialized, developing countries have predominantly agricultural economies supported by rural dwelling populations with little education. Access to clean water and modern medical services is comparatively low, with infant mortality, child malnutrition, and maternal mortality very high in the less developed areas. Life expectancy is considerably lower, and fertility is much higher.

Research on health behavior in developing countries differs markedly from its counterpart in developed countries, for several reasons. First, child health and survival is the most important public health problem in the Third World because of the predominance of youth in the population (a product of high fertility) and because mortality in this age group exceeds adult mortality. Second, infectious and parasitic diseases are more prevalent in developing countries than are chronic, noncommunicable diseases, and environmental risk factors for these health problems are more important than individual health behavior. Third, whereas health behavior research in developed countries tends to be organized around particular behaviors (e.g., smoking, exercise, diet, use of seat belts), behavioral research in developing countries is largely centered around biomedically defined diseases and organized efforts to control them (e.g., malaria, AIDS, tuberculosis, diarrhea). Fourth, governments and families in developing countries have fewer resources to invest in lifestyle change, and individuals have less choice and control of their health-related behavior than is typical of developed countries. Thus, behavioral research on health in developing countries is shaped by the dominant health goal of reducing child mortality from preventable infectious diseases, whereas in developed countries the emphasis is on reducing adult morbidity from chronic diseases, primarily through lifestyle modification.

TABLE 11.1   Indicators of Health in Developing and Developed Areas

Indicator	Developing Areas	Developed Areas
Infant mortality rate	100	10
Under-5 mortality rate	175	13
Maternal mortality rate	500	11
Life expectancy	53	75
Total fertility rate	5	2
Population urban (%)	30	73
Adults literate (% male/female)	53/33	97/90
Access to clean water (%)	37	95
Ratio of expenditures for health/defense	4/33	50/50

METHODOLOGICAL ISSUES

Overreliance on Aggregate Data

The most serious methodological issue of concern to this review is the pau-city of available research conducted in developing countries on specific health-related behaviors. The bulk of the literature focuses on epidemiologic trends, mortality patterns, availability of services, evaluation of programs, and policy issues such as the relative merits of alternative strategies for improving health. Much of the research relies on aggregate data, vital statistics, broad population indicators, and the like, with little attention to individual-level data, which allows analysis of the predictors of health behavior. For example, much of the health transition research is based on national statistics comparing different societies on indicators such as life expectancy, infant mortality, education of women, and per capita income. Studies that do focus on individual behavior have been largely concentrated on utilization of health services and, to a lesser extent, performance of health-promoting actions in the home. Comparatively little research has addressed personal attributes such as beliefs, expectations, motives, values, perceptions, and other cognitive elements. Studies that have addressed these kinds of factors derive primarily from operational research on externally funded programs aimed at high-profile health problems affecting children and childbearing women. Thus, available research is skewed toward issues important to donor agencies that fund large-scale public health initiatives.

Knowledge, Attitudes and Practices Surveys

Research on individual health behavior in developing countries has been heavily focused on the standard Knowledge, Attitudes and Practices (KAP) Survey, which segments behavior into discrete elements such as knowledge of disease risk factors, use-nonuse of a health practice/service, and perceptions of therapeutic efficacy. The KAP Survey served as the standard for applied behavioral research in the Third World, providing quantifiable, demographic data and behavioral indexes amenable to statistical analysis (Hursh-Cesar, 1988). For example, KAP-type variables (e.g., contraceptive prevalence, breast-feeding rate, and use of oral rehydration therapy for diarrhea) are often measured in large-scale surveys such as the Demographic and Health Survey and the World Fertility Survey. The utility of the KAP Survey method for understanding health behavior has been criticized on several grounds, including the validity of responses (Schopper, Doussantousse, & Orav, 1993), the limited explanatory power of survey items, and the moderate impact on policy that expensive national surveys have achieved (Davis, 1987).

Qualitative Methods

In contrast with the KAP Survey approach, anthropological research on health behavior traditionally has relied on qualitative ethnographic methods and small-sample community studies. Both theoretically oriented and applied research on ethnomedical beliefs and practices have followed this approach. This tradition has stimulated the development of specialized methodologies variously referred to as *rapid ethnographic assessment, rapid anthropological procedures,* and *focused ethnographic studies,* which share a basic grounding in qualitative methods applied to a specific domain of inquiry (Manderson & Aaby, 1992). These methods aim to collect in-depth data on the cultural construction of health problems and identify local patterns of prevention and treatment. Rapid assessment grew out of the need of applied researchers to provide policy-relevant information about how people think and act in a relatively short time frame. In addition, the qualitative data complemented KAP Studies by addressing questions such as why people acted as they do and by providing insights into the social context of behavior.

With the popularization of social marketing approaches to behavior change in Third World settings in the past decade, group interview methods—focus groups in particular—have gained prominence in health behavior research (Coreil, 1995). Like its ethnographic cousin, the "consumer" approach to research seeks to illuminate how people think about a health issue, but it is more explicitly oriented toward uncovering values and motives that underlie behavioral decisions and choices. Identifying barriers and incentives to behavior change is an important process in this endeavor, with the aim of applying the information to program design.

Integration of Qualitative and Quantitative Methods

Contemporary discussions of methodological issues in applied behavioral research reflect a growing consensus that an integration of qualitative and quantitative data provides the most powerful analysis, and multimethod approaches increasingly are viewed as the standard for applied research in developing countries (Yach, 1992). For example, it is common for community-based studies to include a household survey, focus group interviews, key informant interviews, and participant observation as complementary sources of data to address a research problem.

THEORETICAL PERSPECTIVES

Health behavior research in the United States has focused primarily on individual behavior change, drawing on conceptual frameworks from social psychology and health education such as the Health Belief Model, Social Learning Theory, the Precede Model, and the Transtheoretical Model (see Chapter 4, this volume). In contrast, behavioral research on health in developing countries has been much less conceptually oriented. The literature is heavy on empirical studies organized around an essentially biomedical/epidemiologic framework of disease-focused studies that seek to identify specific determinants of health practices. Much of the research is purely descriptive with no stated theoretical underpinnings. Overall, the field is less focused on individual behavior and more oriented toward family and community contexts of behavior. In line with this, anthropological and culture change perspectives have figured importantly in research traditions, and in recent decades economic models have gained increasing prominence.

Health Communication Models

In the 1970s, innovation theory gained popularity as researchers sought to explain why some people adopt healthy behaviors more readily than others and to identify the characteristics of people who try new behaviors early versus late in the culture change process (Valente & Rogers, 1995). This approach was applied to a variety of public health problems, including family planning, breast-feeding, dietary change, and, more recently, oral rehydration therapy and condom use. Early anthropological research in this vein tended to conceptualize the issues in terms of determinants of culture change, with traditional cultural patterns often assumed to serve as barriers to successful innovation, or "acculturation," if it involved a culture-contact situation. However, the outcomes of change studied were usually specific behavioral practices (Paul, 1955). What was described as directed culture change programs in that era would appropriately fall within the field of applied health communication in the 1990s. Health communication models have continued to evolve over the years, experiencing a burst of development in the 1980s and 1990s as social marketing intervention strategies gained importance (Ling et al. 1992). In the 1990s, variants of the health communication/innovation/social marketing/behavior change models were found in a wide range of international health projects.

Ecological Models

Much of the anthropological research conducted on health behavior in developing countries uses, either explicitly or implicitly, an ecological conceptual framework that situates human behavior within a broadly defined physical, biological, and sociocultural environment (Pelto, Bentley, & Pelto, 1990), one similar to the Social Ecology of Health model used in this volume. Decision making about treatment choices (often involving an array of modern and traditional alternatives) is analyzed in terms of the influence of factors such as climate and seasonal conditions, subsistence patterns, social organization (including household dynamics), and ethnomedical systems (e.g., illness beliefs and treatment options). Behavior is conceptualized as "adaptive" in the sense of being the best solution to a given set of circumstances, resources, and constraints in a particular situation. The unit of analysis in most ecological studies has been a defined population or community.

Since the 1980s, researchers have developed microlevel ecological models that focus on the household or family as the unit of analysis, an approach we described in Chapter 5 as the household production of health (Bentley & Pelto, 1991; Berman et al., 1994). For example, Harkness and Super's (1994) *developmental niche* framework focuses on the domestic context of child care. Derived from studies of children's behavior and development in different cultural contexts, the developmental niche framework builds on recent theoretical advances in anthropology, psychology, and biological ecology and reflects current thinking in developmental systems theory. In this view, the child and his or her environment are viewed as interactive systems, and "the household, as the center of early human life, is seen to be the focal mediator of this relationship, working largely through culturally constructed mechanisms" (p. 218). The developmental niche is conceptualized in terms of three integrated subsystems: the physical and social setting in which the child lives; culturally regulated customs of child care and childrearing; and the psychology of the caretakers. Health-related behavior is analyzed in terms of the influence of these interacting subsystems on care provided to the child.

Still other approaches encompass a much broader sociocultural context of health behavior, such as those that rely heavily on political economic analysis of social inequality and differential access to power and resources as explanations for individual behavior (Turshen, 1989). For example, political economic analysis of AIDS risk behavior has underscored the effects of gender relations and limited employment opportunities, which constrain the degree of control women have in sexual relationships (Miles, 1993).

Cultural Construction of Health and Illness

A large number of studies have been conducted on health beliefs and practices and use of services in different cultural settings of the developing world. Very often, the notion of "cultural differences" is invoked to explain observed patterns of behavior. Sometimes, more specific cultural concepts are applied to the problem, such as the notion of explanatory model of illness, folk illness or culture-bound syndrome, indigenous categories of illness, and preferred traditional methods of treatment. What this broad field of study has in common is an underlying assumption that how people think about, make sense of, and act on illness is profoundly determined by the shared understandings and interpretations given the raw events of sickness, that is, how the events are culturally "constructed" to be meaningful. For example, numerous studies that sought to explain why people choose modern versus traditional medicine for treatment of different episodes of illness have stressed the importance of perceived etiology in determining appropriate treatment. Early work of this nature emphasized a dichotomy between natural, biomedically defined illnesses and supernatural or folk illnesses, with the former perceived to fall within the realm of modern medical treatment and the latter within the traditional domain. Later studies described a more complex system integrating multiple kinds of therapies within single illness episodes. Although a large part of such studies have been conducted by anthropologists, many health and social scientists have implicitly or explicitly invoked a constructivist paradigm to explain health behavior. For example, numerous studies examine local perceived causes of illness as explanatory constructs for understanding behavioral response to illness episodes. Because of the disease focus of international health research, often such studies examine local ethnomedical models of a single illness category with an implied comparative framework, and a few projects have been designed as multicultural comparative studies of particular illness problems (e.g., Weller, Patcher, Trotter, & Baer, 1993).

Analytic Frameworks for the Study of Child Survival

In the mid-1980s, international attention became increasingly focused on understanding the determinants of child survival as many countries adopted interventions identified as "selective primary health care," an approach aimed at reducing the major diseases contributing to child mortality (Walsh & Warren, 1979). An influential model that guided the research of many investigations of this nature was Mosley and Chen's (1984) Analytic Framework for the Study of Child Survival in Developing Countries, a model that is similar to the Causality Continuum described in Chapter 3 of this volume. A key component of the model was a set of proximate determinants that directly influence the risk of morbidity and mortality in children, grouped into five categories: maternal factors, environmental contamination, nutrient deficiency, injury, and personal illness control. The category of personal illness control is the component that incorporates health behavioral factors, including practices that are both preventive (e.g., antenatal care, immunization, malaria prophylaxis) and curative (e.g., medical treatment). Cognitive variables such as beliefs about disease causation are grouped with socioeconomic determinants, which are viewed as operating through the proximate determinants to affect child survival.

Operational Research Model

A great deal of international health research, including health behavior studies, is conducted within the context of specific health programs sponsored by local governments, bilateral and international agencies, private foundations, and other organizations. Research components are built into the overall project with very specific, problem-focused aims of providing practical information applicable to the design and evaluation of such programs. Studies of this nature are referred to as *operations* or *operational* research to reflect their direct links to actual program operations and objectives. The delineation of research questions tends to be based on narrowly defined, pragmatic needs of decision makers and administrators rather than on theoretical models of human behavior (although some concepts and theory might be used selectively in designing the research).

Consequently, a large number of health behavior studies follow what can be called the operational research model, one that gives primacy to program needs and practical use of findings in selection of methods, analysis, and reporting of information. Operational research begins with the central question "What do we need to know about the behavior of our target population to most effectively achieve the aims of the program?" Subsequent decisions about who, what, where, and how to collect data flow directly from this basic question.

More than any other category of behavioral health research in developing countries, operational research tends to be documented in the "gray literature" of project reports, monographs, agency publications, and other nonindexed sources, as opposed to books and peer-reviewed journal articles. Another characteristic of this type of program-specific study is the use of structured data collection guides, which usually are focused on a single health domain or problem (as are programs), and sometimes involving cross-national comparisons. A number of manuals have been developed to guide the collection of ethnographic data by researchers working in different cultural settings to provide standardized indexes for comparison (Herman & Bentley, 1992).

HEALTH BEHAVIOR ACROSS THE LIFE SPAN

Because the kinds of health problems afflicting individuals in all societies are so closely linked to age and life course, this chapter uses a life span perspective to structure the discussion of health behavior in developing countries. The review addresses health issues in three broad categories: infancy and childhood, the reproductive years, and the adult and older age groups. The focus of the discussion is on determinants of health behavior and utilization of modern health services. Not systematically addressed are the related issues of the social and behavioral consequences of disease, the relative merits of alternative intervention programs to prevent or control disease, and the use of traditional and alternative medical services.

Infancy and Childhood

By necessity, a discussion of health behavior in relation to the youngest age group must focus on the perceptions and actions of the caregivers on whom infants and children depend for their survival. In large measure, this boils down to understanding the behavior of mothers, who hold primary responsibility for the care and feeding of their children. Indeed, because within international health so much emphasis is accorded the well-being of children, the bulk of research on health behavior in developing countries in fact focuses on mothers as the subjects of study. A large literature exists on mothers' knowledge and practices regarding child health issues, including infant feeding, child care, home management of diarrhea, preventive services (immunization, growth monitoring), and therapeutic responses to acute respiratory infections. This body of research seeks to identify the characteristics of mothers and their households that are associated with desirable behavior. As noted previously, maternal education has been consistently correlated with positive health practices. Other predisposing factors include exposure to health information, positive experiences with the modern health care system, social support (e.g., the availability of substitute caregivers), economic roles and resources, and personality characteristics. Some studies also have given attention to child variables that affect health, such as gender differences in family response to illness, and how infant behavior can influence feeding practices. To illustrate some of these issues, selected studies are reviewed in the areas of breast-feeding, immunization, and home management of diarrhea. These interventions make up three of the four cornerstone child survival interventions subsumed under the acronym GOBI (growth monitoring, oral rehydration, breast-feeding, and immunization) that have dominated child health programs in developing countries since the early 1980s.

Breast-feeding. Of the child survival interventions, breast-feeding promotion has the longest history in international health research because recognition of its importance for the developing world predates child survival programs per se. Very often, behavioral studies of breast-feeding have been conducted within the broader context of infant feeding and weaning practices. A review by Brownlee (1990) of behavioral issues in this area highlights several problems that are common in many developing countries. First, there are detrimental feeding practices, such as discarding colostrum, giving prelacteal feeds before breast milk comes in, introducing supplemental food too early or too late, improper preparation of breast milk substitutes, and use of weaning foods with inadequate nutritional value. Second, infant feeding practices are influenced by sociocultural variables such as social networks, urbanization and social change, women's work patterns, household income, gender biases (e.g., differential feeding of female babies), maternal health and nutrition, and advertising of commercial infant formula. Third, interventions to promote optimal infant feeding practices must address the problem at the levels of the community, health institutions, national policy, and regulation of the commercial sector.

Although breast-feeding rates have fallen in some developing countries, in most Third World settings the most serious problem is not the total abandonment of breast-feeding but the premature introduction of supplementary foods and liquids in the infant's diet, leading to suboptimal nutrition and exposure of the infant to infectious agents (World Health Organization [WHO], 1981). Although the choice of bottle-feeding is strongly correlated with urban residence, exposure to mass media, economic status, and maternal employment, the decision to introduce supplementary foods is attributed to mothers' beliefs about the perceived adequacy of their milk production. The most common reason given by women for introducing other foods is insufficient milk, whether caused by their own inadequate diet, stress, illness, or deviation from behavioral norms (e.g., sexual misconduct). The insufficient milk explanation probably subsumes a variety of psychosocial mechanisms, including poor understanding of lactation, lack of social support for breast-feeding, and stressful life situations that undermine lactation (Huffman, 1984).

Immunization. In developing countries, routine childhood immunizations are recommended for six preventable diseases: diphtheria, pertussis (whooping cough), tetanus, polio, measles, and tuberculosis. The study of immunization behavior is conceptually significant because it encompasses a constellation of factors germane to understanding the use of preventive health services in general (Coreil, Augustin, Holt, & Halsey, 1994). It requires multiple occasions of seeking care at a health facility in the absence of child illness and involves complex knowledge and costs in the process. Research on the determinants of immunization use has identified both "user" and "service delivery system" variables operating in different settings (Heggenhougen & Clements, 1987; Pillsbury, 1990). On the user side of the equation, studies have pointed to barriers such as maternal time constraints and competing priorities, socioeconomic factors, lack of knowledge, low motivation, fears, and community opinion. On the service delivery end, factors related to accessibility, availability, acceptability, affordability, education, and communication have received attention. Overall, the immunization literature has stressed the importance of parental knowledge about the kinds and schedule of recommended vaccines and the difficulties families face in seeking care. Many parents have a very sketchy understanding of how vaccines work; some even think they cure the illnesses in question. Others have difficulty making time to get away from work and family demands. Clinic schedules are often not compatible with the time availability of clients, and the way parents are treated by clinic staff often discourages utilization. Analysis of successful immunization programs has underscored the importance of education, outreach, monitoring, and client-friendly delivery systems in overcoming these obstacles (Sherris, Blackburn, Moore, & Mehta, 1986).

It should be noted that these barriers to immunization use and the ways found to overcome them in developing countries are very similar to those relevant for the industrialized world (Orenstein, Atkinson, Mason, & Bernier, 1990). It appears that the behavioral issues important in preventive health service utilization transcend national differences in economic development. Indeed, the advances made by developing countries in immunization coverage in the 1980s and early 1990s have prodded industrial countries like the United States to mount comprehensive public health initiatives to improve access to immunization services, which draw on the experience of Third World nations.

Management of diarrhea. One outcome of the worldwide attention given to control of diarrheal diseases during the 1980s has been the accumulation of a large body of comparative research on local perceptions of digestive disorders and home management of diarrhea, including use of oral rehydration therapy and other home-based remedies (Sukkary-Stolba, 1990). Research on the cultural construction of diarrhea has shown that in most settings there exist several named categories of illness that include the symptom of watery stools in their definition, often discriminated into simple and complicated types, and that there may be multiple etiologies for similar illness categories, each variant perceived to have a unique pathophysiology and appropriate set of treatment guidelines (Coreil & Mull, 1988). For example, cross-cultural studies of diarrhea have identified etiologic beliefs related to hot and cold body states, intestinal worms, teething, diet, indigestion, germs, sorcery, violation of taboos, evil eye, fallen fontanel, and numerous folk medical conditions. Perceived severity, prognosis, and appropriate care may vary considerably across illness categories. These insights have highlighted the importance of elucidating culturally valid definitions of terms used in investigations of knowledge and behavior related to any illness.

Discussions of the help-seeking process in management of diarrhea have accorded considerable attention to the domestic domain of care, in part because much of the research was aimed at understanding and promoting the use of oral rehydration therapy in the home. Here, the key role mothers play as therapy managers for sick children was highlighted, including the importance of maternal characteristics and knowledge, gender roles, and economic factors such as maternal time availability (Leslie, 1989). Household variables also received attention in these analyses, such as studies that documented the importance of family structure and resources in therapeutic response patterns. To understand how the new therapy could be integrated into traditional practices, researchers identified a range of indigenous treatments for diarrhea, including dietary modifications, herbal remedies, purgatives, massage, ritual practices, and pharmaceutical medicines. Findings from studies of traditional dietary management of diarrhea contributed to the shift in WHO policy emphasis away from home use of oral rehydration therapy as the first response to diarrhea and toward the recommendation of continued usual feeding and giving of locally available fluids (WHO, 1995).

Reproductive Years

Health issues related to the reproductive years overwhelmingly concern women, mostly because of the high rates of maternal mortality found in developing areas. Although infant mortality is roughly 10 times greater in developing countries compared to developed countries, maternal mortality is 50 times greater or more. There are a number of factors that account for this, including the disadvantaged social and economic status of women in the Third World, their poor nutritional status, maternal depletion from frequent childbearing, and inadequate access to maternity services. Furthermore, unlike most health problems of the developing world—which are largely avoidable through environmental improvements, good nutrition, preventive care, and early detection—maternal mortality can be reduced significantly only through access to technological interventions for complications of pregnancy and childbirth (Freedman & Maine, 1993). Attempts to identify risk factors for the four main complications—hemorrhage, eclampsia, infection, and obstructed labor—have been unsuccessful at providing early detection criteria. Thus, it is the availability of emergency acute care for these problems that makes a difference in whether women die from childbirth, and it explains the profound maternal mortality differential between industrial and preindustrial societies.

Family planning. Although not directly practiced for prevention of maternal deaths, family planning can lower current maternal mortality by 25% (Freedman & Maine, 1993) through birth spacing, prevention of unsafe abortions, and reduction of the severity of the maternal depletion syndrome. In addition to this advantage, family planning, again through birth spacing, promotes improved child health and nutrition and reduces the economic and social demands that high fertility exerts on families, communities, nations, and the world.

Earlier research on family planning focused on the cultural acceptability of different methods of contraception (Polgar & Marshall, 1978). Current discussions are more concerned with the factors that favor the practice of family planning in general (McNicoll, 1992). The prevalence of modern contraceptive use is 32% in the developing world, excluding China (Robey, Rutstein, Morris, & Blackburn, 1992). The demographic factors associated with contraceptive use are maternal age, number of children, urban residence, and maternal education. As would be expected, older women with more children are more likely to seek to delay having additional children, and women with more education and who live in urban areas are more likely to limit their family size. However, in countries where the fertility transition is well advanced (e.g., Sri Lanka and Thailand), education has much less impact on family planning use; in these areas, women of all educational levels seek to limit their fertility.

The emphasis on education and other demographic factors in explanations of contraceptive behavior reflects the influence of economic models of fertility change that have dominated this field, particularly in the past two decades. These analyses are guided by the "rational actor" model of human behavior, which assumes that decisions are based on assessments of costs and benefits, opportunities and constraints, factors largely accounted for by demographic transition processes. However, some researchers have argued that both cultural change and the diffusion of contraceptive technology (i.e., health transition processes) also are important variables in explaining change in contraceptive practice (Pollak & Watkins, 1993). Much attention has been focused on explaining the so-called KAP-gap, that is, the disparity between measures of the number of reproductive-age women who do not desire more children or who wish to delay childbearing and the rate of contraceptive practice. Planners use this as an indicator of unmet need for family planning services, and there has been much discussion of the validity of the methods used to calculate this need. To the extent that some unmet need exists, researchers have investigated the reasons for nonuse of modern contraceptives, with their results pointing to behavioral factors such as fears of side effects or health concerns, disapproval of contraceptives by women or their partners, and religious beliefs (Nair & Smith, 1984; Williams, Baumslag, & Jelliffe, 1994).

Use of maternity services. In contrast to its low impact on maternal mortality, prenatal care can significantly improve child health outcomes in developing countries, and there are maternal health advantages, as well. Assuming that prenatal services are, in fact, available, what are the behavioral determinants of their use? Studies consistently have found an inverse relation between age and parity on one hand and use of formal antenatal care. Given that age and parity are strongly intercorrelated, this suggests that older women with greater experience having children are less likely to use services, perhaps because their prior experience increases their confidence. However, evidence from the Philippines indicates that it is the presence of other children that restricts high-parity women from seeking care and has little to do with age (Leslie & Gupta, 1989). It is probably that other situational factors as well interact with maternal age in its influence on service utilization.

There is substantial evidence that indicates that education is positively correlated with use of maternal health and nutrition services for both urban and rural areas of developing countries (Leslie & Gupta, 1989). A later section addresses possible explanations for the relation between education and mother's health behavior. Related to education, income also has been found to influence use of prenatal health services positively (Timyan, Brechin, Measham, & Ogunleye, 1993). Apart from its obvious importance for expensive services, income level can affect utilization of free services as well because of the opportunity costs associated with the time demands of care seeking, which are particularly acute among poor women. How income is distributed within a family also can affect its availability for health care, and competing demands on women's time have been reported to influence use of prenatal care (Leslie & Gupta, 1989). Moreover, the aggressive promotion of family planning in the Third World has made some women suspicious of all health services; in some areas, for example, women report that they avoid going to clinics for fear of being sterilized.

In the domain of reproductive health behavior, childbirth practices in developing countries have been the least responsive to the forces of modernization. If one ranks the different types of maternity care help seeking, curative and emergency care is utilized most often, prenatal care is second, and childbirth services are sought least often (Royston & Ferguson, 1985). For normal, uncomplicated pregnancies, women prefer home deliveries attended by family members or traditional midwives. Roughly 80% of deliveries in the Third World take place at home, but the percentage attended by trained midwives varies greatly across areas. Although medical institutions are perceived as providing help with complications, the normal birth process is perceived to be a natural event that is best managed within the context of home care, where the attention of loved ones and midwives provides emotional and spiritual support during labor and delivery (Jordan, 1990). Hospitals are avoided because of the stark, unfriendly environment, the frequently dirty wards and beds, and the technologically invasive procedures that typify modern obstetrics. Also, the risk of infection is often greater in crowded hospitals that lack hygiene, supplies, and personnel. Traditional birthing practices allow the parturient woman to maintain greater control over the birth process, such as allowing her to move around in a familiar setting during labor and to deliver the baby in a manner that is comfortable and that protects her privacy (Pillsbury & Brownlee, 1989).

Adult and Older Years

Although child and reproductive health has been the dominant focus of public health research and policy in developing countries for many decades, there has been increasing concern about the neglected needs of the growing adult population (Mosley, Jamison, & Henderson, 1990). Adult mortality from chronic diseases is increasingly becoming a serious public health problem in Third World countries, but not because the rates for these diseases are escalating, as is commonly believed. Age-specific mortality from noncommunicable diseases actually is decreasing, but the magnitude of the problem has increased because adults make up a growing proportion of the adult populati on (Phillips, Feacham, Murray, Over, & Kjellstrom, 1993). Although tropical diseases and other communicable diseases are a significant cause of morbidity and mortality in developing countries, the leading causes of adult death are cardiovascular diseases, cancer, and unintentional injuries.

AIDS-related behavior. Research on AIDS-related behavior has had more of a purely behavioral orientation than research on other health problems in developing countries, primarily because prevention is so strongly dependent on deliberate individual action. Consequently, there has been comparatively greater attention directed at developing theoretical models focused on AIDS-related behavior. For example, the Applied Behavior Change Model (Smith & Middlestadt, 1993), the AIDS Risk Reduction Model (Catania, Kegeles, & Coates, 1990), and other adaptations of behavior change theory have been applied in studies of AIDS prevention behavior. Whereas early research focused primarily on the association between predictor variables and HIV risk factors, more recent work addresses the psychosocial and cultural influences on decision making and outcomes at different stages of the behavior change process. At the same time, others have directed our attention to the social structural and political conditions that create so-called high-risk groups, such as the economic pressures that force poor, marginal women into formal sex work or multiple sexual partnerships to survive (McGrath et al., 1992; Miles, 1993).

Like research on contraception discussed earlier in this chapter, behavioral research on AIDS faces all the challenges posed by research on socially sensitive topics, in this case sexual behavior associated with a highly stigmatized disease. Many of the studies rely on KAP Surveys for measures of sexual activity, but there can be problems with the accuracy and validity of reported information (Schopper et al., 1993). In light of such potential problems, anthropological research has figured importantly in the AIDS literature, because of its attention to cultural sensitivity and social context of behavior; however, even anthropological research cannot be used uncritically (Standing, 1993). Indeed, a diversity of methodological approaches has been applied to the study of AIDS-related sexual behavior, including complex mathematical modeling of sexual contacts (Anderson, 1992).

Among the developing areas of the world, Africa is the most severely affected by the AIDS pandemic. In Africa, women are at greater risk for exposure to the human immunodeficiency virus than are men, not so much because of their own behavior but because of the sexual behavior of men. Males report a higher number of female sexual partners, and they tend to have relations with younger women, who form a larger cohort within the population. Consequently, the prevalence of HIV infection is higher among females in this region, and this has implications for maternal-infant transmission (Decosas & Pedneault, 1992). Women traditionally have been the target group of public health interventions; likewise, AIDS prevention programs have aimed safe sex messages at women, but in reality they have little control over the risk behavior of their male partners.

Tropical diseases and behavior. A distinctive component of health behavior in developing countries is the importance of individual, household, and community activities related to tropical diseases. Although not the leading causes of adult mortality, tropical diseases such as malaria, yellow fever, filariasis, schistosomiasis, dengue fever, dracunculiasis (guinea worm), onchocerciasis, and trachoma account for a significant amount of morbidity and mortality in developing areas. These infectious and parasitic diseases are closely tied to environmental conditions, including poverty and inadequate water and sanitation, and many of the available control strategies are community-based public health interventions. However, large-scale public works such as improved water supply and chemical vector control often require a level of funding and infrastructural development that is beyond the reach of local governments. In the wake of unsuccessful efforts at environmental control, behavior change has gained increased attention in the control of tropical diseases in recent years. Depending on the disease in question, the specific behavioral control measure often involves a technologic aspect (e.g., prophylactic pills for malaria, bed nets for dengue fever, water filters for guinea worm) or a hygienic practice (face-washing for trachoma, latrine use for schistosomiasis). Efforts to encourage people to adopt such measures often encounter complex socioeconomic and cultural constraints that hinder the incorporation of recommended behavior change into everyday activities. Intensive health education and community organization efforts are required to support the behavior change (Gordon, 1988).

Studies of the transmission of tropical diseases have identified various human behaviors (e.g., water, habitation, and subsistence-related activities) associated with exposure to disease vectors. The theoretical models guiding behavioral research on tropical disease, not surprisingly, have had a strong ecological orientation, with emphasis on environmental influences and individual adaptive response. In recent years, researchers have integrated household production perspectives with the traditional ecological approach to tropical diseases. For example, Castro and Mokate (1988) analyze the individual, household, and community determinants of malaria in Colombia, highlighting the importance of variables such as work and water collection patterns that regulate exposure to mosquito bites. Similarly, Coreil, Whiteford, and Salazar (1997) apply a model for studying the household ecology of disease transmission to dengue fever in the Dominican Republic, examining aspects of the biophysical, social, and cultural environments that affect risk behavior, transmission behavior, and risk protection for mosquitoes.

In their review of the social patterning of schistosomiasis, Huang and Manderson (1992) identify schistosomiasis as a *behavioral* disease, in which exposure to the snail vector is conditioned by factors such as gender, age, occupation, and religion. While acknowledging the political context of development projects that propagate the vectors, the reviewers note the importance of women's roles that bring them into greater contact with water than men or religious proscriptions that produce the reverse gender effect. Furthermore, knowledge and perceptions of the illness have been found to influence exposure to risk as well as treatment-seeking behavior, an important component of disease control because chronic sufferers can infect others through water contact.

Cross-cultural studies of malaria have documented the importance of indigenous explanatory models for various fevers, of which malaria is often one type, in local responses to control measures (Oaks, Mitchell, Pearson, & Carpenter, 1991). There are usually multiple perceived causes for malaria-type fever, some of which are perceived to be beyond the control of individuals (e.g., hard work, getting cold); thus, communities often remain skeptical about the possibility of preventing this infection.

RESEARCH ISSUES

Although the preceding review has focused on separate health problems across the life stages, it is useful to examine some of the recurrent issues that weave common threads across the disparate domains of investigation. Though by no means an exhaustive discussion, I briefly address the issues of maternal education, time allocation, and future directions for health behavior research in developing countries.

Maternal Education

Although the education-health behavior link is significant for both mothers and fathers in developing countries, the effects of maternal education are most striking in their impact and scope. Moreover, the effects of maternal education have been shown to be independent of economic factors and access to health services. The preceding review highlighted its influence on child health-promoting behavior (immunization, breast-feeding, management of diarrhea) and reproductive practices (family planning, use of perinatal services). Discussions of possible mechanisms linking maternal education and positive health actions have suggested a variety of pathways of influence (Caldwell, 1990; Cleland & van Ginneken, 1988). First, education is likely to alter a person's worldview such that the more educated are more receptive to new ideas and novel ways of responding to life situations. Education probably enhances one's sense of control over the outside world, fostering confidence in one's ability to seek out resources and manipulate the social environment. Important communication and management skills are undoubtedly learned through formal schooling that can be applied in diverse situations. These factors may account for the increased propensity of educated mothers to seek services for themselves and their children. A related argument stresses the empowering role of education for women within their families and communities, leading to more assertive action in favor of health (e.g., allocation of household resources). Second, there may be direct benefits of education apart from perceptual changes. For example, women may acquire specific knowledge and skills related to hygiene, health, nutrition, and availability of services through school experiences. Educated mothers may be better able to recognize the signs and symptoms indicative of health problems needing professional attention. Also, literate persons may receive better treatment by medical personnel, and they may be more able to understand the educational messages imparted by health workers in clinical settings. Third, it is likely that the effects of education interact with other societal factors to influence health behavior. For example, in settings where it is normative for females to attend school, the general status of women is probably enhanced such that women's roles favor a more active involvement in public life, including interactions with organized health institutions. In addition, aspects of the social environment, such as father's behavior and support from other family members, may enable mothers in such settings to provide better care to children.

Cleland and van Ginneken (1988) summarized the potential mechanisms whereby maternal education may influence positive behavior by listing six hypotheses. Compared to the uneducated, educated mothers may

- attach a higher value to the welfare and health of children;
- have greater decision-making power on health related and other matters;
- be less fatalistic about disease and death;
- be more knowledgeable about disease prevention and cure;

- be more innovative in the use of remedies;
- be more likely to adopt new codes of behavior which improve the health of children though they are not perceived as having direct consequences for health. (p. 1364)

Although the effects of maternal education on different kinds of health behavior have been fairly well documented, there have been few attempts to elucidate which of the hypotheses previously set out account for the observed relations. Focused studies are needed to illuminate the mediating links to guide policy development that goes beyond the obvious need to strengthen educational opportunities for women in developing countries.

Time Allocation

In a manner similar to maternal education, the importance of women's time constraints has emerged as a recurrent determinant of health behavior in Third World settings. Here, the discussion has focused on the effects of competing demands on women's time deriving from multiple role functions in the economic and domestic spheres of family life. Analysis of barriers to use of health services as well as home-based interventions repeatedly have cited the time costs of engaging in the desired action, as reflected in the review presented in this chapter. A number of issues have surfaced in the discussion of maternal time allocation for health, including the opportunity costs of time lost from income-generating activities; the increased time demands of new health technologies introduced through child survival programs; and the relative impact of expanded economic roles (e.g., in agricultural development), which increase women's financial resources but take them away from home for greater lengths of time.

Recognition of the deterrent role that maternal time constraints place on health behavior has led to surprisingly little discussion of ways to ameliorate the situation. Where solutions have been addressed, attention has been focused primarily on altering domestic organization such as improving child care resources in mothers' absence (Engle, 1989). Although researchers have cited the need for changes in service delivery systems to accommodate maternal time limitations, a responsive call to action at this level is not evident. In fact, comparatively little attention has been directed toward ways that the health establishment, which includes sociomedical researchers, can redefine its mission to respond to the needs of populations being served.

Future Directions

Looking to the future of health behavior research in developing countries, the most important new trends likely will be linked to changes in disease patterns within the growing adult and older populations. Increased attention to behavioral factors in chronic and noncommunicable diseases can be expected over the next few decades.

Men, risk behaviors, and lifestyle. Although women have been the focus of attention in the past because of their pivotal role in child and reproductive health, men soon will have their day as the "target" of research, policy, and planning in the Third World. One area in particular where males will take center stage is within the arena of personal health behavior or lifestyle patterns. Take, for example, the problem of tobacco use in developing countries, which shows signs of becoming a public health problem of equal or greater magnitude than found in the developed world. Although cigarette consumption has declined in industrial countries, it has shown an alarming rise in the world's poorer countries, where transnational tobacco companies have been intensively marketing their products (Stebbins, 1990). People in the Third World currently consume between one third and more than one half of the world's tobacco, a proportion likely to increase if cigarette marketing continues to flourish with the limited restrictions typically imposed in developing countries. Moreover, it is primarily men who are taking up the smoking habit in developing countries, where, in general, about 50% of males and 5% of females use tobacco (Crofton, 1984). The impact of male smoking on lung cancer rates is already evident in several countries and will surely magnify over succeeding decades. This, in turn, will prompt researchers to study the social and behavioral factors that influence cigarette use in these populations.

Unintentional injuries. Another repercussion of the ongoing epidemiologic transition in developing countries is the rise in unintentional injuries, most notably from motor vehicle accidents and occupational risks, which, like tobacco use, affect males disproportionately (Smith & Barss, 1991). Death and disability from other injuries, such as drowning, poisoning, burns, and falls, variably affect age and sex groups and will become increasingly important public health problems as countries modernize. Few studies of risk behaviors and preventive measures have been conducted on unintentional injuries in Third World settings; thus, a new item will be added to the agenda of behavioral research.

Adherence to regimens. Implicit in the vast literature on health behavior in developing countries is the underlying premise that the goal of research is to identify the factors that enhance or impede the performance of desirable actions that improve health and prevent disease. In the broad sense, research on compliance with recommended health actions has been conducted on a wide range of health behavior in developing countries. In the more restricted sense of patient adherence to therapeutic regimens, however, the literature is sparse for the developing world (Homedes & Ugalde, 1994). As Third World societies undergo health transition processes that entail increasing use of modern medical services, there will be a need for empirical research on factors affecting patient response to prescribed medical treatment, the use of pharmaceutical medicines, and the ability to sustain healthy lifestyle changes. Adaptations of traditional approaches to the study of compliance will be needed to ensure that concepts and methods are appropriate for diverse cultural settings, health care systems, and patient characteristics.

Self-care and elderly populations. Given the scarcity of resources for health care in developing countries, particularly because of the introduction of economic structural adjustment measures in the late 1980s, there will be greater interest in promoting self-care, another fertile ground for health behavior study. This will be especially important for the growing elderly populations in Third World areas, where social welfare programs are much less developed than in industrial countries (Koseki & Reid, 1991). The entire field of research on elderly health behavior in developing countries undoubtedly will develop in coming years as the public health needs of older persons grow in priority on national planning agendas.

Commonalties and differences. As the Third World is transformed by the various demographic, epidemiologic, and health processes discussed in this chapter, we can expect to find a convergence of problems and trends in global health behavior. Future studies may increasingly emphasize the commonalties in determinants of health behavior across variously developed countries, in contrast to the differences stressed in this review. However, it remains to be seen to what extent the health transition will unfold in predictable ways in the developing world or take uncharted paths resulting in heterogeneity of behavior patterns. Whether the transition leads to less differentiation or not, it will be important to study the processes and outcomes to profit from the lessons such research will have for understanding health behavior generally.

12

Food and Society

United States consumers are aware of the importance of nutrition for maintaining good health, as evidenced by the rapid growth of the health food industry, the emphasis on nutrition in mainstream marketing, and sales of weight loss and other nutrition products (American Dietetic Association, 1997). Surveys show that about half of American adults know that eating too much sugar may contribute to diabetes mellitus and eating too little fiber may cause bowel problems. Even more men and women know that excessive intakes of fat increase a person's risk of developing hypertension and coronary heart disease.

Most North Americans also report that they are concerned about what they eat and are making changes in an effort to eat a more healthy diet. The dietary goals cited most frequently are increased fruits and vegetable consumption (78%) and decreased consumption of fat (71%), red meat (35%), and junk food (24%) (Food Marketing Institute, 1997; Schwartz & Borra, 1997). More than half of American shoppers say they read labels the first time they buy products and seek out foods claiming to be "low fat," "low cholesterol," "natural," or "low salt."

Despite these efforts, most Americans continue to consume a diet too rich in fat, calories, sodium, and simple carbohydrates and too low in vegetables, complex carbohydrates, fiber, and calcium. Consider Americans' excessive fat consumption. Although the proportion of energy derived from fat has declined from 37% to 34% over the past decade, the actual amount in grams has remained basically the same—80 grams per day. The decreased proportion results from an actual increase of 300 calories in the diet's total energy intake (Hill & Peters, 1998). High fat and calorie intakes, combined with a sedentary lifestyle, have contributed to an increased prevalence of weight problems. The proportion of adults who are overweight increased from 24% in 1961 to 35% by 1994 (Sigman-Grant, 1997). According to the National Health and Nutrition Examination Survey conducted between 1994 and 1998, the crude prevalence of overweight and obese adults over the age of 20 was 59% for men, 51% for women, and 55% overall (Flegal, Carroll, Kuczmarski, & Johnson, 1998). *Overweight* is defined as a Body Mass Index equal to or greater than 27.8 for men and 27.3 for women, which corresponds to the 85th percentile values on the Metropolitan Life tables or about 120% of the ideal body weight for women and 124% of ideal body weight for men. *Obesity* is defined as a Body Mass Index equal to or above 30 for men and 28.6 for women (Flegal et al., 1998).

Other widespread dietary problems are inadequate intakes of fruits, vegetables, grains, and calcium-rich foods. Only 40% of American adults eat five or more servings of fruits and vegetables per day, and only 52% eat the recommended six servings of grain products. The recommended intake of calcium is consumed by only 18% of female adolescents, 38% of females aged 20 to 49, and 24% of older women. Consumption of milk has decreased 16% since the late 1970s, whereas soft drink consumption has increased by the same amount. The per capita consumption of soft drinks has reached 53 gallons per capita, making it Americans' favorite beverage and the source of two thirds of the sugar consumed in the United States.

These trends carry costs. North Americans' dietary patterns have been linked to four of the leading causes of death in the United States—coronary heart disease, stroke, some types of cancer, and Type 2 diabetes mellitus—accounting for nearly two thirds of the deaths in the United States. Diet also plays a role in other health conditions, such has hypertension and osteoporosis. It is estimated that diet-related diseases cost society more than $200 billion annually in medical costs and lost productivity. Osteoporosis contributes another $13 billion to $18 billion to the nation's medical bills each year.

Why does a society with an apparent interest in nutrition as a way to improve health and longevity continue to consume a diet that places its population at increased risk for chronic disease and premature death? To answer this question, we must look at how social groups choose the items that make up their diet and the complex relation among the food system and other aspects of social life. This chapter examines how physiological, environmental, and social factors influence human dietary practices and the sociocultural context in which food is produced, distributed, purchased, and consumed.

BIOLOGICAL IMPERATIVES
AND PHYSIOLOGICAL LIMITATIONS

First and foremost, a successful diet must be compatible with human biological needs: it must provide enough energy and the 45 essential nutrients necessary for the body to function properly. Nutrients are substances the body cannot produce or cannot make in sufficient amounts to meet its needs. These substances include carbohydrates, proteins, fats, water, vitamins, and minerals (Smolin & Grosvenor, 1997). If the diet fails to meet these basic nutrient needs, the group—and its unsound dietary practices—eventually will die out.

Allergies and digestive intolerances limit the diets of some people. For example, approximately two thirds of the world's population becomes lactase-deficient by the time they reach adulthood. Because individuals who are lactase-deficient lack the enzyme necessary to digest the sugar in milk, moderate amounts of milk products containing lactose can produce gas, cramps, bloating, and diarrhea.

In general, however, humans enjoy tremendous nutritional versatility. They can obtain needed nutrients from a wide range of plant and animal substances, a feature that has contributed to the species' ability to inhabit much of the earth. Because of the adaptive value of finding new nutrient sources, people may have a natural interest in variety and seeking out novel food items. This curiosity, however, must be balanced with caution; many potential food sources are toxic or contaminated. Referred to as the "omnivores' paradox," human's interest in new and varied food sources (neophilia) is balanced by their fear of new food items (neophobia), especially those that taste different from foods already determined to be safe (Rozin, 1982). As we see in the next section, biological taste preferences and rapid acquisition of taste aversions may be important strategies for dealing with this dilemma (Armelagos, 1987).

TASTE PREFERENCES

Taste is consistently ranked as the top consideration when selecting food, outranking health concerns and all other reasons (Schwartz & Borra, 1997). *Taste* refers to the perception of flavors using smell and sensations in the mouth. Taste buds on the tongue, palate, uvula, and throat have the ability to distinguish between sweet, salty, sour, and bitter. These basic taste sensations are combined with an ability to detect an almost infinite variety of food odors to produce flavor and the ability to detect chemical irritation.

Children are born with a preference for sweet substances and a strong aversion to bitter and sour substances. Humans also appear to have an innate preference for meat, its fat, or both. These taste preferences may have developed because of the selective advantage they offer; a preference for sweetness and fat directs people to fruits that have ripened toward greater nutritiousness and foods rich in calories, and an aversion to bitterness protects them from potentially poisonous plants (Duffy & Bartoshuk, 1996).

Genetic variation creates significant differences in people's taste sensations. Some people, for instance, inherit the ability to taste a bitter substance, called phenylthiocarbamide, found in some vegetables and other foods (Duffy & Bartoshuk, 1996). In general, women have superior bitter detection than men. Bitter sensitivity increases during pregnancy and varies across the menstruation cycle, possibly because it helps protect women from consuming poisonous foods when pregnant (Duffy & Bartoshuk, 1996; Than, Delay, & Maier, 1994). The ability to detect bitterness affects the pleasure of eating and may affect food choices. For instance, the ability to taste bitterness has been associated with a preference for strong cheeses and, in women, for a dislike of sweets and fats (Looy & Weingarten, 1992). In one study, women with enhanced bitterness perception were thinner and had lipid profiles reflective of lower cardiovascular disease risk (Luchina, Bartoshuk, Duffy, Marks, & Ferris, 1995).

People's innate taste preferences are soon overwhelmed by learned preferences. Studies with young children show they usually reject new foods, especially those that are not sweet or salty. However, repeated exposure (tasting a food 8 to 10 times) often leads to acceptance and liking (Birch & Fisher, 1996). The implications for parents is obvious: Although their children's reluctance to try novel foods is understandable, they are wise to encourage their children to taste new foods repeatedly so that, over time, they can learn to enjoy a varied diet. In fact, with time, people learn to like many types of foods that are innately unpalatable or irritating, such as bitter foods, burnt foods, quinine water, and irritants. Although Mexican children are born with an innate preference for sweets and an aversion to hot, spicy foods, they quickly acquire an appreciation for chili peppers. By age 6 or 7, about half will select a spicy, hot snack over a sweet one (Rozin, 1996).

Experience with foods also can result in robust and long-lasting taste aversions (Schafe & Bernstein, 1996). People often develop a strong dislike of a food eaten just before becoming ill and will avoid foods with that taste in the future. Many college students, for example, report aversions to specific alcoholic beverages associated with nausea and vomiting after excess consumption. Known as *taste aversion learning,* this type of conditioned response has obvious adaptive value for the omnivore who is exploring new food sources.

FOOD AVAILABILITY

Another important determinant of food choice is availability: People can eat only what is available. Climate, geography, and other aspects of the environment determine the availability of edible animals and plants. Even today, social groups living in the tropics are more likely than those living in Siberia to consume fruits and vegetables on a regular basis. People also consume more produce when they are in season locally. Food availability, however, is modified by culture in several important ways. First, culture restricts availability by determining which of the biologically compatible substances present in the environment are considered edible. Although humans eat just about everything physiologically possible—including a wide range of poisonous plants, clay, blood, and rotted meat—no group has used all available nutritious substances for food (Foster & Anderson, 1978, p. 265). Everywhere, people have overlooked valuable resources, failed to develop technologies to raise nutritious plants and animals, and rejected highly nutritious items. Even hunters and gatherers living in harsh environments select only a portion of what is available to eat. The !Kung Bushmen derive 90% of their vegetable diet from only 23 of the 85 available edible species. Of the 223 local species of animals known to the Bushmen, 54 species are classified as edible and, of these, only 17 species are hunted on a regular basis.

Americans, too, overlook many valuable food resources. Insects, for example, far outnumber any other animal on earth, both in the number of species and the number of individuals, and offer a calorically rich source of protein, fat, carbohydrate, water, vitamins, and minerals. In contrast to most social groups who enjoy the taste of insects, North Americans and Europeans do not consider them edible. In fact, there are so many nutritious items that we do not consider edible—cats, horses, dogs, small birds, salamanders, sea urchins, octopus, seaweed, acorns, armadillos, rattlesnakes, and many wild plants—that a well-balanced diet could be made of foods most Americans never eat (Foster & Anderson, 1978, p. 265).

Second, technological advances in the marketplace enhance food availability by manufacturing new products. In North America, shoppers can now select from a vast array of nutrient-modified and bioengineered products, including soy milk and cheese products, rice milk products and Tofurkey, a nicely browned, meatless centerpiece dish made from bean curd with fermented-soy drumsticks. The number of items stocked in most large supermarkets in the United States now exceeds 15,000.

Third, the past 50 years have seen a revolution in the world's food system, characterized by delocalization and increased interdependency among a global network of producers, distributors, and consumers. Improved agricultural techniques, transportation, refrigeration, and food processing make it possible to ship food just about anywhere. This system is in sharp contrast to that of traditional societies, in which most foods were consumed within a few miles from where they were produced. Food, energy, and services that once were provided within a local setting have been transformed into commodities exchanged in the global marketplace. Complex social, political, and economic factors regulate the flow of food through this distribution system, and international commercial and political organizations act as gatekeepers, controlling the type and amount of food that is imported or exported in any given community.

The consequences of delocalization have varied. In industrialized nations, delocalization has brought people access to a food supply characterized by remarkable quality, quantity, safety, and convenience. The number of items imported from distant countries has grown, and many people can now enjoy fresh produce and exotic foods all year long.

In developing nations, delocalization has had very different consequences. Traditionally, most communities maintained localized food systems, even though their economies were tied into international markets. Most foods consumed were locally produced, and those not consumed by the producers were distributed within local markets. With delocalization, most food producers are encouraged to replace subsistence crops with commercial products (cash crops) to trade in international markets. Delocalization has contributed to migration to urban areas, where people work in large-scale industrialized food processing or other sectors of the economy. As these societies shift from subsistence food crops to cash crops, their diets change radically, usually with deleterious effects. The shift to a cash economy means that a large part, if not the majority, of food is purchased instead of produced. As a result, the variety of foods consumed has decreased, and many people have replaced traditional foods with less nutritious, processed foods. The high cost of purchased protein-rich foods often makes them prohibitive, forcing people into an affordable high-carbohydrate diet deficient in many vitamins and minerals as well as in protein. Not only have people's diets deteriorated, but their means of production have become highly dependent on international forces—trade agreements, tariffs, subsidies, and food aid—over which they have little or no control (Beardsworth & Keil, 1997; Pelto & Vargas, 1992).

Another factor affecting food availability at the consumer level is personal income. More than a century ago, Ernst Engel (1882) demonstrated that the proportion of expenditure devoted to food decreases as the standard of living in a household rises. Wealthier families spend a lower percentage of their income on food than do those less well off. In Great Britain, for example, the poorest families (lowest quintile) spent approximately 24% of their income on food in 1992, compared to only 14% of those families in the highest quintile bracket (Warde, 1997).

As incomes rise, consumption of foods also increases. Referred to as *price elasticity*, this relation is expressed in terms of the percentage change in demand with income changes of 1%. Demand for specific types of food also changes as families' incomes rise. In industrialized countries, increased income is accompanied by increased demand for fruit and other expensive items but a decreased expenditure on staples. In contrast, increased wealth in poorer nations results in increased demand for staples as well as other foodstuffs (Krondl & Coleman, 1986).

Focus: Obesity

Unfortunately, rising incomes and an abundant food supply have contributed to obesity and increased prevalence of chronic disease. Designed to enable people to survive in environments with fluctuating food supplies, the human body is equipped with efficient mechanisms for accumulating body fat and excellent defenses against the depletion of these energy stores. These biological mechanisms place people with access to an abundant food supply at risk for gaining excessive amounts of weight (Hill & Peters, 1998).

Technological advances also have reduced the amount of physical activity people need in daily life. The appeal of television, electronic games, and computers has increased greatly the time spent in sedentary pursuits. More than 60% of adults do not get the recommended amount of physical activity—30 minutes of vigorous exercise at least 5 days a week. Twenty-eight percent of adult males and 44% of females report they rarely or never engage in vigorous exercise (see www.barc.usda.gov/bnrc/foodsurvey/96result.html). Half of people aged 12 to 21 do not engage in regular physical activity. Youth spend an average of more than 20 hours a week watching television, a pastime shown to be associated with both unhealthy eating habits and excessive weight gain (Andersen et al., 1998). Another contributing factor is the elimination of mandatory physical education programs in many public schools (Hill & Peters, 1998). The percentage of students engaged in daily high school physical education declined from 42% in 1991 to 25% in 1995 (U.S. Department of Health and Human Services, 1996).

Once a problem prevalent only in developed nations, obesity is also becoming a problem in many low-income countries. As these nations industrialize, incomes among the upper and, to a lesser extent, middle classes are increasing. The total caloric intake, the percentage of energy from fat, and obesity rates also are increasing rapidly. In China, for instance, the proportion of people who are overweight increased in all groups except for low-income women between 1989 and

1991. In the English-speaking Caribbean, more than 50% of adult women are obese. Similar dietary changes are reported for upper-income groups living in Africa and South America (Popkin, 1994).

SOCIAL FACTORS

People choose food not only because it is nourishing, tastes good, or is readily available but also because of the important social functions it plays in their lives. Food allows people to express their social identities and acts as an important means for building and solidifying social ties.

Food and Social Identity

Because food practices often differ among social groups, they symbolically mark social boundaries and the inclusion or exclusion of people in specific groups. In many societies, food practices are an important means of communicating one's social identity. Food can serve as a symbol of one's gender, position in the life cycle, or status within the socioeconomic hierarchy.

Food and gender. Gender variation in diets dates back to prehistory (Ross, 1987). As we have seen already, food production and distribution reflect and reinforce status and power differences between men and women in foraging societies, when women gathered vegetables and fruits while men hunted. Among horticulturalists, women typically plant, weed, and do most of the harvesting, while men clear the land and fence it in. In industrialized societies, food-related work is also divided between the sexes. Most women are responsible for meal planning and preparation, despite dramatic changes in women's roles in the formal work sector (approximately 76% of mother-headed households and 64% of mothers in "dual worker" households are employed outside the home) (U.S. Census Bureau, 1996). A 1994 survey of U.S. families found that men were far less involved in meal planning and preparation than were women. Only 23% of men, compared to 93% of women, were involved with meal planning. Thirty-six percent of men, compared to 88% of women, shopped for food, and 27% of men, compared to 90% of women, cooked. Even in families with children and a mother who was employed full-time, only 31% of men participated in meal planning, 39% assisted with food shopping, and 39% prepared meals (Harnack, 1998).

Food is also distributed unequally between men and women. In many societies, men eat first, children eat next, and women consume the leftovers. Taboos prohibiting consumption of rich protein sources are directed primarily at women of childbearing age. These prohibitions may play a role in diverting scarce food sources to men in the event such sources become available. These practices are commonly explained as a way to ensure adequate intake for men whose workload is greater, even though the woman may be pregnant or lactating (Ross, 1987). Sex discrimination in North America is often more subtle: In some families, meals are based predominately on the father's food preferences. He also may be given special privileges, such as getting the best cut of meat or having the first chance at second helpings.

Another way food is tied to sex status concerns the types of foods considered appropriate for men and women. In Western societies, alcohol and red meat are widely linked to masculinity, and salads are associated with femininity (Caplan, 1997). One study found that obese men prefer meat dishes and other combinations of fat and protein, and obese women prefer sweet desserts and other mixtures of sugar and fat. A similar pattern was noted among adults who were not overweight (Nestle et al., 1998).

Finally, dieting and diet disorders are more common among women than men, reflecting different norms and values placed on body imagery and other aspects of gender identity. Although explanations of the high incidence of anorexia and other eating disorders among Western women abound, many scholars believe they reflect cultural norms on thinness. Some feminists also argue that anorexia nervosa reflects misogynistic societal norms and values that demean women by objectifying their bodies. The anorexic's decision to lose weight is seen as a symbolic protest against these values (Banks, 1992).

FOOD AND THE LIFE CYCLE

In every society, people pass through a life cycle marked by birth, puberty, marriage and/or reproduction, and death. Rituals typically mark a person's passage from one age status to another. These practices give communal recognition to the new or altered relationships people experience as they pass from one position in the social structure to another. In most places, dietary practices vary throughout the stages that make up life and symbolically reinforce these important social boundaries.

Infancy and Childhood

Most societies view infancy and childhood as a period requiring special nutritional attention. Breast milk is considered safe; many adult foods are considered dangerous for newborns. Breast milk provides optimal nutrition; protection from infection; and more than 77 hormones, enzymes, neurotransmitters, and other molecules needed for optimal development of the brain, gastrointestinal system, and growth. These protections give human infants an important selective advantage. Unfortunately, many groups have adopted artificial breast milk substitutes, placing their children at increased risk of gastrointestinal and upper respiratory infections, otitis media, Chron's disease, diabetes, and leukemia (Lawrence & Lawrence, 1999).

In the United States, children's diets are selected to provide sufficient quantities of protein, calories, and other essential nutrients needed to support growth. Foods are also chosen based on their digestibility by the still-developing digestive tracts of infants and children. Because infants and children are considered too young to tolerate some items, they are not given the entire repertoire of adult foods. Parents are usually advised to withhold solid foods until 4 to 6 months of age, potentially allergenic foods such as egg whites and cow's milk until 1 year, and coffee and alcohol until adulthood. Childhood is also viewed as an important time for establishing future food habits that will sustain good health. Children are encouraged to "clean your plate," "take three bites of everything," and "eat your vegetables."

Some societies mark a child's transition from the critical early days or months of life into a period when the child's survival is more assured. One example comes from peasant villagers in West Bengal, Bangladesh, where infant food restrictions are ritually regulated. A special rice-feeding ceremony, the *mukhe bhat*, is held when the child has passed through the dangerous first 6 to 12 months (when most infant mortality occurs). The ceremony is quite elaborate and requires the presence of all extended family members to give the child their blessings and presents. Up until the ceremony, foods that are considered unhealthful to infants (called *shokori* food) are restricted. The child may not be given rice, fish, eggs, meat, or a variety of other foods that are considered dangerous (Jelliffe, 1957).

The Teenage Years

About the time of puberty, the rights and responsibilities of children begin to change. In much of the world, adolescence is a brief period with a clearly defined and ceremonially observed end. Traditional initiation rites usually involve a change in diet and the relaxation of childhood taboos (Farb & Armelagos, 1980).

In contemporary North America, the situation is quite different. Adolescence is a long, and, for some, difficult period when rights and responsibilities are ambiguously defined. Adolescence is a time for expressing independence, developing a distinct personality, and gaining social acceptance. In North America, the fast-paced, independent lifestyle of teenagers affects their dietary habits significantly. Skipped breakfasts, increased snacking on empty calories, irregular meals, and frequent dining at fast-food restaurants are characteristic. An increased concern with physical attractiveness and body image are also seen in the relatively high incidence of fad dieting, anorexia nervosa, bulimia, and the use of hormones to increase muscle mass.

As teenagers become more independent, they assume greater control over what they eat. They tend to change their eating habits, rejecting foods their parents served them and eating even more fast foods and soft drinks. One study conducted in Canada found that teenagers tend to divide food into two categories—junk food and nutritious food. Even though they know junk food contributes to weight gain and fear it will cause skin problems, they eat it because of what it represents: "freedom from parental restraint and good times with their friends" (Caplan, 1997, p. 6). In an attempt to express their individuality, some teenagers sometimes deliberately try new things that are different from their parents' ways of life. About 33% of girls aged 12 to 15 and 48% of girls aged 16 to 17 think vegetarianism is "in," according to a study by the National Restaurant Association conducted in 1995. By college age, 15% of students eat vegetarian on a typical day (Walker, 1995).

Given the special nutritional and social circumstances of adolescence, it is not surprising that the diets of many North American teens fall below the recommended daily allowance for some nutrients. As noted previously, most teenage girls do not get enough calcium. Deficiencies in other vitamins and minerals are not uncommon. Because of increased consumption of empty calorie snack foods and processed meals, many teens consume excessive amounts of fat, cholesterol, sodium, and sugar, and too few fruits and vegetables. In one study, more than 40% of high school students ate no fruits or vegetables the day before they were surveyed. Of course, not all teenagers eat poorly. Some people become particularly interested in nutrition during this time in their lives and eat quite well.

Reproduction

Reproduction is another phase in the life cycle frequently marked by special dietary habits. Many societies recognize that eating habits of pregnant women affect the development of their babies and prescribe special foods or avoidance of certain foods for the prenatal period. Another common practice is to avoid foods thought to explain birthmarks or deformities, and women are advised to avoid foods that mimic the color or shape of birthmarks or have odd-looking features.

In many societies, pregnant women are allowed to eat more than other people do. In the United States, women are advised by health care providers to increase their calories, protein, calcium, phosphorous, magnesium, folic acid, and other vitamins and minerals to meet the increased nutrient needs of pregnancy and ensure a birth weight greater than 5½ pounds. Milk is presented by many nutrition educators as a "superfood" necessary to obtain the recommended daily allowances for calcium, whereas alcohol and coffee are to be avoided. Some women in the United States are warned by friends and relatives to avoid eating or even looking for long periods of time at strawberries, because they can cause red birthmarks. Beliefs, poverty, lack of prenatal care, or lack of exposure to nutrition advice, as well as a host of other circumstances, interfere with the observance of these dietary recommendations. In general, however, the pregnant woman is considered to be eating for two, weight gain is desired, and her cravings for pickles, ice cream, or other foods are accepted.

In contrast, women in some societies try to control weight gain by restricting their diets. They know a smaller weight gain during pregnancy will produce a smaller, easier to deliver baby that can be especially important in populations that experience stunted growth and development due to nutritional inadequacy. The short stature and small pelvis of many poor women makes the birth of large babies extremely dangerous.

Many women experience intense food cravings and aversions during pregnancy. The most commonly craved foods are sweets and dairy products, whereas alcohol, coffee, and meats are the most common aversions. There is obvious advantage to avoiding alcohol and coffee during pregnancy, but other cravings and aversions make less nutritional sense. One common craving that has received a great deal of attention is pica—the consumption of nonfood items such as clay, laundry starch, and ice. Compulsive cravings for many other items—burnt matches, hair, charcoal, and many other inedible substances— also have been recorded (Worthington-Roberts & Williams, 1989).

Focus: Geophagia

Geophagia, or clay eating, is practiced by a wide variety of people around the globe—West Africa, New Guinea, the Philippines, Guatemala, and the Amazon Basin. One of the most well-studied groups are poor African Americans living in the South (Johns, 1991). However, geophagia has been reported among U.S. whites, Mexican Americans, and Native Americans as well. For most people who eat clay, only particular types of clay are acceptable. In Ghana, for example, certain sites are held in high regard for the quality of their edible clay. The clay is formed into egg shapes and marketed throughout East Africa. In the southeastern region of the United States, some women collect clay from select sites for sale or home consumption. The clay is sent to farmers' markets, where it is sold in shoe boxes (Farb & Armelagos, 1980; Johns, 1991). Some eat clay plain, and others add salt and vinegar and bake it to impart a smoked flavor. Others, unable to obtain good clay, have used laundry starch as a substitute. Despite its resemblance to clay (the texture is similar), laundry starch has none of the minerals found in the clay.

Many reasons have been proposed for the widespread practice of pica. First, it may be stimulated by dietary deficiencies, such as iron deficiency anemia, and can be corrected by nutrient replacement therapy. Samples of clay eaten by people in West Africa are rich in calcium, magnesium, potassium, iron, copper, and zinc. Clays from some sites in California and Sardinia contain large amounts of calcium and may have been an important nutrient source. Second, pica is a cultural phenomenon passed from generation to generation. Women teach their daughters and nieces to eat certain clay or other substances as a way to ensure a healthy pregnancy. Third, pica may be a way to cope with unpleasant physiological changes associated with pregnancy. Clay and laundry starch absorb the excessive amounts of saliva produced during pregnancy, and some women who practice pica say that eating clay or starch reduces nausea during pregnancy just as soda crackers do. Fourth, pica is seen as a way of solidifying social ties during a stressful period in life. Clay is sometimes given as a gift to pregnant women and new mothers while they are recovering from childbirth. Fifth, pica may be a way to satisfy the appetite. Clay and starch are very filling. A 1-pound box of laundry starch provides 1,800 calories, making it an inexpensive source of energy.

Finally, and perhaps most compelling, is the theory proposed by Timothy Johns (1991). Johns examined clay eating by men, women, and children in a variety of societies. He believes clay eating originated as a way to detoxify foods containing poisonous substances. Because clay binds to the toxins, rendering them less harmful, clay eating provides people with an important adaptive advantage—greater flexibility in the foods they consume. In the Andean mountains, natives eat wild species of potatoes that contain toxic glycoalkaloids that cause stomach pains, vomiting, and even death. These natives are able to consume large quantities of these potatoes by dipping them into slurry clay gruel that binds to the glycoalkaloids. Similar practices are observed elsewhere. The Pomo Indians of Northern California mix clay with the ground meal of acorns, and the natives of Sardinia mix clay with boiled acorns to make bread. In these cases, the clay does not bind to the toxic tannins but rather alters the structure of its molecules, rendering it capable of binding to the gut wall. In each society, natives explain their customs as a way to eliminate the bitter taste; however, the survival advantage comes from the clay's ability to actually detoxify the food and make it available for consumption. Over time, Johns argues, the practice of eating clay became a cultural norm and was practiced by later generations after the diet no longer contained toxic substances. Even when other members of the society no longer practice geophagia, pregnant women may continue the custom because it helps them counter the nausea and vomiting that result from hormonal metabolites released into the small intestine during pregnancy. Indeed, many women say they eat clay or laundry starch (Argo in the Blue Box) to settle their stomachs (Worthington-Roberts & Williams, 1989).

Clay eating and other forms of pica usually have relatively little nutritional impact. Ingestion of some clays may decrease iron levels by binding to dietary iron, making it unavailable for absorption. Although laundry starch does not bind to iron, if eaten in large quantities, it can replace more nutritious foods. Some people have reported eating up to 2 pounds of laundry starch per day (a total of 3,600 calories), leaving little room in the diet for nutrient-rich foods. Fortunately, most people who practice pica do so on a limited basis, and serious complications are uncommon (adapted from *The Cultural Feast*, Bryant, Courtney, Markesbery, & DeWalt, 1985).

Old Age

In some societies, elders are highly esteemed for their wisdom and extensive life experience. Among foraging groups, the group's informal leader is chosen from the oldest men in the group. Older women are also respected. In Chinese culture, the best foods are often reserved for the elders. However, old age is not highly esteemed in all cultures. In industrialized societies, for example, elders are often stereotyped as sickly and lonely, receiving relatively little respect from younger people.

Aging brings many biological changes that place the elderly at nutritional risk. Metabolism decreases, so fewer calories are needed. Some older people produce less saliva, digestive acids, and enzymes than younger people do. This may make some foods difficult to eat and digest. Taste sensations also may diminish with age, so that some elderly people increase their use of salt, sugar, and other seasonings.

In some social groups, the elderly are expected to modify their diets. Some foods are eliminated because they are perceived as "too strong" or "too hard" for the elderly, other foods are eaten in greater quantities because they have attributes considered desirable for older people. Coffee and red meat are deemed by some as inappropriate in large quantities, and prunes and foods high in roughage may be eaten to prevent constipation. As in other age groups, many food beliefs reflect an awareness of physiological changes and special nutritional needs.

Death

The last transition of the life cycle is death. With rare exceptions, societies mark this event ceremonially.

> Death is an occasion when the routine of life is broken not simply for the deceased, but also for many other people. Kinship ties must now be re-shaped, inheritances distributed, and new roles assumed by the survivors. Recognition by the community of this upheaval has its effect on the one activity common to everyone: the preparation and distribution of food. The disruption of community life is often symbolized by basic changes made in the customs of eating-fasting, temporarily extinguishing the hearths, placing new taboos on foods, and special offerings of food to the gods. (Farb & Armelagos, 1980, p. 93)

As in other phases of the life cycle, some dietary practices associated with death have important nutritional implications. The Tsembaga of New Guinea mark the passage of a warrior with a ritual pig slaughter. Several pigs are sacrificed, and the pork is consumed only by close relatives. Though the Tsembaga perform these rites primarily for ideological reasons, the consumption of a high-protein food such as pork during times of stress makes good nutritional sense as well in this essentially vegetarian population. Moving closer to home, in the United States, friends and neighbors take food to families who are mourning the death of a relative. This custom provides relief from cooking and shopping when family members are preoccupied with making funeral arrangements and grieving.

FOOD AS A SYMBOL OF PRESTIGE

Some foods become symbols of prestige, often because they are made of expensive or rare ingredients, take a great deal of time to prepare, are consumed only on special occasions, or are consumed only by members of privileged groups. Because the poor have limited access to expensive items, certain foods become associated with the rich and the poor.

Consumption of prestige foods can be used to communicate one's social status or facilitate movement up the social ladder. Whereas the principal sign of wealth was once the absence of work, today people must display their wealth through conspicuous consumption of foods and other commodities (Veblen, 1925). In a 1998 survey of Americans, 67% of respondents considered eating at expensive restaurants a sign of wealth (Goldman, 1999). Another vehicle for this display is the contemporary *nouvelle cuisine,* with small portions of exotic, fresh foods beautifully prepared and presented. As Warde (1997) noted,

> Such cuisine is exclusive, both because of its very high cost, its inaccessibility, its unfamiliarity, and its anti-popular ethos. The widespread popular reaction to *nouvelle cuisine,* puzzlement that anyone should pay so much money for so little food, is predictable. Nothing could be more extravagant. Nothing is further from the notion of value for money. Such behavior is precisely conspicuous waste. (p. 103)

As abundance and prices change, so do the specific foods considered prestigious—lobster was once associated with poverty, and chicken was once a luxury. Usually, food products lose their prestigious appeal after they appear regularly in supermarket shelves and become affordable by the majority of people.

FOOD AND ETHNICITY

People who share an ethnic heritage are likely to share some common food habits based on the traditional cuisine of the group. These traditional practices and specific foods enjoyed by the group function as symbols of ethnic identity. They serve as boundary markers, setting the group apart from the larger society. A study of Italian Americans in a Mormon Utah community (Raspa, 1984) found that consumption of foods like goats' meat, goats' heads, and other items unacceptable to Mormons served as powerful symbols of ethnic identity and difference, even though some of these practices were invented instead of traditional. Foods easily recognized by ethnic members and outsiders as boundary markers include Italian pasta and spaghetti sauce, Polish sausage, Jewish matzah, German bratwurst, and English tea and crumpets. Besides the obvious emotional benefits that come with renewed ethnic pride, these boundary maintenance activities also build group solidarity. Traditional foods play a central role in the nostalgic enactment of identity (Raspa, 1984) and reinforce ties with ethnic heritage.

Despite the importance that dietary practices play in unifying and distinguishing members of an ethnic group, a great deal of variation exists within ethnic groups. One cannot assume that the food preferences and meal patterns of one Italian American are like that of his or her Italian American neighbor. As in all communities, ethnic food practices are a mix of traditional and nontraditional customs. All ethnic groups are exposed to the cultural traits and lifestyle of the larger society, and, like other aspects of culture, food habits change as a result of this contact. Other sources of change and intracultural variation are unavailability of traditional foods and food processing techniques, work and leisure cycles, the entrance of women into the labor force, the effects of mass media, and meals shared with people outside the ethnic group.

CREATING AND MAINTAINING SOCIAL TIES

Food brings people together, promotes common interests, and stimulates the formation of bonds. Almost everywhere, a food offering is a sign of affection and friendship; to accept food from someone signifies the acceptance of his or her offer and the reciprocity of the feelings expressed. Likewise, withholding food may be seen as an expression of anger or a form of punishment and rejection of a food offer as a rejection of the givers' kindness or an expression of hostility. Eating creates a sense of belongingness, and people go to great lengths to eat with those they love.

Meals eaten together strengthen family relationships and promote unity. In all societies, the family has important economic functions related to food production. Carrying out these activities and distributing food within the family strengthens kinship ties. Family members usually share the major food-getting and food-preparation tasks. Food is shared with the entire family and is not just for the individual members who purchased or produced it. In a classic study of British families, Charles and Kerr (1988) found that feeding a family was an important vehicle for nurturing family members. Preparation of a proper meal—a meat and two vegetables—was viewed as a way to maintain or produce family ties. Others also have argued that meal preparation by women is a symbol of their domesticity, femininity, and inequality. Women who fail to carry out their responsibilities have failed in their roles as wives and mothers (Beardsworth & Keil, 1997).

Family mealtime may be particularly important for youth and adolescents. Teens who eat with their families five times per week or more tend to be at decreased risk for poor adjustment—depression, drug use, and low school motivation (Bowden & Zeisz, 1997). Although the relation between family mealtime and decreased risk for negative outcomes remains to be elucidated, it does appear that family mealtimes may aid teens in coping with the pressures of adolescence. For example, mealtime may be the only time during the day when the family has a chance to sit down and talk. Food etiquette is also taught to children along with ways to combine foods, colors, textures, and flavors into the cuisine of the family and larger society. The importance of food and family meal sharing is evident in the strong sentiments attached to favorite family dishes and customs.

Mealtime patterns have changed dramatically in the United States. First, Americans eat fewer meals. Only 49% follow the American norm of eating three meals a day. Fifteen percent eat just two meals, and another 26% eat two meals and one or two snacks. The others eat one meal and snacks or other combinations of meals and nonmeals (Mogelonsky, 1998). The number of meals cooked and eaten at home also has decreased dramatically. Once reserved for special occasions and travel, meals are eaten outside the home at least twice a week by approximately one third of American families. Even those eating at home often rely on food prepared elsewhere. Although a 1997 survey of shoppers conducted by the Food Marketing Institute found that 90% usually eat their main meal at home, most shoppers say they rely on prepared foods for at least a portion of that meal. More than half of shoppers buy precut, cleaned, and ready-to-cook vegetables, and nearly as many purchase bagged, ready-to-eat salads. Forty percent of shoppers buy frozen main dishes, and one third buy precooked or preseasoned meat or other main dishes (Food Marketing Institute, 1997). The food and restaurant industries have responded to Americans' time-starved, mobile lifestyle by creating many new foods that can be eaten in the car or while working on the computer. By 1996, three fourths of U.S. supermarkets offered some home "meal replacement" products. As Americans rely more heavily on the burgeoning meal replacement industry, important cooking skills are being lost; however, some companies are trying to counter this trend by teaching children to cook from basic ingredients (Mogelonsky, 1998).

Food also helps establish or solidify ties with neighbors and friends. Sharing food has the ability to create new relationships and bind people together who already know each other. In the United States, an invitation for drinks or dinner may signal the desire to start a relationship; many close friends share meals together on a regular basis.

Throughout history, food has been used cross-culturally to build economic and political alliances between groups. Elaborate state dinners for visiting dignitaries are a common occurrence in North America as well as in many other societies. Serving food before, during, and/or after political meetings is a sign of respect and a desire to overcome tension found in arriving at major political decisions (Leininger, 1970).

Many governments also use food aid to build political ties. In the United States, the use of food to strengthen ties with other countries is clearly articulated in Public Law 480, the Food for Peace Act. This legislation has four basic goals: to provide humanitarian assistance, to spur economic development, to develop markets for U.S. agricultural products, and to promote U.S. foreign policy objectives.

Another form of building alliances is gift giving. Despite the giver's contention that it is a free presentation of goods that involves no obligation, gift giving is part of a network of distribution that is often intentional. Gifts serve to solidify social ties and build economic alliances. Friendship, kinship, and other relationships are reinforced and validated by the exchange of gifts. Food is an appropriate gift for many occasions and, as such, serves to distribute wealth and strengthen social ties. Asking the boss over for dinner has economic as well as social implications. Soft drinks, beer, and snacks are offered to friends who help with residential moves or other labor-intensive projects. Grateful patients sometimes supplement their cash payments to physicians with food from their gardens or kitchens.

RELIGIOUS BELIEFS

Religious beliefs also influence food selection in most societies. Despite great variation in specific beliefs and practices, special dietary practices serve many of the same functions in all religions. First, religion provides people with explanations for illness, death, and natural disasters and offers ritual practices for controlling supernatural forces. By establishing an orderly relationship between people and the supernatural, people use religion to make sense of the inexplicable and reduce anxieties associated with the unknown. Religious rituals that involve prescribed foods or food avoidances are often used to reduce uncertainty. We already have seen that milestones throughout the life cycle often are marked with special feasts and may be accompanied by food proscriptions designed to diminish the dangers associated with passage to a new stage of life. Almost everywhere, pregnant and lactating women avoid certain foods believed to be harmful. The Mbum Kpau women of Chad avoid antelopes with twisted horns for fear that eating them will deform their offspring. In many places, pregnant and lactating women are proscribed foods high in protein and other nutrients needed to support fetal growth and development. Not all food proscriptions are nutritionally beneficial. Some may be deleterious, such as those that limit women's intake of certain nutrients. Most religious dietary proscriptions, however, have little nutritional impact. Many of the prohibited foods are consumed infrequently anyway, and other items containing the same nutrients can be eaten in their place. For example, Mbum Kpau women avoid eating chicken and goat in an effort to minimize labor pains. Although this taboo restricts them from eating a source of protein, these goats are butchered only rarely for ceremonial occasions, and other equally rich protein sources are permitted. Regardless of their nutritional effects, these proscriptions serve an important function—they give women a sense of security that they are protecting their unborn children from harm (Farb & Armelagos, 1980).

Religious ritual practices also are used to relieve anxiety about adequate food supplies. Communal hunting and agricultural rituals are practiced to ensure fertility of animals or soil, to bring rain, or to make game more willing to be captured. Although all people recognize the need to work to obtain food, there is still sufficient room for uncertainty about the availability of game and about fluctuations in rainfall and other weather conditions needed for successful outcomes. Religious rituals serve an important function—they reduce the food producer's anxiety about his or her ability to secure an adequate food supply. By reducing anxiety, efficiency may actually improve: The hand is steadied, movements become more skilled, behavior becomes more flexible, and members cooperate more willingly in team endeavors. The Netsilik Eskimo observe numerous taboos concerning hunting and butchering designed to respect the souls of their prey. The systematic and ritualistic character of these taboos provides a defense against uncontrollable dangers. By following them carefully, the Netsilik gain a sense of control and reduced anxiety (Balikci, 1970).

A second function served by religion is to enhance a feeling of unity and social solidarity. Religious ceremonies bring people together to participate in a common activity in an atmosphere heavily charged with emotion. Through this communal activity, people renew and reinforce their identification with the social unit and gain a heightened sense of social cohesion. Religious ceremony and feasting is a familiar theme in many religious traditions. In Christianity, the Last Supper and its derivative Holy Communion are sacred meals in which participants share symbolically the flesh and blood of the Divinity. By partaking of Communion, religious followers reaffirm their faith and reinforce their sense of oneness with each other. Church picnics, potluck suppers, and sharing prayer before meals are other examples of activities practiced in the Christian religion that serve to solidify the group. A study of the relation between religious participants and diet patterns of the aged (McIntosh & Shiffleet, 1984) found that elderly people who participate frequently in religious activities have higher essential nutrient levels and eat meals more regularly than those who do not.

A third function of religion is to reinforce cultural values and standards of behavior. Common goals and rules of conduct are embedded in religious codes such as the Five Pillars of Islam and Buddhism's Noble Eightfold Path. Rituals and symbols, many of which involve food practices, are used to evoke a sense of commitment to the moral order. Almost everywhere, religious codes restrict some foods, and several (e.g., Hinduism, Judaism, and Islam) include elaborate dietary laws. The Seventh-Day Adventist religion restricts meat, tobacco, tea, coffee, and alcohol. Overeating is discouraged, and a variety of whole grains and vegetables are recommended. These dietary practices have been associated with decreased incidence of cancer, heart disease, and other chronic illnesses (Kittler & Sucher, 1989).

Finally, many religious practices contribute significantly to a society's adaptation to the physical environment. The adaptive functions may not be obvious to members of a society; people follow these practices for religious, not ecological, reasons. Nevertheless, they are important to public health professionals who might introduce changes that could inadvertently disrupt the ecological balance established by traditional religious customs. For example, Hindu doctrine forbids the slaughter and consumption of beef. For many years, Western economic planners recommended that the Indian government improve the country's animal husbandry techniques and promote the consumption of cattle—a source of high-quality protein. They noted that a large proportion of the Indian population subsisted on inadequate calorie and protein rations, and the Hindu avoidance of beef endangered many Indians' health status. After careful study of the role cattle played in the country's ecology, Marvin Harris (1987) proposed an alternative view: The Hindu doctrine making cattle sacred has several important advantages. By scavenging throughout the streets and countryside, cows convert many items of little or no direct human value (such as grass) into products of immediate human utility: draft labor, dung, and milk. Cattle serve an important role in agriculture by pulling plows and carts. Even the most scraggly and barren breasts provide manure that is collected and used as cooking and heating fuel (a highly valuable product in a largely deforested country) or fertilizer for crops. Milk products play an important role in the Indian diet, and a considerable amount of beef is consumed by lower castes that eat cattle that have died from natural causes. The taboo placed on cows protects this valuable source of agricultural power, fuel, and fertilizer from being consumed during famines. If Indians were to eat their cows, they would have no way to produce crops when the next season began.

HEALTH BELIEFS AND DIETARY PRACTICES

Food practices often are viewed as an effective means of preventing illness and maintaining health and vigor. Nearly all societies consider certain foods to be endowed with special strength or health-giving properties.

One of the most widespread belief systems about preventing and curing diseases involves the proper balance of bodily humors identified by Hippocrates—blood, phlegm, black bile, and yellow bile. According to this theory, each humor has two opposing qualities; blood is defined as hot and wet, phlegm as cold and wet, and so forth. According to this model, illness results from a humoral imbalance that causes the body to become too hot, cold, dry, or wet.

As this belief system was introduced to other parts of the world, the wet-dry dichotomy was dropped and the hot-cold dimension emphasized. In South Asia and many other parts of the world, some people still view the body in these terms and believe illness results from allowing the body to become too hot or too cold. An important feature of this system is the classification of foods, beverages, and medications as having "hot" or "cold" qualities that affect bodily balance. Typically, the categorization of food is determined by its effect on the body, its medical use, or its association with natural elements rather than observable characteristics or the physical temperature of the substance. Although most South Asians do not routinely select foods based on the hot-cold distinction, they may modify their diets when sick, pregnant, or lactating to maintain the desired balance between hot and cold (Sekhon, 1996). In Malaysia, for instance, the hot-cold dichotomy remains an important feature in folk medicine. People consume foods classified as hot when they are chilled or have illnesses considered cold, and use cold foods to alleviate conditions classified as hot, such as rashes, fevers, and constipation (Manderson, 1987).

In many societies, foods and herbs are used as folk remedies. Many of these plants contain pharmacologically active ingredients that correspond with their native use. Onions, garlic, apples, and radishes contain antibacterial properties. Grain stored in clay pots and mud bins can produce a tetracycline-like mold. Epazote, a spice used to fight intestinal worms, contains chenopodium graveolens, an effective anthelminthic. Many plants used by African tribes to treat malaria contain effective antimalarial ingredients (Etkin & Ross, 1983).

Focus: Herbal Extracts in the Treatment of Malaria: A Case Study of Artemisinin

Many traditional folk remedies have been shown to have active pharmaceutical properties that produce the effects claimed by native healers. Wormwood (*Artemisia mexicana*) contains a helminthic agent (santonin) and a camphor (a mild stimulant and colic reliever), for example, that has been used in rural Mexico since the time of the Aztec Indians as a tonic to aid digestion and treat intestinal parasites. The bark of willow trees (*Salix lasidpelis*) also was used by the Aztecs to relieve pain and treat fevers. It contains a salicylic acid, an aspirin-like substance effective in lowering fevers and relieving pain.

Western scientists are now investigating many traditional folk remedies in hopes of identifying plants that contain compounds effective in treating disease.

The plants selected for study are usually those used by local healers and for home remedies widely reputed to be effective. The World Health Organization (WHO) sponsors research in this area. Studies usually begin with precise botanical identification of the plant species used in herbal remedies and continue with the isolation and extraction of compounds believed to have therapeutic value. Laboratory studies, animal studies and human case studies are used to identify the extract's physiological effects. Clinical trials are then conducted with humans to assess the compound's effectiveness in combating specific diseases. Plant extracts found to be effective are then used to make new drugs, or their molecular structures are used as templates for designing synthetic analogues (Warrell, 1997). An illustration of the tremendous potential herbal remedies offer for identifying new therapeutic agents is the development of new antimalarial drugs.

Malaria is one of the world's most insidious infectious diseases, killing between 1.5 million and 2.7 million people each year and affecting at least 300 million people worldwide. Two fifths of the world's population live in areas where they are exposed to mosquitoes that carry malaria parasites. Four parasites cause various forms of malaria; however, the most severe species is *Plasmodium falciparum*. Found in Africa, parts of Southeast Asia, and Latin American, this parasite can cause severe anemia, kidney failure, and cerebral malaria. If untreated, it often results in death.

One of the greatest public health challenges in malaria control is the increasingly widespread multidrug-resistant strains of *Plasmodium falciparum*. The parasite's resistance to standard drugs, such as chloroquine and quinine, has prompted the search for alternative agents. Funded by the WHO and other sponsors, the search has led to the identification of an impressive array of substances that may have potent antimalaria activity. Many of these substances are derived from herbs and other plant sources traditionally employed by the local population for the treatment of fevers and other symptoms of malaria. The Yanomami Indians living in the Amazon and Orinoco basins of Brazil use more than 90 species of plant to treat malaria. Initial screening of extracts from these plants suggests that many contain substances effective in relieving malaria's symptoms and/or attacking the malaria parasite (Milliken, 1997). On the continent of Africa, in Hurumi Nigeria, the Hausa use 126 different plant species to treat fevers. Laboratory investigations of these plants revealed that at least 22 of the species have demonstrated in vitro activity against *Plasmodium falciparum*. In some cases, the plant extract elevates red blood cell oxidation, creating an environment antagonistic to the malaria parasite's growth. In other cases, the compound attacks the parasites through other mechanisms, some of which are not yet understood. Interestingly, many of these plants are also used as food by the Hausa and may explain why this group has relatively fewer and less severe infections than other groups living in the region (Etkin & Ross, 1983).

Although hundreds of plants are used worldwide to treat malaria, perhaps the most impressive and widely recognized antimalarial compound is artemisinin, extracted from *Artemisia annual L.*, a member of the *Compositae* family. Called *quinhao* in China, the herb's therapeutic use dates back to the Maw Ang Dui Hang Dynasty, more than 2,000 years ago (Warrell, 1997). Quinhao also was described as a remedy for fever in the Chinese *Handbook of Prescriptions for Emergencies* in the 4th century C.E. (Warrell, 1997). However, it was not until 1972 that its active ingredient, artemisinin, was isolated and clinical studies initiated in China demonstrated its effectiveness in treating malaria. China soon began growing the herb and developed injectables, tablets, capsules, and suppositories.

Although the drug was quickly adopted in Southeast Asia, where it has dramatically reduced malaria associated morbidity and mortality, the WHO and Western medicine in general were slow to respond, in large part because of concerns about production quality and toxicity standards (Warrell, 1997). By the 1990s, however, they had sponsored large clinical trials demonstrating the extract's efficacy in other malaria endemic settings. A review of 23 trials in *The Lancet* (Hien & White, 1993) showed that artemisinin derivatives decreased parasites and reduced fever more rapidly than intravenous quinine—a standard antimalarial. Also, semisynthetic derivatives, arteether and artesunate, were developed from the plant extract that are less expensive, have more antimalarial activity than other derivatives, and have been subjected to the pharmacokinetic studies required to be registered in Western countries (Kirby, 1997).

Despite their many advantages, artemisinin derivatives rely on extracts of the herb quinhao, a plant with a low yield. Therefore, enormous areas would have to be planted in quinhao to meet world demand for artemisinin. To reduce reliance on the botanical source, researchers are now trying to synthesize analogues of artemisinin's molecular structure from commercially available products. At least four compounds developed at Johns Hopkins University have displayed antimalarial activity in vivo (Brennan, 1998). The development of several synthetic alternatives is a potential source of less costly and more effective ways to treat malaria and may provide the diversified armament needed to combat drug resistance by the malaria parasite.

CONCLUSION

In Western societies, health is a dominant value that has gained importance as a determinant of food choice. As noted at the beginning of this chapter, many North Americans have made dietary changes to be healthier. Other changes that reflect a concern with preventive nutrition are increased sales of vitamin and mineral supplements and the growing popularity of many alternative medical treatments. In 1997, American consumers spent more than $76 billion on foods, dietary supplements, and other "nutraceuticals"—foods and other ingestible products used to provide health benefits beyond basic nutrition, such as disease prevention and treatment, sleep, or mood elevation (Wellner, 1998).

In many Western societies, especially the United States, values placed on health and youthfulness are manifest in a preoccupation with body size and shape. Over the past 30 years, the ideal body image for women has become slimmer, and the distance between the ideal and average body size has increased. Norms regarding body image vary by ethnicity and socioeconomic status; however, preoccupation with body image, slimness, and dieting are pervasive and probably contribute to the rise in eating disorders during the same period of time (Beardsworth & Keil, 1997).

Interestingly, the growing concern with healthy eating has been accompanied by increased use of food for indulgence. In a study of recipe columns in women's magazines in Great Britain, Warde (1997) found that preoccupation with managing the body through dietary regimens was mixed with increased use of food to indulge oneself. Between the mid-1960s and early 1990s, explicit recommendations and implicit references to health and indulgence increased significantly in recipes, food columns, special articles, and feature sections devoted to cooking and food.

Several factors have contributed to today's counterpressures between health and indulgence. First, it may not be coincidental that glorification of slimness and dietary restraint are promoted at the very time the food system offers an unprecedented availability of sweet and fatty items designed to appeal to human taste preferences. Self-discipline is not necessary when occasions for overeating are rare. As we have noted already, the human body has adaptive features that equip it to cope with cycles of feast and famine, but it lacks mechanisms to defend itself from overconsumption. When faced with a steady supply of delicious and novel foods, dietary rules and self-restraint take on new importance.

Another factor contributing to people's concerns about nutrition and health is their regular exposure to government and commercial messages warning them of the dangers of excessive dietary consumption and the need to exercise regularly. The U.S., Canadian, and British governments have published dietary guidelines since the 1970s. Government efforts to promote moderation are combined with commercial advertisements glorifying a slim figure and promising consumers they will become more sexually attractive and healthier if they select nutritious, low-fat, low-cholesterol, and low-sodium food products. These messages have motivated consumers to change their food practices; they also have induced anxiety, guilt, and self-loathing in many of those who fail to follow the recommended rules (Lupton, 1995).

Some scholars argue that the current preoccupation with bodily appearance and health reflects the importance of the body as a vehicle for conveying self-identity and the assumption that people are personally responsible for regulating their bodies properly (Warde, 1997). The ideal body today, what Lupton (1995) calls the *civilized body*, is regulated and self-controlled. People restrain themselves from overeating and push themselves to exercise as part of a conscious effort to produce a slim, trim, youthful-looking body. The regulated body is a sign of success and mastery. As Lupton (1995) wrote, "This mastery, it is believed, is what sets humans apart from animals: the more an individual can display self-control, an unwillingness to 'give in' to the desires of the flesh, the more civilized and refined that individual is considered" (p. 8). In contrast, bodies that are allowed to become overweight are seen as repulsive, undisciplined, and evidence of moral failing.

Strict dietary and exercise regimes, however, have created a counterpressure—the desire to relax the rules and indulge. People fluctuate between selecting foods that make them healthier and food that comforts and provides emotional security and pleasure, as explained by Warde (1997):

> The motivational complex that keeps this antinomy in existence is in some respects a vicious circle. Anxiety about bodily appearance requires regimes of severe self-discipline; self-restraint creates the sense of being unfree, but also of being "displeased," being deprived of pleasures; hence the temptation to indulge, to transgress the rules of the dietary regime; and thus, again, a renewal of a sense of guilt and anxiety about bodily virtue. This is a potentially distressing antinomy, made worse because of the emotional significance of food and one which affects educated middle-class women more than other sections of the population—partly explaining the uneven incidence of eating disorders. (p. 94)

This cycle and the myriad other factors that influence food choice may help explain why many North Americans continue to consume excessive amounts of calories, fat, and sugar despite their understanding of nutrition and the value they place on health promotion and disease prevention. When faced with a wide range of foods to choose from, their selection will be determined by the interaction of biological, environmental, and sociocultural factors. Because food plays many functions in peoples' lives, their food choices only can be understood when a multiplicity of factors are considered within the larger sociocultural context in which food is produced, distributed, purchased, and consumed.

In sum, an understanding of the multiple factors that influence human dietary practices is essential for health professionals who want to improve the public's health and nutritional status. Without an appreciation of the many functions food can play, the public health professional may introduce dietary practices that are more nutritious but that do not replace the social or religious functions provided by traditional customs. Sensitivity to the sociocultural context of human food systems—a society's dietary norms, beliefs, and values and the assumptions they make about food—enables the public health professional to identify change strategies compatible with the broader culture and to propose more easily accepted dietary modifications.

13

Public Mental Health

Melinda S. Forthofer

HISTORY OF THE PUBLIC HEALTH MOVEMENT

The history of public mental health reveals a series of recurring struggles over how and by whom mental health problems should be addressed. During the Middle Ages, the treatment of persons with mental illnesses could be characterized as extreme neglect. Then, in the 18th century, as public health measures focused more on the health of the society and less on the health of the individual, efforts to manage persons with mental illnesses resulted in large, inhumane institutions designed to protect the populace from contact with the mentally ill.

At the turn of the 19th century, the "Moral Treatment" movement emerged, with the goal of returning persons with mental illness to normal function. Experts came to believe that this goal would be best accomplished by establishing small, locally administered institutions characterized by high levels of staff-patient interaction. In many instances, staff lived in the institutions with their patients to foster staff-patient contact. The fantastic successes reported by some exceptional facilities at that time contributed to the perception that full recovery was an attainable goal for all patients. Nonetheless, the quality of care provided at these sundry institutions varied greatly, and the vast majority of institutions did not enjoy the success rates heralded by a select few. Lower than anticipated success rates led many experts to become disillusioned with their earlier belief that all patients could be "cured." As the disillusionment became widespread, the conditions in mental institutions began to decline steadily, eventually reaching a level of care no more humane than that of the large institutions that they replaced.

By the mid-19th century, strategies for diagnosing the mentally ill had evolved to the point that the mentally ill could be distinguished from other socially marginal persons. Yet, the limited availability of psychiatric specialists prevented many persons with mental illness from receiving expert treatment. The Great Reform Movement, led by Dorothea Dix, came to the aid of persons with mental illnesses. Dix advocated for state administration of centralized hospitals for the mentally ill. Dix was convinced that mental patients could be collected and efficiently treated by qualified specialists in such facilities. Many of Dix's goals were achieved; however, as the nation became distracted by the Civil War, many asylums grew more crowded and were faced with diminishing resources. Gradually, the capacities of psychiatric institutions to serve human needs eroded.

Toward the end of the 19th century, Freudian psychology became very popular, and optimism about the prevention and curability of mental illness returned. Amid growing interest in mental health issues, mental health disciplines grew, contributing to unprecedented availability of private mental health services and a reduction in the social stigma associated with mental illness. Not surprisingly, private facilities were available only to those individuals with resources to pay for services.

By the mid-20th century, the epidemiology of mental health was beginning to provide valuable scientific data on the prevalence and distribution of mental illness (see Table 13.1 for a summary of the historical development of the epidemiology of mental health in the United States). Gradually, these studies also began to examine the determinants and consequences of mental illness. One of the most influential early studies of psychiatric epidemiology was conducted in New Haven, Connecticut, by Hollingshead and Redlich (1958). This study revealed substantial social inequalities in mental health status and in service utilization.

Soon after Hollingshead and Redlich (1958) published their findings, two additional studies were completed. Srole and his colleagues expanded on the New Haven Study to use a sample representative of the general population in their Midtown Manhattan Study. Srole, Langner, Michael, Opler, and Rennie (1962) found that approximately 20% of the population had serious mental illness and that mental illness was associated with subsequent declines in socioeconomic status (SES), supporting an explanation for social inequalities in health that has come to be known as the "Social Drift Hypothesis." Leighton (1959) conducted a study commonly referred to as the "Sterling County" study in an eastern province in Canada. The results of the Sterling County study were consistent with those of the Midtown Manhattan Study.

TABLE 13.1   The Historical Development of Mental Health Epidemiology in the United States

Study	Findings
Generation 1	
Prior to the mid-19th century	General practitioners were the primary source of information about the prevalence and determinants of mental illness
Generation 2	
New Haven Study (Hollingshead & Redlich, 1958)	Documented social inequalities in mental health status
Midtown Manhattan Study (Srole, Langner, Michael, Opler, & Rennie, 1962)	Prevalence of serious mental illness: Approximately 20% Found evidence for Social Drift Hypothesis
Sterling County Study (Leighton, 1959)	Prevalence of mental illness: As high or higher than was found by Srole et al. (1962) Found an association between community disorganization and mental illness
Generation 3	
Epidemiologic Catchment Area Study (Robins & Regier, 1991)	Current prevalence of mental disorder: 20% Lifetime prevalence of mental disorder: 32%
National Comorbidity Survey (Kessler et al., 1994)	12-month prevalence of mental disorder: 29% Lifetime prevalence of mental disorder: 48%

During the period in which Hollingshead and Redlich and Srole et al. were conducting their studies, a trend toward the deinstitutionalization of the mentally ill was gaining momentum. Rapidly declining censuses in state mental hospitals were erroneously viewed as indicative of success rather than a of failure of the system to provide continuity between state hospitals and community mental health services. With good—albeit misinformed—intentions, many advocates for the mentally ill argued that state hospitals were excessively restrictive and "too institutional" for the mentally ill. As funding for state hospitals declined without proportionate increases in funding for community mental health centers, many mentally ill persons were forced to live in substandard facilities or on the streets.

The 1970s saw the publication of a report from the President's Commission on Mental Health (1978) that concluded that the most pressing concern regarding mental illnesses in the United States was a lack of information regarding (a) the prevalence of mental disorders in the United States, (b) the major risk and protective factors for mental disorders, and (c) patterns of utilization of mental health services. Moreover, as research on the social patterns of mental disorders became relatively widespread in the 1980s, debates over explaining those patterns flourished.

The 1990s saw the development of rigorous epidemiologic studies designed not only to estimate the prevalence and distribution of mental illness but also to identify both long- and short-range risk factors and consequences of mental illness. The Epidemiologic Catchment Area (ECA) Study (Robins & Regier, 1991) was funded in response to the report of the President's Commission (1978), and its results were first published in 1991. Then, the National Comorbidity Survey (NCS) (Kessler et al., 1994) was conducted to improve on the methodology employed in the ECA and to obtain more specific information about the risk factors for mental illness and the mechanisms for their influence.

PUBLIC HEALTH SIGNIFICANCE OF MENTAL HEALTH PROBLEMS

Recognition of the public health significance of mental health problems has grown steadily in the latter half of the 20th century, for two reasons: (a) the availability of sound epidemiologic research on the scope of mental health problems and the existence of widespread social disparities in mental health status, and (b) increasing evidence of the interrelations between mental health and physical health.

Our best available data on the prevalence of mental disorders in the United States come from the NCS (Kessler et al., 1994) and suggest that nearly 50% of the population have at least one lifetime disorder and that nearly 30% of the population have had an active disorder within the past 12 months. Approximately 14% of the population have a history of three or more major mental disorders, reflecting especially severe psychopathology. The most commonly reported disorders were major depressive episode, alcohol dependence, social phobia, and simple phobia. Results of the NCS also provide evidence of gender, age, and cohort differences in the prevalences of psychiatric disorders, with affective and anxiety disorders more prevalent among women (Kessler et al., 1994), substance use disorders and antisocial personality disorder more prevalent among men (Kessler et al., 1994), rates of disorders declining with age (Kessler et al., 1994), and disorders more prevalent among recent cohorts (Kessler et al., 1994; Warner et al., 1995; Wittchen, Zhao, Kessler, & Eaton, 1994). Results from the NCS revealed that fewer than 40% of those with a lifetime disorder had ever received professional treatment. For most mental disorders, rates of disorder decline as SES increases.

In the 1960s and 1970s, several studies documented an inverse relation between SES and a particular mental disorder (e.g., Dohrenwend & Dohrenwend,

1969). Then, William Rushing and Suzanne Ortega (Ortega & Rushing, 1983; Rushing & Ortega, 1979) conducted a comprehensive analysis of admissions to six Tennessee state mental hospitals. Their results revealed that the relation between SES and mental illness was much stronger for organic disorders and schizophrenia than for depression, neuroses, and personality disorders. This variation across types of disorders in the strength of the relation between SES and rates of mental illness is somewhat consistent with recent findings from the NCS (Mutaner, Eaton, Diala, Kessler, & Sorlie, 1998). In the NCS, the association between income and the 12-month prevalence of anxiety disorders was stronger than the associations between income and the 12-month prevalence of affective or substance use disorders. Such inequities may be compounded by the fact that individuals with low incomes and high mental morbidity are less likely to receive mental health services than are persons with high incomes and low mental morbidity (Katz, Kessler, Frank, Leaf, & Lin, 1997). Consistent with these findings, the results of a recent prospective study conducted in Great Britain suggest that SES may be associated with the course of episodes of mental illness rather than with the onset of episodes of mental illness (Weich & Lewis, 1998).

Moreover, social scientists and epidemiologists have long observed associations between mental or physical illness and social location, particularly with respect to sex and marital status. Generally, married individuals enjoy better mental health than their unmarried counterparts, and, among married people, men are healthier than women (e.g., Bloom, Asher, & White, 1978; Eaton, 1980; Kessler & McRae, 1984; Morgan, 1991; Siddique & D'Arcy, 1985). Much of the previous research on associations between marital status and mental health has been based on samples primarily comprised of whites (Takeuchi & Speechley, 1989). Nonetheless, evidence beginning to accumulate suggests that the patterns of marital status differences in mental health that have been documented are not consistent across ethnic groups. The association between mental health and marital status may be weaker among blacks (Brown, 1996; Williams, Takeuchi, & Adair, 1992) and may be nonsignificant among Japanese Americans and Filipino Americans (Takeuchi & Speechley, 1989).

In addition to evidence that social factors are associated with the onset and course of mental illness, we also have increasing evidence that many aspects of mood and individual disposition, in turn, are associated with physiologic factors. For example, optimism, explanatory style, and self-esteem are positive aspects of individual disposition that have been shown to suppress the effects of stressful life events. Through this mechanism, optimism and self-esteem may be considered resilience factors, factors that explain who stays healthy despite high levels of risk.

Similar evidence exists regarding the effects of negative aspects of individual disposition on physiologic processes. For example, hostility, anger, emotional distress, and exhaustion have been shown to be important in the etiology of cardiovascular diseases. Likewise, emotional distress has been associated with immune function and, subsequently, cancer incidence and/or mortality. Neuroticism magnifies the effects of stressful life events; in this way, neuroticism represents a vulnerability factor that explains individual differences in outcomes among persons who experience the same level of exposure to stressors. Finally and perhaps most important, negative mood is associated with increased reporting of physical symptoms. Independent of biological risk factors, perceived health is a strong predictor of mortality. In fact, there is so much evidence that perceived health predicts mortality that many health researchers would measure perceived health only if forced to select only one predictor.

CONCEPTUALIZATION OF MENTAL HEALTH AND ILLNESS

Psychiatric and social science approaches to conceptualizing mental health and illness are quite distinct from one another. In the psychiatric approach, a mental disorder is defined in the third edition of the *Diagnostic and Statistical Manual of the American Psychiatric Association* (*DSM*):

> [A mental disorder is] a clinically significant behavioral or psychologic syndrome or pattern that occurs in an individual and that is typically associated with either a painful symptom (distress) or impairment in one or more important areas of functioning (disability). (American Psychiatric Association [APA], 1980)

The current guide for defining mental illness used by clinicians is the *DSM-IV*, the fourth edition of the *DSM* (APA, 1994). The diagnostic criteria outlined in the *DSM-IV* are the result of extensive documentation and review of evidence. The goal for *DSM-IV* was to achieve a balance between historical tradition's compatibility with the International Classification of Diseases (World Health Organization, 1992); evidence from reviews of the literature, unpublished data, and field trials; and consensus of members of mental health professions. Rather than relying on a single conceptual framework, the diagnostic criteria presented in the *DSM-IV* were intended to be atheoretical and appropriate for use in varying conceptual frameworks.

Many social scientists would argue, to the contrary, that the very act of establishing diagnostic criteria for mental disorders represents the use of a particular conceptual framework, one in which mental health and mental illness are viewed as discrete, conceptually distinct states. Nonetheless, despite a fair amount of agreement among social scientists that the use of "cut-points" for definitions of mental illness is oversimplified, there is little consensus among social scientists as to alternative conceptualizations. Thus, a review of the social science literature on mental health reveals a wide range of approaches to its definition.

For example, at the crux of one social science approach to defining mental health is the notion that maintaining balance or equilibrium during periods of high exposure to stress represents mental health. This conceptualization, heavily based in theories of stress and coping processes, would suggest that symptoms of mental illness are manifested only when one's coping resources have proved insufficient for dealing with one's personal circumstances.

Another social science approach, derived in large part from Maslow's theories of self-actualization, bases its conceptualization of mental health on the idea that self-acceptance of one's positive and negative attributes reflects positive health. The concepts of self-esteem, locus of control, and self-efficacy are closely linked with this conceptualization of mental health.

Yet another way that mental health has been conceptualized by social scientists focuses not on one's response to stressful experiences or on self-acceptance but on the degree of congruence between perceptions and reality. Within this approach, an individual whom we might describe as "in denial" regarding some objective fact would be viewed as lacking in mental health. The results of recent empirical studies by Shelly Taylor and her colleagues at UCLA would suggest that optimism, and even a moderate amount of self-illusion, can be important protective factors against poor health outcomes (Segerstrom, Taylor, Kemeny & Fahey, 1998; Taylor & Armor, 1996). As a result of these findings, definitions of mental health that focus on the congruence between the objective and subjective may be declining in use among social scientists.

APPLYING THE SOCIAL ECOLOGY MODEL TO PUBLIC MENTAL HEALTH

Applying the Social Ecology of Health Model to mental health and illness quickly brings to mind the conceptualization of mental health as successful adaptation to stressful experiences. Strong evidence of the influence of geography and community-level factors on exposure and reactivity to stressors would support the use of an ecological approach to the prevention of mental disorders.

Perhaps the most striking lesson to be learned from the existing body of literature on exposure to stressors is that not all individuals who are exposed to the same stressor experienced that stressor in the same way. Models of the impact of personal attributes and stress on adjustment fall into three broad categories (Luthar & Zigler, 1991): (a) *compensatory models*, (b) *protective versus vulnerability models,* and (c) *challenge models.* Compensatory models (analogous to social causation models of differential exposure) assume simple additive, counteractive relations, wherein stressors or exposure to risks tend to lower levels of competence, and personal attributes help to improve adjustment levels. According to these models, those who escape the hazardous consequences of negative experiences may have fewer or less severe adversities, or negative experiences may be counterbalanced by a sufficient weight of compensatory positive experiences (Rutter, 1985). Compensatory models do not fully account for individual differences, underscoring the need for different mechanisms and different models that address both protective factors and interactive processes. Accordingly, protective versus vulnerability models (analogous to social causation differential vulnerability models) assume an interactive relation between stress and personal attributes in predicting adjustment. If a particular trait is protective, individuals with high levels of the trait are relatively unaffected by increasing stress, whereas those with low levels of the trait show declines in competence with increasing stress levels. A vulnerability exists when individuals with high levels of a certain attribute are more susceptible to increasing stress than those with low levels of the attribute. For example, risk factors may not be negative experiences in the absence of another stressor; rather, they may be factors that sensitize individuals to the effects of other stressors. Likewise, protective factors may not always be experienced as positive experiences in the absence of another stressor. In contrast, challenge models specify a curvilinear relation between stress and adjustment, so that stressors can have "steeling" influences and enhance competence, provided that levels of stress are not too high.

APPLYING THE HEALTH IMPACT MODEL
TO PUBLIC MENTAL HEALTH

In previous chapters, the health impact model has been discussed as a process surrounding discrete illness or health events. When we consider the health impact model with respect to mental health issues, we are more likely to think in terms of a process surrounding one or more stressful life events rather than the onset of a mental disorder. Beginning with the influence of Hans Selye's (1956) work in the latter half of the 20th century, distress and mental disorders were commonly thought to be the result of ineffective adaptation to stressful life experiences. According to this view, social patterns in the prevalence of mental disorders were attributed to social patterns in exposures to stressful life experiences (e.g., job loss, divorce, poverty). More recently, common knowledge about the relations between life events and mental disorders takes into consideration the fact that exposure to stress explains only a portion of the variation in mental health status (Dohrenwend, 1998; House, Lepkowski, Kinney, Mero, & Kessler, 1994; Turner & Lloyd, 1995). A vast body of empirical evidence now available reveals that responses to "risks" are not the major determinant of mental health status. In this regard, the Health Impact Model does not provide an adequate explanation for mental disorders.

This is not to say that the Health Impact Model is irrelevant to the application of social and behavioral factors to mental health. The model is particularly relevant to understanding processes that influence use of health services in response to psychiatric symptoms, a complex area of study that is outside the focus of this chapter. Furthermore, the Health Impact Model becomes particularly relevant to examinations of public mental health when we consider the interface between mental health and physical health. Given the evidence cited previously that negative personal disposition and symptoms of mental illness can play the role of vulnerability factors and that positive personal disposition and manifestations of positive mental health can play the role of resilience factors, mental health cannot be overlooked as a potentially relevant factor in any use of the Health Impact Model.

For example, many studies of health promotion employ the Health Impact Model to predict change in one or more health behaviors. Often, these studies have as a primary objective the evaluation of some intervention program's effectiveness; many such studies rely on self-reports of health status or the enactment of health-promoting behaviors. Mental health and illness may be an often-overlooked component of receptivity to health promotion interventions. Moreover, mental health status is likely to influence individuals' perceptions of their physical health status (Farmer & Ferraro, 1997).

Alternatively, mental health may be an important predictor of other health behaviors or outcomes. Consistent with this reasoning are the results of a study conducted by Forthofer, Janz, Dodge, and Clark (1999); self-esteem was identified as an important predictor of improvement in health functioning of older women with cardiac disease, even after adjusting for the effects of other known predictors (i.e., demographic factors, disease severity, treatment compliance).

The study assessed the associations of perceptions of self-esteem, social support, and stress with subsequent total, physical, and psychological health functioning among 502 older adults with cardiovascular disease, controlling for demographic characteristics and clinical factors. Stress, self-esteem, compliance with medication regimens, and marital status were significantly associated with subsequent maintenance or improvement in functioning among women, whereas only age and stress were significantly associated with functioning among men.

APPLYING THE CAUSALITY CONTINUUM
MODEL TO PUBLIC MENTAL HEALTH

Most commonly used in large-scale mental health research today (particularly research on the epidemiology of mental disorders), the Causality Continuum Model provides an excellent framework for our attempts to understand the mechanisms through which mental illness emerges as well as for our attempts to understand the social consequences of mental illness. The most informative studies of risk and protective factors that influence the onset of mental disorders are those that take a multidimensional developmental approach, incorporating consideration of genetic and early childhood factors, other developmentally specific factors, and community-level factors.

It is also important to note that the criteria for diagnosis of major mental disorders vary somewhat in the relative importance of distal factors (i.e., genetics and early childhood adversities) and proximal factors (i.e., life events and contemporary social factors). Nonetheless, most experts would agree that most, if not all, mental disorders have a complex etiology that includes the combined influences of distal and proximal factors.

Case Example: The Role of Basic Research
from the NCS in Theory Development

As discussed earlier in this chapter, numerous studies conducted since the late 1960s have reported evidence to support the notion that married persons experience more positive mental health status than unmarried persons. The consistency of this pattern across study methodologies, populations, and time has motivated a great deal of theorizing about the reasons for the observed patterns. Explanations of the mechanisms responsible for gender and marital status differences in rates of mental illness focus either on social selection processes or on social causation processes.

Social selection models are based on the premise that individuals who are free of negative psychological symptoms are more likely to choose and attract appropriate partners, maintain positive social relationships, and cope with the dissolution of their relationships than are individuals who exhibit such symptoms (Bloom et al., 1978; Johnson, 1991; Morgan, 1991). Persons with mental illnesses are believed to be less emotionally stable and more disagreeable and unpredictable. During the intimacy of courtship, even subtle differences between potential mates can be recognized, and those with psychiatric illnesses may be rejected as prospective partners (Eaton, 1980; Merikangas, 1982). These models assume that our society sorts individuals into different social locations based on physical and mental health, levels of social competence, and so forth (Turner, Wheaton, & Lloyd, 1995). In general, individuals with histories of psychiatric disorders are expected to be less likely than individuals without prior psychiatric disorders to marry (see Figure 13.1), and if they do marry, they are expected to be more likely than individuals without prior psychiatric disorders to experience marital dissolution.

Proponents of social selection models argue that social selection effects on the basis of mental health should be stronger for men than for women. Traditionally, men are expected to assume more active roles in courtship processes (Gotlib & McCabe, 1990). Moreover, physical attractiveness is customarily emphasized for women as potential mates, whereas potential performance as a breadwinner is important for men (Eaton, 1980). Accordingly, it is expected that men with psychiatric disorders are less likely to get married and more likely to get divorced than women with psychiatric disorders.

Several researchers also argue that gender differences in the selection effects on the basis of mental health status may be contingent on the type of psychiatric disorder—the symptoms associated with different psychiatric disorders may be more or less socially accepted when manifested by men than when manifested by women. For example, externalizing disorders (i.e., alcohol abuse, conduct dis-

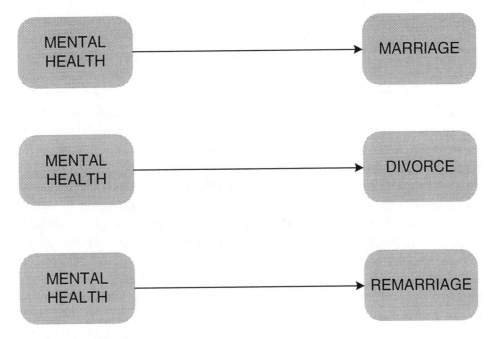

Figure 13.1. Social Selection Processes

order) may be more compatible with the traditional male sex role, whereas internalizing disorders (i.e., depression, agoraphobia) may be more compatible with the traditional female sex role (Rosenfield, 1982). According to this view, selection effects among women are expected to be stronger for externalizing disorders, whereas selection effects among men are expected to be stronger for internalizing disorders.

Social causation models assume that the occupation of certain social locations influences psychological functioning (Johnson, 1991). These models can be differentiated into those that view certain transitions or the occupation of specific social locations as associated with persistent life strains that result in increased levels of psychopathology and those that view the transitions into these statuses as crises that are characterized by an elevation in stress, after which the individual returns to precrisis levels (Booth & Amato, 1991; Moos & Schaefer, 1986). Models of social causation processes that view social locations as the mechanisms responsible for differences in mental health status (see Figure 13.2) conceptualize two possible processes through which differences in mental health status result: differential exposure to stressors (Brown & Harris, 1978; Kessler & Essex, 1982) and differential vulnerability to stressors (Bloom et al., 1978). In contrast, models that view transitions as the mechanisms responsible for differences in mental health status conceptualize differences in mental health status as a result of differential vulnerability to stressors.

Social causation models that view social locations as the mechanisms responsible for differences in mental health status consider the status of being married and living with a spouse to result in a number of benefits that operate to reduce vulnerability to a wide variety of stressors, diseases, and/or emotional disorders, thereby exerting a protective effect (Bloom et al., 1978). These benefits include factors related to differential exposure to stressors: reduced economic strain resulting from greater economic resources and reduced social isolation as a result of being a member of an intimate relationship. Other benefits derive from differential vulnerability to stressors: emotional security and self-esteem, having a confidant and source of support in times of stress, having a stable sexual relationship, and engaging in health-promoting behaviors. According to this perspective, mental health status differences between never-married individuals and previously married individuals are attributable to a dose-response relation between exposure to marriage (marriage duration) and mental illness or to the fact that divorce exposes individuals to persistent life strains. However, research in this area has not documented the expected inverse relation between length of marriage and morbidity (Tucker, Friedman, Wingard, & Schwartz, 1996) or that levels of distress endure among previously married individuals (Booth & Amato, 1991).

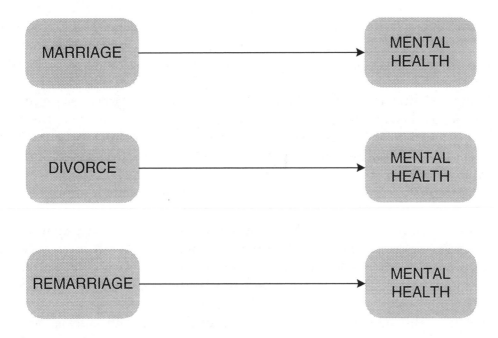

Figure 13.2. Social Causation Processes

The literature on social causation models that focus on social locations as the mechanisms responsible for differences in mental health status provide both theory and empirical evidence for gender differences in the benefits of marriage as a result of differences in both exposure and vulnerability to stressors. Social role theorists (Gove & Tudor, 1973) argue that women, to a greater extent than men, are limited to the family as a single source of gratification. Furthermore, they argue that the demands associated with women's social roles are more stressful and less gratifying than those associated with men's social roles. In contrast, men have outside employment as well as the family as sources of gratification, without the double burden faced by wives. According to this perspective, marriage does not reduce exposure to stressors as much for women as it does for men. Moreover, evidence that the relation between marital satisfaction and overall life satisfaction is much stronger for women than for men (Brown & Fox, 1979) suggests that marriage may not reduce vulnerability to stressors as much for women as for men, especially in marriages with high levels of marital distress. Gender differences in stress levels are primarily viewed as a result of differential exposure to stressors (Brown & Harris, 1978; Kessler & Essex, 1982); recent research on gender differences in social stress suggests that more than half of the gender difference is due to differential vulnerability, whereas only approximately one fourth of the gender differences are attributable to differential exposure

(Turner & Lloyd, 1995; Turner et al., 1995). There also exists considerable evidence that women experience adverse economic outcomes following marital dissolution, whereas men often experience economic gain (Holden & Smock, 1991).

Some studies have provided indirect evidence that social selection processes and/or social causation processes exist and/or that social causation processes are stronger than social selection processes (Gove, 1972; Nolen-Hoeksema, 1987; Turner et al., 1995). The author's previous research (Forthofer, Kessler, Story, & Gotlib, 1996; Kessler, Walters, & Forthofer, 1998) built on the large body of previous literature documenting associations between marital status and well-being to investigate the actual mechanisms or processes (social selection and/or social causation) that may be responsible for the widely cited patterns in mental health status. Prior to this work by Forthofer and colleagues, few if any investigations had considered the possibility of combined effects of social selection and social causation processes. Methodological advances in the design of the NCS enabled an empirical test of social selection and social causation processes.

The results suggested that psychiatric disorders are significantly associated with the subsequent probability and timing of marriage and marital dissolution (evidence for social selection processes). In particular, the results concerning social selection processes reveal that psychiatric disorders are positively associated with early first marriage. Psychiatric disorders are negatively associated with on-time and late marriage, especially among first marriages. Psychiatric disorders are positively associated with marital dissolution, especially among first marriages and younger birth cohorts. The associations of prior psychiatric disorders with marriage do not differ significantly for males and females. However, the associations of prior histories of psychiatric disorders with marital dissolution are, in general, slightly stronger among males than among females. The results also revealed that marriage is associated with substantial protection against the onset of psychiatric disorders (evidence for social causation processes). The protection provided by marriage seems to be strongest and most widespread among those who married prior to age 19 and for those in first marriages. Marriage provides stronger protection for childless individuals than for parents against anxiety and affective disorders, whereas marriage provides more protection against addictive disorders for parents than for childless persons.

These results underscore the importance for future research of considering both social selection and social causation processes when investigating the associations between marital status and mental health. Furthermore, these results may enable continued theory development, as investigators seek to understand in detail how it is that social selection and social causation processes influence the production of social disparities in mental health status.

EMERGING STRATEGIES TO PREVENT MENTAL ILLNESS

A growing number of well-designed research programs has provided us with the cumulative knowledge of the risk and protective factors that affect the onset of mental disorders. Moreover, there is strong evidence that the risk factors associated with the onset of many mental disorders can be reduced through preventive interventions. Advances in the scientific knowledge base regarding risk factors for mental disorders have contributed to an appreciation that many risk factors occur in multiple life domains; fortunately, examples of successful multidomain interventions are now available. Increasingly, a developmental epidemiologic framework is employed—one that combines the strengths of developmental psychology, epidemiology, life course theories, and prevention science to examine multiple causes of mental illness (Kellam, Koretz, & Moscicki, 1999)

Several types of preventive interventions show particular promise as avenues for the reduction of risk factors and, eventually, the incidence of mental disorders. Perhaps the most promising intervention strategies are reflected in programs aimed at young children designed to enhance social skills and to create appropriate norms regarding social behavior. For example, work by Beardslee et al. (1997) with families of depressed parents has shown that participation in a clinician-facilitated group to promote understanding of parental affective disorder can affect parental outcomes as well as prevent depression among children. Another example of a very promising avenue for translation of research into practice is work by Olds and colleagues (Olds, Kitzman, Cole, & Robinson, 1997; Olds et al., 1998), who have provided evidence that prenatal and infancy home visitation can reduce risks for early-onset antisocial behavior among children.

CONCLUSION

This chapter began by reviewing the history of public mental health and the public health significance of mental health problems today, including attention to the interface between mental and physical health. Major conceptual perspectives on mental health and illness also were discussed. The section highlighted the applicability of the Social Ecology, Health Impact, and Causality Continuum Models to public mental health through an exploration of the roles played by social and behavioral factors as determinants and/or consequences of mental health and illness. The importance of mental health research for the development and refinement of social and behavioral science theory was illustrated through a case example from the author's research. Results from the NCS provide an example of how basic research informs the development of theories to explain social disparities in mental health status. The chapter concluded with brief examples of interventions aimed at primary prevention or at reducing the negative consequences of mental illness for families.

14

Public Health and Aging

The New Imperative

Never before have so many people lived for so long. Yet, public health and aging is one of the newest constructs of the public health paradigm. The culture of public health has a century-long history focusing on the survival of infants, health of mothers, and vaccinations against epidemic disease. Of all the specialties of public health, only one is age-specific, and it is typically known as "maternal-child health."

Today, the demographics of the American and international populations literally create an imperative for the inclusion of aging as an integral part of the public health mission. In fact, in 1978, a few American Public Health Association members initiated a special interest group titled "Gerontological Health." Now, there is a rapidly growing interest in the development of this topic as reflected in new and specific curricular and text offerings in public health and aging in colleges of public health across the nation.

Longevity in communities of all kinds is a multifaceted phenomenon. For instance, long life cannot be assumed desirable if the quality of life is low. This is reflected in the prescient work of the first director of the National Institute of Aging, Robert Butler, who titled a 1975 book on aging, *Why Survive: Being Old in America* (Butler, 1975). There was then and is now a gap between longevity and high quality of life for most people in their eighth and ninth decades. As a former president of the American Public Health Association, Dr. Walter Bortz, has said, "We live too short and die too long" (Bortz, 1991). However, it should be known that most people in their 60s and 70s consider their lives to be reasonably high in quality (Stewart & Hays, 1997; von Mering, 1996). Yet, the 85-year-and-over cohort is the fastest growing and holds the greatest lifetime risk for major manifestation of chronic diseases coupled with severe functional loss. These diseases include cerebrovascular accidents, cancer, and brain disease (Kausler & Kausler, 1996; Williams & Temkin-Greener, 1996).

The corrective for the problems of public health and aging are just as multi-faceted as the phenomenon itself. Although there are apparently fixed biologic parameters regarding a person's longevity and disease risks, there are also known behavioral "interventions" that can be employed in early and midlife to provide some protection in late life. For example, early optimal nutrition and brain development are clearly linked (Greenspan, 1997; Huttenlocher, 1994). Also, risk for skin cancer in late life is a function of early-life experiences of sunburn (Brookbank, 1990; Ham, Holtzman, Marcy, & Smith, 1983). Lifetime attention to cardiovascular health, such as hypertension, also may contribute to protection from strokes (Brookbank, 1990; Kane, Ouslander, & Abrass, 1984). Finally, Alzheimer's disease may be symptomatically moderated in those with large brain reserve capacities due to inheritance and lifetime cognitive stimulation (Mortimer, 1995). Research also has indicated that estrogen replacement therapy may delay the clinical manifestations of dementia in women (Barrett-Conner & Kritz-Silverstein, 1993; Rowe & Kahn, 1998).

In terms of medical advances, the cures for chronic disease probably will remain elusive, but the symptomatic management of them probably will increase in effectiveness. For example, diabetes management is currently being improved with nasal inhalants so that behavioral obstacles are significantly reduced (Marks, 1998). Also, rheumatoid arthritis sufferers continue to have more efficacious drugs available with fewer side effects. Even Alzheimer's disease continues to have more advances in drugs to combat the loss of neurons and to improve the cognitive capacities of victims so that more symptom-free years will be a reality.

Educationally, those in health sciences training and practice have increased amounts of scientific literature and continuing education available. The U.S. Public Health Service has developed a geriatric initiatives division in its Bureau of Health Professions branch. One result is the development of several Geriatric Education Centers (GECs) across the nation. These GECs also have a strong responsibility toward attention to aging in a culturally diverse world (Klein, 1998).

Policy issues for improving the health of elderly people in communities include new methods of financing and delivering long-term care. A primary part of such a scenario is the development of support for in-home care as a means to reduce the use of institutional care, which is the most costly of all long-term care types (Binstock, Cluff, & von Mering, 1996). Also, less obvious matters must be considered. For example, the National Institute on Aging is now conducting experiments to determine the most effective means by which to train at-home caregivers to Alzheimer's disease victims (Ory & Schulz, 1996). Most people know the name of the disease but little else, and certainly not the specifics of providing care to confused and forgetful adults.

The most obvious connection of public health and aging is not connected to age segmentation. It is most productive to examine public health and aging from a life span perspective (Morgan & Kunkel, 1998). Gerontology, although seemingly defined as specific to old age, is actually an examination of the process of aging. The process of aging is a lifelong phenomenon. This life span conceptual base leads to the concept of *preventive gerontology* (Balsam & Bottum, 1997). Preventive gerontology accounts for the health-relevant events of presenescent life in terms of risks for deleterious outcomes in senescence.

DEMOGRAPHICS

Old is new. This means that although there have always been some people who have lived well into their 60s and 70s or even beyond, the magnitude of this longevity today is a very recent development among the human species. If age at death is plotted for the human evolutionary line beginning about 3 million to 5 million years ago, most hominids were dying in their teens and 20s. By the time the first *Homo sapiens* of the Neanderthal subspecies were around, human life averaged about 30 to 38 years. The date was 100,000 years ago. By 50,000 years ago, the first *Homo sapiens sapiens* were present and lived on average into their late 30s and early 40s. It is true that some lived into their 60s, but only a few. By 10,000 years ago, humans had discovered how to grow plants and tend herd animals for an improved food supply. Yet, longevity stayed basically the same as it had been for the last 40,000 years. The probable cause for the ceiling effect on longevity was the lack of control over infectious disease (Harrison, Weiner, Tanner, & Barnicot, 1977; Moore, 1987).

It was not until the 20th century that human longevity began to climb to its current extent of 75-plus years for most people in technologically developed societies. In 1900 C.E., the average age of death was 49 years, due primarily to problems of high infant mortality. However, by the mid-century mark, the rapid ascent of human longevity was well on its way. It has not yet stopped climbing. Today, public health is practiced in the face of an unprecedented demographic event marked by common and extreme longevity.

The desire for escape from the negative effects of longevity has produced many myths of very long-lived populations (Holmes & Holmes, 1995). These "Shangri-Las" are mythic. For example, one putative case for extreme longevity is the Abkhasians of current Azerbaijan (Brookbank, 1990). In fact, one American yogurt manufacturer used this myth to sell its yogurt. In one commercial for television, a distinctly elderly looking man appears on the screen touting the benefits of this yogurt, claiming that it was responsible for his long life, and that his dear old mother was to thank for her encouragement to eat yogurt. His mother must be long dead given his apparent age. Then, his mother walks into the picture with him! She must be *very* old to still be living. The problem is that the scenario is not true.

Among the Abkhasians, age exaggeration is common, whereas in the United States, age reduction is common. The status of elders among the Abkhasians is highly desirable, and many strive for it, even including efforts to look older! Also, birth records were not well kept and introduced the window for opportunistic age exaggeration. What is worth noting is that many of these people of both genders do hard physical labor in the fields well into their seventh decade. But, a society of centenarians it is decidedly not.

In 1990, there were 31.6 million people over age 65 in the United States, and they make up 13% of the U.S. population. By the year 2050, this number will more than double to 68.5 million and constitute 23% of the total population (Angel & Hogan, 1994). For those surviving to age 65, men will live another 15.2 years and women another 19.1 years (Haley, Han, & Henderson, 1998). The fastest-growing age segment is the 85-and-over group (Kausler & Kausler, 1996; Williams & Temkin-Greener, 1996). It is exactly this group that is at highest risk for becoming symptomatic for several chronic diseases.

Among all older adults, the Hispanic population is the fastest-growing of the so-called ethnic minority groups, with a projected increase of 91% by 2030. African American elders will increase by 159% and Native Americans by 294% (Haley et al., 1998). In 1990, about 10% of persons 65 and older were considered minority; this will increase to 21% in 2050 (Angel & Hogan, 1994).

The geographic distribution of the older adult population is uneven. By population numbers, California ranks first, New York second, and Florida third (Reynolds-Scanlon, Reynolds, Peek, Polivka, & Peek, 1999). However, by percentage, Florida ranks first, with 18.3% of its population over age 65 compared to the nation's 12.6% over age 65 (Reynolds-Scanlon et al., 1999). Within states, there can be great variation, too. In Florida, for example, the west coast counties average 34% of elders over age 65, whereas the inland adjacent counties are at about the national average (West Central Florida Area Agency on Aging, 1990).

AGING AND HEALTH EFFECTS

There are several conditions for which increased risk occurs as a function of advancing years of life. These include the major diseases of mortality, such as cardiovascular diseases, cancers, brain injuries like strokes, metabolic disorders like diabetes mellitus type II, osteoporosis, and dementing diseases like Alzheimer's disease and vascular dementias. There are no absurd illusions that health science will eliminate death, nor would this be desirable. However, there are very good chances of moderating the direct effects of these chronic diseases at the population scale, as well as pushing their onset into the future. The result is that although the disease is not eradicated, its effects are postponed. Consequently, the value of the couplet of longevity and quality of life is vastly improved.

The upper limit of human aging is about 110 to 115 years (Sidell, 1995). This is determined by studies of various animals' metabolic rates related to their body mass. The index figure generated by this calculation is plotted against the species-specific life span of several animals, including humans. For example, dogs' species-specific life span years correspond to about 12 to 15 chronological years, whereas horses correspond to about 40 to 45 chronological years. At an extreme, some tortoises map onto the chronological year line at about 175 years. In this mix is the human group that maps onto the line at about 110 to 115 years. The biological lesson is that longevity is predetermined at the species level (Brookbank, 1990). The question then becomes, How much of the biological upper limit of years of life will be attained in the context of running the gauntlet of life?

Current research into the biology of aging suggests that it may be possible to extend artificially the species-specific upper limits of longevity. This possibility becomes clear given the understanding of the effects of telomere shortening over the life of an organism (Campesi, Dimri, & Hara, 1996; Chang & Harley, 1995; Hoffman, Hromas, Amemiya, & Mohrenweiser, 1996). Telomeres occur at the ends of chromosomes and serve as a means to preserve the integrity of the chromosome body. As each replication occurs, some of the telomere length is lost, which causes imperfect replication. The imperfection of replication and subsequent functioning of cells is a significant cause of the aging process, characterized by reduction of optimal body performance.

Telomere loss can be slowed by adding telomerase, an enzyme that assists in the regeneration of the telomere. The body produces telomerase but does not completely replenish the amount lost at each replication. Over the course of many years, the net loss of telomere is enough to result in imperfect replication and loss of body function, with the effects commonly thought of as aging.

HEALTH CHARACTERISTICS OF OLDER ADULTS:
THE GERIATRIC PATIENT PROFILE

Public health is generally concerned with community-level and population-level health. However, it is always true that the aggregate is comprised of individuals. It is helpful to understand the unique attributes of older adults in terms of health so that clear conceptual distinctions in function can be made across the life span. Also, large-scale programs for older adults can profit from understanding the changes in health functioning of individuals.

Physiological changes in functioning in old age have been cataloged by Wallace (1997) to show that, collectively, the older person is increasingly vulnerable to the ordinary insults of life and are due specific medical consideration (Wallace, 1997). Wallace notes that pathogenesis of some diseases is altered with age. Compromised immune system function often found in old age can cause greater chance of disease onset in later life compared to early life. Also, disease risk and severity may be altered due to environmental exposures. For example, hypothermia is a greater risk for older adults than for younger adults because their homeostatic regulation is suboptimal (Brookbank, 1990). Compounding this risk is the reduced sensitivity to awareness of warning signs in older persons themselves. Sensory sensitivity causes awareness of simple heat and cold to be "triggered" later than in a younger person, with the effect that tissue damage can occur before the person takes corrective action.

Older adults as patients have several characteristics that collectively produce the need for a unique knowledge base and set of skills to provide care for them optimally. First, the older adult is more likely than other age groups to express symptoms atypically (Ham et al., 1983; Wallace, 1997). The "atypical presentation" of symptoms occurs at all ages; however, in old age, it is more common. A propensity for atypical presentation of symptoms introduces the risk that clinicians will miss important symptoms or misinterpret them (Ham et al., 1983). For example, older adults may not have high temperatures in the presence of significant infectious disease. Also, myocardial infarction may be "silent"—medical texts usually describe the patient's complaint as a "crushing substernal chest pain with possible radiation into the left arm" and often cue the clinician to watch for the patient to place their fist over their chest in the vicinity of the heart in reaction to the severe pain typical of the classic "MI." Yet, the older adult may show none of these classic signs. They often present with very vague reports of general malaise, no particular pain, some nausea, and may walk into the hospital and not seem to be in a medical crisis.

Mental health conditions such as depression also can be expressed atypically. The "masked depression" is more common among older adults, posing a challenge for clinicians to detect the altered signs (Kausler & Kausler, 1996). For example, typical signs of significant depression can include sadness of affect; expression of despair; changes in appetite; changes in sleep; and a general slowing of motion, reflexes, and movement. Among older adults, the depressed person may not clearly show any of these signs. Masked depression may present with a cheerful person who is involved in various social activities without signs of obvious distress. However, this same person may have loss of appetite; sleep disturbance; a cognitive awareness of sadness, loss, or despair; and inadequate energy to feel comfortable in conducting ordinary activities of daily living (ADLs). The problem is that some of these signs of masked depression are considered to be a normal part of the aging process. The older adult may not eat as much as they had in the past, may have sleep pattern change, may move generally slower, and may have less energy than in earlier life. Still, the clinician alert to the increased probabilities of masked depression in older adults must distinguish between normal age-related change and those associated with underlying depression.

The older adult population also has increased instances of "multiple pathologies" (Brookbank, 1990; Ham et al., 1983). This means that older adults often have several diseases at any one time. Many of these are chronic diseases for which there is no cure, only symptom management. However, it is very important to recognize that the older person with multiple pathologies may be quite able to perform his or her ordinary daily activities because having several diagnosed diseases does not necessarily produce a net effect of noxious disability.

Related to the phenomenon of multiple pathologies, the older adult population is more at risk of "polypharmacy" than their younger counterparts (Brookbank, 1990; Ham et al., 1983; Kane et al., 1984). Clinicians treating multiple diseases and conditions prescribe medications to ameliorate the older adult's symptoms or improve function. However, some of the prescribing may occur among several clinicians who may not be aware of each other's actions. Even so, when one clinician treats one older adult patient, there is increased risk of noxious interactive effects and several predictable side effects. The collective experience of this by the older adult patient is that although their disease lab values may be improved, their overall sense of good health, well-being, and daily excitement about life may be reduced as a result of health care intervention.

"Impaired homeostasis" is another characteristic of older adult life that affects health care interventions (Ham et al., 1983). The ability of the older adult to maintain and/or recover from alterations to normal functioning is reduced in both speed and absolute terms. For example, tests of sway that measure the sensitivity of imbalance and recovery show that normal older adults will tilt out of balance a slightly further distance before sensing the tilt and recovering from it compared to younger adults. Although the older adult may not fall and the sensory sensitivity of the antigravity centers of the brain still function, the speed of reestablishing homeostasis is slower. Also, bed rest can produce loss of muscle tone very rapidly compared to younger adults. Some have suggested that 1 day of bed rest is equivalent to 3 days of bed rest for younger adults in terms of muscle tone and possible atrophy. Even the occurrence of acute disease such as the flu can take the older adult much longer than younger adults to recover to baseline functioning and subjective sense of wellness.

Iatrogenic disease is a type of malfunctioning due to the application of medical care. The term *iatros* derives from the Greek root word for physician. The current use of iatrogenic disease does not always, however, mean specifically the physician, but, rather, exposure to the health care system as a whole or to individual practitioners, resulting in compromised health (Ham et al., 1983; Kane et al., 1984). All people are at some unavoidable risk, such as from postsurgical or other nosocomial infections acquired during hospital care. However, older adults are at heightened risk for several reasons. First, they have more diseases, physician visits, and hospital days than younger adults, which increase their exposure to such risks. Second, they have increased vulnerability to medication problems due to polypharmacy. Third, ageism in health care can lead to undertreatment or unrecognized problems due to atypical presentation.

Collectively, these characteristics of older adults as patients constitute a clear statement of the need for a specific set of conceptual and practice skills to provide optimal treatment for older adults. Public health and aging must account for these unique factors in all types of population-based interventions, ranging from primary to tertiary prevention. To ignore the unique attributes of older adult health commits the "one size fits all" fallacy and, worse, heightens the vulnerability index already applicable to older adults and particularly to very old adults.

PUBLIC HEALTH AND AGING: THE ROLE OF PREVENTION

Prevention, moderation, and treatment of disease in older adults can be seen from at least two viewpoints. One is the "prevention in remaining years" view, and another is the "preventive gerontology" or life span view (U.S. Administration on Aging, 1994). First, it is simply wrongheaded to ignore the current elderly population in terms of prevention during late life. Although many effects of prolonged unhealthy lifestyles cannot be obliterated, they can be modified (Ham et al., 1983). It is necessary to remember that longevity today and in the future means that older adults can expect decades of life after reaching 65 years of age. In fact, it may be all the more important to attend to prevention at this stage of life due to the increased health vulnerability common to longevity. For example, primary prevention in the form of vaccinations against influenza for older adults is even more important in older age compared to earlier years because the risk of death from the flu is now higher. In youth, the main risk for not getting vaccinated is getting the flu and experiencing much discomfort. Although the "discomfort index" is very high, the "mortality index" is comparatively low. In old age, both indexes are high for influenza.

Smoking and physical activity also have been found responsive to modification in old age. For example, in a study of 70- to 79-year-olds who had no cognitive dysfunction, no functional limitations, and one or no chronic disease, those who currently smoked had a doubling of risk of death within 3 years compared to those who never smoked (Schoenfeld, Malmrose, Blazer, Gold, & Seeman, 1994). It is also clear that smoking is related to reduction in physical activity and functioning over the course of the lifetime. Moreover, reduction in physical activity has numerous and rapid negative effects on the functional status of a person simply due to disuse of the body. For example, immobility or disuse of the body can have compounding effects that introduce the risk of serious morbidity and even mortality. The cascade of smoking, physical inactivity, and increased immobility can lead to a linked scenario such as gait unsteadiness, fear of falling, more immobility, actual falls, skeletal fractures, surgical repairs, hospital stays, infection, pneumonia, and death. The human and fiscal costs of such a cascade are huge and, largely, preventable.

Preventive gerontology seeks to identify the universe of toxic exposures and unhealthy behaviors (and, somewhat futuristically, perhaps genetic loads for certain diseases) in youth and middle age so that efforts can be made to reduce exposures and improve healthy behaviors (Oshansky & Rudberg, 1997). The outcome is expected to be a healthier life experience in old age. This would include a reduction of hospital days, sick days, and long-term care with a much more robust physical function capacity. Longevity may increase due to fewer premature mortalities as a result of healthier cardiovascular systems and less cancer risk, but the real importance is the improvement in functional status so that ADLs are adequately performed. Emotional health is also improved in the presence of persistent function rather than inexorable loss.

Functional status decreases among today's older adults. Although this may be universally true, the extent to which decline in function is related to inherent changes of aging and/or to lifestyles is difficult to determine (Kosorok, Omenn, Diehr, Koepsell, & Patrick, 1992). Ethnic minority status also has been seen to drastically affect health and function within the older age cohort. African Americans report their functional status on ADLs as fair or poor much more often than do whites (Harlow & McDonald, 1991). These functional losses are the pathways to dependency requiring assistance in the form of specialized long-term care and/or personal surveillance in one's own home.

Most older persons have at least one chronic condition, and many have multiple chronic conditions, which is consistent with the characteristic of multiple pathologies (Mezey, 1996). In 1991, per 100 population, for men arthritis ranked first, heart disease second, hearing impairments third, hypertension fourth, and orthopedic impairments fifth. For women, arthritis ranked first, hypertension second, heart disease third, orthopedic impairments fourth, and diabetes fifth (Reynolds-Scanlon et al., 1999).

The Institute of Medicine compiled a list of conditions common in old age for which there is some primary or secondary prevention (Berg & Cassells, 1992). The list includes hypertension, osteoporosis, medications, sensory loss disability, oral health, cancer, nutrition, smoking, physical inactivity, social isolation, falls, and depression (Berg & Cassells, 1992). It is obvious that there are many late-life conditions of significance for which there are productive individual and community-level interventions.

The IOM report omitted Alzheimer's disease and Parkinson's disease, for example, because they were considered nonresponsive to primary or secondary prevention. The same is true for the highly prevalent conditions of osteoarthritis and rheumatoid arthritis. Yet, the mental health conditions associated with social isolation and the multiple levels of depression are considered either preventable or treatable and so are included in the list. The topic area of psychosocial problems or dysfunction are potentially treatable with both pharmacologic and nonpharmacologic interventions (Berg & Cassells, 1992).

Community-level intervention for social isolation can take the form of day care center participation or the incorporation of the person into a network of phone callers or visitors. For depression, both psychosocial and drug intervention may be appropriate because older adults respond well to antidepressant medications. Of course, case ascertainment and compliance with issues of mental health can be difficult with older adults, who tend to view such matters as stigmatizing. Still, there are numerous cases of very successful mental health intervention in older populations (Berg & Cassells, 1992).

Over time, there is a way to gauge the success of health interventions in older adults. One approach is to compare the ages at which chronic disease becomes apparent and limits function relative to ages at death. The current curve shows that after age 65, the number and seriousness of functional limitation increases significantly while the person still has many years of expected life to live. This leads to the need for long-term care. However, if there is some success in the efforts of health promotion and disease prevention, the effects may be manifest in late life by compressing the time of chronic disease and functional limitations to many fewer years prior to death. Overall, people live long and healthier, at least as measured by physical health and functional status (Fries, 1980; Sidell, 1995).

Case Study: Dementia in an Oklahoma Choctaw Woman

Mrs. Mary Maytubbee (a pseudonym) is extremely angry and yelling at her husband to stop having sex with that African American woman right in the living room in front of everyone. A granddaughter reassures her grandfather by saying, "That's not her," meaning that normally his wife would not talk to him like that. Another granddaughter will not visit the house again because the grandmother had recently noticed her come into the room and then loudly asked, "Who's that Jersey cow over there?"

In fieldwork done by one of this volume's authors (JNH), some Choctaw families have an explanatory model for forgetfulness and confusion in old age that is radically different from the usual medical model. American medicine views brain function as normal or, as with Alzheimer's disease, pathological, because there is a deteriorating brain observable at the microscopic level. However, the behavioral symptoms of forgetfulness and confusion are open to cultural interpretation. Interpretations could create a pathological, normal, or, in the case here, "supernormal" explanation for observed behaviors like hallucinations or getting lost.

Mrs. Maytubbee, who is 84 years old, lives in a remote part of Oklahoma where the greatest density of monolingual Choctaw speakers reside. This community is a holdover from the early 1800s, when the Choctaws were forced from Mississippi to Indian Territory. The community is identifiable by two wood-framed stores with a gas pump in front of one. The pavement from the main road stops a mile from "town," leaving the front of the stores opening onto dirt streets. It is common to see horses being ridden, and often there are fewer cars than horses. Yet, for all its pristine isolation, there are satellite TV dishes and VCRs everywhere.

Mrs. Maytubbee lives with her husband in a two-bedroom house. The husband is generally well, with good functional status. He does not work any longer. However, he does not respond well to his wife's condition. He says that any time he tries to help her, she screams and is always upset with him. Mrs. Maytubbee's social network mainly consists of her husband and her granddaughter, who is a Community Health Representative (CHR) for the tribe. CHRs are paraprofessionally trained members of the tribe who provide health promotion, health education, screening, and transportation to health care sites. There are great-grandchildren, but they are too young to be of direct assistance. Another granddaughter is estranged from her but lives nearby.

Mrs. Maytubbee "sees things that aren't there," according to her CHR granddaughter. Over the last year, Mrs. Maytubbee has been getting cognitively worse. Her current status is a score of 12 out of 30 points on the Folstein Mini Mental State Exam (Folstein, Folstein, & McHugh, 1975). She also constantly wants to go home because she thinks she is in the hospital, possibly due to her bed being equipped with side rails. She also cries a lot. She frequently reports seeing her dead parents riding by on their horses and doing various gardening chores. The patient's daughter, who lives about 20 miles away, considers her mother's hallucinations to be evidence of her preparing to go to the "other side." She speaks somewhat reverently about this, although she seldom visits or provides support in any way.

Further questioning revealed that, when the Choctaw language was being used to talk about the forgetfulness and confusion, the word for brain (*lopee*) was never used. However, the concept that the "mind" was experiencing problems was common, such as the statement that the person's "mind was not good" (*imanokfila achukma keyu*) or the "mind was lost" (*imanokfila kanea*). These phrases reflect a separation of the "brain" and "mind" and allows for the brain to be considered normal while the mind is quite confused and forgetful (Haley et al., 1998).

Mrs. Maytubbee's behavior was interpreted as different from others, but not deviant or socially stigmatizing, as is common among American society. The belief was that the different behavior was due to her communicating with the "other side" while no one else knew what was being "said" to her and, therefore, could not judge the correctness of this one part of a multifaceted communication. It would only *seem* deluded. The awe and honor accruing to this behavior was connected to the vaguely understood other side, which was being at least partly confirmed by the presence of Mrs. Maytubbee interacting with it.

This "supernormal" explanatory model for allopathic medicine's Alzheimer's disease can be best understood in the context of a culture that has strong beliefs about supernatural phenomena, like the "little people" who are present in the surrounding woods but who are seldom seen. There is also a multicultural religious belief system common to groups who have undergone forced acculturation. Little people are mixed into beliefs about the "Holy Ghost," with no disruption of the integrity of either system.

Mrs. Maytubbee and her family are experiencing an effect of new life spans among American Indians. The longer people live, the greater their chance of experiencing symptoms of forgetfulness and confusion. For the Choctaws, the growing number of tribal people living longer lives means that a new wave of "lived experience" is occurring. Explanations for this new wave of lived experience are being constructed in the context of old ways of being.

PUBLIC HEALTH AND AGING IN THE FUTURE

The future of public health and aging is driven by a demographic and political engine (Kodner, 1996). Components of this engine include the effects of the aging baby boomers and an epidemiologic transition of increased chronic disease. Older adults in the future will be better-educated and wealthier, work longer prior to retirement, and be more politically assertive. Yet, they will experience highly diverse family support systems due to family composition change related to divorce, remarriage, or remaining single.

Kodner (1996) points out that, today and in the future, there is a national tendency to value a restrained governmental role in public welfare issues. This includes social security, Medicare, and Medicaid, which continue to be threatened targets for tax cuts. In spite of this, the need for expensive long-term care increases. In-home long-term care does not mean "free" long-term care; rather, it shifts the expenditures of dollars for caring for dependent elders. The future of long-term care will involve new ways of financing and possibly involve more interest in preventing the need for it during the earlier years of a person's life.

What is unknown is the effect of technological breakthroughs on diseases of old age that today are seemingly resistant to medical cure. For example, osteoporosis was long considered a near-normal part of aging for many women. As it was more appropriately conceptualized and biologically understood, the "cure" was the long-term pathway of early life nutrition and physical activity to ward off the risk of bone fracture by building a reserve capacity of high bone density (Prince, 1997). Now, it is also known that estrogen replacement therapy helps maintain bone mass (Berg & Cassells, 1992; National Institute on Aging, 1998). Medication is also available that not only stops bone loss but also helps to rebuild it, even in old age (Berg & Cassells, 1992). Although this does not suggest that early life nutrition and physical activity are unimportant, it serves as an example of the continued wish (and occasional reality) to find technological fixes for human ailments.

Another example is the near frenzy of research on Alzheimer's disease to treat or prevent its devastating effects in which brain cells are killed, leaving people confused and in need of supervised help. It is inevitable that more cases of Alzheimer's disease will occur simply because more people are living into the decades of greatest risk. Yet, recent genetic studies are helping to understand the etiology of Alzheimer's disease and to create potential predictive formulae for determining probabilities of occurrence. Also, medications are now available to improve thinking ability during the early stages of the disease. New medications are in experimental trials that will postpone the symptoms by several years. Actual prevention is a goal, but it is not considered to be realistic in the near future. A scenario, unimaginable just a few years ago, includes a person in his or her 20s getting a genetic test, providing a family history relative to dementing disease, and, if considered a high-risk case, beginning to take protective medications in midlife. The intent would be to protect the brain for as long as possible so that the person dies from some other condition before brain function becomes severely compromised.

The future for public health and aging has numerous imperatives. Kodner (1996) enumerated several implications for preparing for the predictable baby boom demographic peak. First, there is a need to prevent disability. This is consistent with the notion that the prevention of death or all disease is absurd, yet, the effects of one's inevitable demise can be much better managed than is seen in the experience of today's cohort of older adults. Next, there is the need to strengthen informal care of older adults. This means that the most expensive long-term care will be drastically reduced by rewarding the use of in-home, non-professional, long-term care. Also required will be better systems of delivering preventive care and final long-term care. The need for properly trained professionals and paraprofessionals is clear. Related to this need is the need for the ordinary citizen to have access to learning how to best manage the needs of a dependent elder, because many middle-aged people today experience "parent care" without benefit of familial models or professional models for such tasks.

CONCLUSION

The immediate and future nature of public health and aging is a mystery. It is a mystery because there has never been a time in this nation's history or in the world that so many people are living so long. There is no precedent or model on which to base action plans for this future. However, there are numerous projections based on thoughtful use of present knowledge that provide some illumination for responding to the needs of an aging society. This includes improved education in the health and social sciences in the topic areas of aging and health. For public health specifically, the importance of prevention is great and capitalizes on the life span perspective. To the degree that public health takes a multidisciplinary approach to health, practitioners of the future can integrate knowledge from across the main public health disciplines to fashion a superior plan of action for national age-related health and well-being. For example, environmental and occupational health specialties can inform aging by virtue of expertise in exposures to deleterious physical environmental and life experience conditions. Epidemiology can contribute to the development of medications and the identification of highly specific risk conditions for the development of disease. Health policy and management can be enormously important in the development of rational plans for cost containment and service delivery systems in long-term care of older adults. Community and family health approaches can be instrumental in the refinement of health promotion and disease prevention strategies in the actual lives of older adults.

Although it is true that all these actions are taking place currently, the immediate future demands their intensification. To "step up" the interdisciplinary effort, there is a need to craft an intellectual culture of cross-disciplinary value beyond the rhetoric common today. This means that although not every professional will be designated a "gerontologist" or "geriatrician," there is likely some connection of their work to this society's aging project. For this reason, public health and aging is highly germane across the health-related professions.

References

Aday, L. A., & Andersen, R. M. (1974). A framework for the study of access to medical care. *Health Services Research, 9,* 208-220.

Aday, L. A. A., & Awe, W. C. (1997). Health services utilization models. In D. S. Gochman (Ed.), *Handbook of health behavior research* (Vol. 1, pp. 153-172). New York: Plenum.

Adler, N. E., Boyce, T., Chesney, M. A., Cohen, S., Folkman, S., Kahn, R. L., & Syme, L. (1994). Socioeconomic status and health: The challenge of the gradient. *American Psychologist, 49,* 15-24.

Adler, N. E., Boyce, W. T., Chesney, M. A., Folkman, S., & Syme, S. L. (1997). Socioeconomic inequalities in health: No easy solution. In P. R. Lee & C. L. Estes (Eds.), *The nation's health* (pp. 15-24). Sudbury, MA: Jones & Bartlett.

African Academy of Sciences. (1994). Statement by the African Academy of Sciences at the Population Summit. *Population and Development Review, 10,* 238-239.

Ajzen, I., & Fishbein, M. (1980). *Understanding attitudes and predicting social behavior.* Englewood Cliffs, NJ: Prentice Hall.

Alter, C., & Hage, J. (1993). *Organizations working together.* Newbury Park, CA: Sage.

Altman, D. G. (1995). Sustaining interventions in community systems: On the relationship between researchers and communities. *Health Psychology, 14,* 526-536.

American Anthropological Association. (1998). AAA statement on race. *American Anthropologist, 100,* 712-713.

American Dietetic Association. (1997). *Nutrition trends survey 1997* (Executive Summary). Chicago: Author.

American Psychiatric Association. (1980). *Diagnostic and statistical manual of mental disorders* (3rd ed.). Washington, DC: Author.

American Psychiatric Association. (1994). *Diagnostic and statistical manual of mental disorders* (4th ed.). Washington, DC: Author.

Andersen, R. (1968). *Behavioral model of families' use of health services.* Chicago: Center for Health Administration Studies, University of Chicago.

Andersen, R. (1995). Revisiting the behavioral model and access to medical care: Does it matter? *Journal of Health and Social Behavior, 36,* 1-10.

Anderson, R. M. (1992). Some aspects of sexual behaviour and the potential demographic impact of AIDS in developing countries. *Social Science and Medicine, 34,* 271-280.

Andreasen, A. (1995). *Marketing social change: Changing behavior to promote health, social development, and the environment.* San Francisco: Jossey-Bass.

Angel, J. L., & Hogan, D. P. (1994). Demographics of minority aging populations. In Gerontological Society of America (Ed.), *Minority elders: Five goals toward building a public policy base* (2nd ed., pp. 9-21). Washington, DC: Gerontological Society of America.

Angrosino, M. V. (1987). *A health practitioner's guide to the social and behavioral sciences.* Westport, CT: Auburn House.

Armelagos, G. (1987). Biocultural aspects of food choice. In M. Harris & E. Ross (Eds.), *Food and evolution: Toward a theory of human food habits* (pp. 579-594). Philadelphia: Temple University Press.

Armelagos, G., & Dewey, J. R. (1978). Evolutionary response to human infectious diseases. In M. Logan & J. E. Hunt (Eds.), *Health and human condition: Perspectives on medical anthropology* (pp. 101-106). North Scituate, MA: Duxbury.

Armstrong, D. (1993). Public health spaces and the fabrication of identity. *Sociology, 27,* 393-410.

Arnette, J. (1990a). Contraceptive use, sensation seeking, and adolescent egocentrism. *Youth and Adolescence, 19,* 171-180.

Arnette, J. (1990b). Drunk driving, sensation seeking, and egocentrism among adolescents. *Personality and Individual Differences, 11,* 541-546.

Avise, J. (1994). *Molecular markers, natural history and evolution.* New York: Chapman & Hall.

Bailey, D. (1992, Winter). Using participatory research in community consortia development and evaluation: Lessons from the beginning of the story. *American Sociologist,* 71-82.

Balch, G., & Sutton, S. M. (1997). Keep me posted: A plea for practical evaluation. In M. E. Goldberg, M. Fishbein, & S. E. Middlestadt (Eds.), *Social marketing: Theoretical and practical perspectives* (pp. 123-146). Mahwah, NJ: Lawrence Erlbaum.

Balikci, A. (1970). *The Netsilik Eskimo.* Garden City, NY: Natural History.

Balsam, A. L., & Bottum, C. L. (1997). Understanding the aging and public health networks. In T. Hickey, M. A. Speers, & T. R. Prochaska (Eds.), *Public health and aging* (pp. 19-21). Baltimore: Johns Hopkins University Press.

Bandura, A. (1986). *Social foundations of thought and action: A social cognitive theory.* Englewood Cliffs, NJ: Prentice Hall.

Banks, C. G. (1992). "Culture" in culture-bound syndromes: The case of anorexia nervosa. *Social Sciences and Medicine, 34,* 867-884.

Barnes, K. C., Armelagos, G. J., & Morreale, S. C. (1999). Darwinian medicine and the emergence of allergy. In W. R. Trevathan, E. O. Smith, & J. J. McKenna (Eds.), *Evolutionary medicine* (pp. 209-244). New York: Oxford University Press.

Barrett-Conner, E., & Kritz-Silverstein, D. (1993). Estrogen replacement therapy and cognitive function in older women. *Journal of the American Medical Association, 269*, 2637-2641.

Barss, P., Smith, G., Baker, S., & Mohan, D. (1998). *Injury prevention: An international perspective.* New York: Oxford University Press.

Beardslee, W. R., Wright, E. J., Salt, P., Drezner, K., Gladstone, T., Versage, E. M., & Rothberg, P. C. (1997). Examination of children's responses to two preventive intervention strategies over time. *Journal of the American Academy of Child and Adolescent Psychiatry, 36*, 196-204.

Beardsworth, A., & Keil, T. (1997). *Sociology on the menu: An invitation to the study of food and society.* Boston: Routledge & Kegan Paul.

Becker, M. H., & Maiman, L. A. (1975). Sociobehavioral determinants of compliance with health and medical care recommendations. *Medical Care, 13*(1), 10-24.

Becker, M. H., & Maiman, L. A. (1980). Strategies for enhancing patient compliance. *Journal of Community Health, 6*(2), 113-135.

Bennett, J. (Ed.). (1975). *The new ethnicity: Perspectives from ethnology.* St. Paul, MN: West.

Bentley, M. E., & Pelto, G. H. (1991). The household production of nutrition: Introduction to the special issue. *Social Science and Medicine, 33*, 1101-1102.

Berg, R. L., & Cassells, J. S. (Eds.). (1992). *The second fifty years: Promoting health and preventing disability.* Washington, DC: National Academy Press.

Berk, R. A., & Berk, S. F. (1983). Supply-side sociology of the family: The challenge of the new home economics. *Annual Review of Sociology, 9*, 375-395.

Berkman, L. F. (1981). Physical health and the social environment: A social epidemiological perspective. In L. Eisenberg & A. Kleinman (Eds.), *The relevance of social science for medicine* (pp. 51-75). Dordrecht, The Netherlands: Reidel.

Berkman, L. F., & Syme, S. L. (1979). Social networks, host resistance, and mortality: A 9 year follow-up study of Alameda County residents. *American Journal of Epidemiology, 109*, 186-204.

Berman, P., Kendall, C., & Bhattacharyya, K. (1994). The household production of health: Integrating social science perspectives on micro-level health determinants. *Social Science and Medicine, 38*, 205-215.

Best Start, Inc. (1997). *The national WIC breastfeeding promotion project: Research report.* Tampa, FL: Author.

Beuttner-Janusch, J. (1966). *Origins of man.* New York: John Wiley.

Binstock, R. H., Cluff, L. E., & von Mering, O. (1996). Issues affecting the future of long-term care. In R. H. Binstock, L. E. Cluff, & O. von Mering (Eds.), *The future of long-term care: Social and policy issues* (pp. 8-12). Baltimore: Johns Hopkins University Press.

Birch, L. L., & Fisher, J. A. (1996). The role of experience in the development of children's eating behavior. In E. D. Capaldi (Ed.), *Why we eat what we eat: The psychology of eating* (pp. 113-143). Washington, DC: American Psychological Association.

Bloom, B. L., Asher, S. J., & White, S. W. (1978). Marital disruption as a stressor: A review and analysis. *Psychological Bulletin, 85*, 867-894.

Bloom, P., & Novelli, W. D. (1981). Problems and challenges in social marketing. *Journal of Marketing, 45*(2), 79-88.

Bogan, I. G., Omar, A., Knobloch, S., Liburd, L. C., & O'Rourke, T. W. (1992). Organizing an urban African-American community for health promotion: Lessons from Chicago. *Journal of Health Education, 23*(3), 157-163.

Booth, A., & Amato, P. (1991). Divorce and psychological stress. *Journal of Health and Social Behavior, 32,* 396-407.

Bortz, W. (1991). We live too short and die too long. *Aging Today, 12,* 1-3.

Bowden, B. S., & Zeisz, J. M. (1997, August). *Supper's on! Adolescent adjustment and frequency of family mealtimes.* Paper presented at the 105th annual convention of the American Psychological Association, Chicago.

Bowman, D. J. (1999). *Stress in the work place.* Retrieved October 29, 1999, from the World Wide Web: www.ttg-consult/guestessay.htm

Bracht, N. (Ed.). (1990). *Health promotion at the community level.* Newbury Park, CA: Sage.

Bracht, N. (Ed.). (1999). *Health promotion at the community level* (2nd ed.). Thousand Oaks, CA: Sage.

Bracht, N., & Kingsbury, L. (1990). In N. Bracht (Ed.), *Health promotion at the community level* (pp. 66-88). Newbury Park, CA: Sage.

Bracht, N., Kingsbury, L., & Rissel, C. (1999). A five-stage community organization model for health promotion: Empowerment and partnership strategies. In N. Bracht (Ed.), *Health promotion at the community level* (2nd ed., pp. 83-104). Thousand Oaks, CA: Sage.

Bracht, N., & Tsouros, N. (1990). Principles and strategies of effective community participation. *Health Promotion International, 5*(3), 199-208.

Braithwaite, R. L., Bianchi, C., & Taylor, S. E. (1994). Ethnographic approach to community organization and health empowerment. *Health Education Quarterly, 21,* 407-416.

Brannon, R. (1976). The male sex role: Our culture's blueprint of manhood, and what it's done for us lately. In D. David & R. Brannon (Eds.), *The forty-nine percent majority* (pp. 1-45). Reading, MA: Addison-Wesley.

Brener, N. D., Simon, T. R., Krug, E. G., & Lowry, R. (1999). Recent trends in violence-related behaviors among high school students in the United States. *Journal of the American Medical Association, 282,* 440-446.

Brennan, M. (1998, March). New anti-malarial drugs move a step further. *Chemical and Engineering News: Weekly News Magazine of the American Chemical Society,* 38-39.

Brightman, J. (1994). What smells like teen spirit? *American Demographics, 16,* 10-11.

Brodwin, P. (1996). *The contest for healing power.* Cambridge, UK: Cambridge University Press.

Brookbank, J. (1990). *The biology of aging.* New York: Harper & Row.

Brown, D. R. (1996). Marital status and mental health. In H. W. Neighbors & J. S. Jackson (Eds.), *Mental health in black America* (pp. 77-94). Thousand Oaks, CA: Sage.

Brown, G., & Harris, T. (1978). *Social origins of depression: A study of psychiatric disorder in women.* New York: Free Press.

Brown, P. (1997, November). *Male gender and health: Cultural and biological perspectives.* Paper presented at the annual meeting of the American Anthropological Association, Washington, DC.

Brown, P., & Fox, H. (1979). Sex differences in divorce. In E. S. Gomberg & V. Franks (Eds.), *Gender and disordered behavior: Sex differences in psychopathology* (pp. 101-123). New York: Brunner/Mazel.

Brownlee, A. (1990). *Breastfeeding, weaning and nutrition: The behavioral issues* [Behavioral Issues in Child Survival Programs, Monograph No. 4]. Washington, DC: U.S. Agency for International Development.

Brownson, R. C., Baker, E. A. & Novick, L. F. (1999). *Community-prevention: Programs that work.* Gaithersburg, MD: Aspen

Brownson, R. C., Riley, P., & Bruce, T. A. (1998). Demonstration projects in community-based prevention. *Journal of Public Health Management and Practice, 4*(2), 66-77.

Bryant, C. A., Coreil, J., D'Angelo, S., Bailey, D., & Lazarov, M. (1992). A new strategy for promoting breastfeeding among economically disadvantaged women and adolescents. *National College of Obstetrics and Gynecology Clinical Issues in Perinatal and Women's Health Issues: Breastfeeding, 3,* 723-730.

Bryant, C. A., Courtney, A., Markesbery, B. A., & DeWalt, K. M. (1985). *The cultural feast: An introduction to food and society.* St. Paul, MN: West.

Bryant, C. A., Davis, M., Unterberger, A., & Lindenberger, J. (1993). *Determinants of prenatal care utilization.* Tampa, FL: Best Start Social Marketing.

Bryant, C. A., Lindenberger, J. L., Blair, C., Brown, C. A., Bustillo, M., Cannon, C., Gaskin, E., Jeffers, J., Pierce, B., & Hurley, K. (1994). *WIC at the crossroads: The Texas WIC marketing study final report* (Tech. Rep.). Austin: Texas Department of Health.

Buchanan, D. R. (1996). Building academic-community linkages for health promotion: A case study in Massachusetts. *American Journal of Health Promotion, 10,* 262-269.

Bunton, R., Nettleton, S., & Burrows, R. (1995). *The sociology of health promotion: Critical analyses of consumption, lifestyle and risk.* Boston: Routledge & Kegan Paul.

Butler, R. (1975). *Why survive? Being old in America.* New York: Harper & Row.

Butter, I. H., Carpenter, E. S., Kay, B. J., & Simmons, R. S. (1994). Gender hierarchies in the health labor force. In E. Fee & N. Krieger (Eds.), *Women's health, politics, and power: Essays on sex/gender, medicine, and public health.* Amityville, NY: Baywood.

Butterfoss, F. D., Goodman, R. M., & Wandersman, A. (1993). Community coalitions for prevention and health promotion. *Health Promotion Research, 8,* 315-330.

Cabanero-Verzosa, C., Bernaje, M. G., Guzman, E. M. D., Hernandez, J. R. S., Rodica, C. N., & Taguiwalo, M. M. (1989). *Managing a communication program on immunization.* Washington, DC: Academy for Educational Development.

Caldwell, J. C. (1990). Cultural and social factors influencing mortality levels in developing countries. *Annals of the American Academy of Political and Social Sciences, 510,* 44-59.

Caldwell, J. C. (1993). Health transition: The cultural, social and behavioural determinants of health in the Third World. *Social Science and Medicine, 36,* 125-135.

Campesi, J., Dimri, G., & Hara, E. (1996). Control of replicative senescence. In E. Schneider & J. Rowe (Eds.), *Handbook of the biology of aging* (4th ed., pp. 134-135). San Diego, CA: Academic Press.

Cannon, W. B. (1929). *Bodily changes in pain, hunger, fear and rage: An account of researches into function of emotional excitement.* Norwalk, CT: Appleton-Century-Crofts.

Caplan, P. (1997). Approaches to the study of food, health and identity. In P. Caplan (Ed.), *Food, health and identity* (pp. 116-144). Boston: Routledge & Kegan Paul.

Cartmill, M. (1998). The status of race concept in physical anthropology. *American Anthropologist, 100,* 651-660.

Cassel, J. (1976). The contribution of the social environment to host resistance. *American Journal of Epidemiology, 104,* 107-123.

Cassidy, C. M. (1996). Cultural context of complementary and alternative medicine systems. In M. S. Micozzi (Ed.), *Fundamentals of complementary and alternative medicine* (pp. 9-34). New York: Churchill Livingstone.

Castro, E. B., & Mokate, K. M. (1988). Malaria and its socioeconomic meanings: The study of Cunday in Colombia. In A. N. Herrin & P. Rosenfield (Eds.), *Economics, health and tropical diseases* (pp. 159-189). Manila: University of the Philippines, School of Economics.

Catalano, R. (1979). *Health, behavior and the community: An ecological perspective.* Elmsford, NY: Permagon.

Catania, J. A., Kegeles, S. M., & Coates, T. J. (1990). Towards an understanding of risk behavior: An AIDS risk reduction model (ARRM). *Health Education Quarterly, 17,* 53-72.

Centers for Disease Control and Prevention. (1998). *Youth risk behavior surveillance—United States, 1997.* Atlanta, GA: Author.

Centers for Disease Control and Prevention. (1999). *National Center for Injury Prevention and Control Division of Violence Prevention.* Retrieved November 12, 1999, from the World Wide Web: http//www.cdc.gov/ncipc/dvp/dvp.htm

Centers for Disease Control and Prevention. (2000). *The behavioral risk factor surveillance system.* Retrieved July 7, 2000, from the World Wide Web: http://www.cdc.gov/nccdphp/brfss/at-a-gl.htm

Chalmers, K. I., & Bramadat, I. J. (1996). Community development: theoretical and practical issues for community health nursing in Canada. *Journal of Advanced Nursing, 24,* 719-726.

Chan, W.-F., & Heaney, C. (1997). Employee stress levels and the intention to participate in a work site smoking cessation program. *Journal of Behavioral Medicine, 20,* 351-360.

Chang, E., & Harley, C. B. (1995). Telomere length and replicative aging in human vascular tissues. *Proceedings of the National Academy of Sciences, 92,* 11190-11194.

Charles, N. K., & Kerr, M. (1988). *Women, food and families.* Manchester, UK: Manchester University Press.

Chesler, M. A. (1990). The "dangers" of self-help groups: Understanding and challenging professionals' views. In T. J. Powell (Ed.), *Working with self-help* (pp. 119-139). Silver Spring, MD: National Association of Social Workers Press.

Chrisman, N. J. (1977). The help-seeking process: An approach to the natural history of illness. *Culture, Medicine and Psychiatry, 1,* 351-377.

Christoffel, T., & Gallagher, S. (1999). *Injury prevention and public health: Practical knowledge, skills, and strategies.* Gaithersburg, MD: Aspen.

Cleland, J. G., & van Ginneken, J. K. (1988). Maternal education and child survival in developing countries: The search for pathways of influence. *Social Science and Medicine, 27,* 1357-1366.

Cohen, J. E. (1995). *How many people can the Earth support?* New York: Norton.

Cohen, M. N. (1989). *Health and the rise of civilization.* New Haven, CT: Yale University Press.

Cohen, M. N., Malpass, R. S., & Klein, H. G. (Eds.). (1980). *Biosocial mechanisms of population regulation.* New Haven, CT: Yale University Press.

Collins, J. G., & Leclere, F. B. (1996). *Health and selected socioeconomic characteristics of the family: United States, 1988-1990.* Washington, DC: National Center for Health Statistics, Vital Health Statistics.

Collins, R. (1993). Why do women live longer than men? *New Scientist, 140*(1896), 45.

Colson, A. C. (1971). *The prevention of illness in a Malay village: An analysis of concepts and behavior* (Developing Nations Monograph Series, Series II, No. 1). Winton-Salem, NC: Overseas Research Center, Wake Forest University.

Committee for the Study of the Future of Public Health. (1992). A history of the public health system. In Institute of Medicine (Ed.), *The future of public health* (pp. 56-72). Washington, DC: National Academy of Sciences.

Conrad, P. (1992). Medicalization and social control. *Annual Review of Sociology, 18,* 209-232.

Coombe, C. M. (1998). Using empowerment evaluation in community organizing and community-based health initiatives. In M. Minkler (Ed.), *Community organizing and community building for health* (pp. 291-307). New Brunswick, NJ: Rutgers University Press.

Coreil, J. (1995). Group interview methods in community health research. *Medical Anthropology, 16,* 193-210.

Coreil, J. (1997). Health behavior in developing countries. In D. S. Gochman (Ed.), *Handbook of health behavior research* (Vol. 3, pp. 179-198). New York: Plenum.

Coreil, J., Augustin, A., Holt, E., & Halsey, N. (1994). Social and psychological costs of preventive child health services in Haiti. *Social Science and Medicine, 38,* 231-238.

Coreil, J., & Behal, R. (1999). Man to Man prostate cancer support groups. *Cancer Practices, 7*(3), 122-129.

Coreil, J., & Mull, J. D. (Eds.). (1988). Anthropological studies of diarrheal illness [Special issue]. *Social Science and Medicine, 27*(1).

Coreil, J., Whiteford, L., & Salazar, D. (1997). The household ecology of disease transmission: Dengue fever in the Dominican Republic. In M. Inhorn & P. Brown (Eds.), *The anthropology of infectious disease* (pp. 145-171). Westport, CT: Greenwood.

Coreil, J., Wilson, F., Woods, D., & Liller, K. (1998). Maternal employment and preventive child health practices. *Preventive Medicine, 27*, 488-492.

Crawford, E. D., Bennett, C. L., Stone, N. N., Knight, S. J, DeAntoni, E., Sharp, L., Garnick, M. B., & Porterfield, H. A. (1997). Comparison of perspectives on prostate cancer: Analyses of survey data. *Urology, 50*, 366-372.

Crocker, D. A., & Linden, T. (1998). *Ethics of consumption: The good life, justice and global stewardship.* Lanhan, MD: Rowan & Littlefield.

Crofton, J. (1984). The gathering of smoke clouds: A worldwide challenge. *International Journal of Epidemiology, 13*, 269-270.

Crombie, I., Kenicer, M., Smith, W., & Tuntstall-Pedo, H. (1989). Unemployment, socioenvironmental factors, and coronary heart disease in Scotland. *British Heart Journal, 61*, 172-177.

Crose, R. (1997). *Why women live longer than men: And what men can learn from them.* San Francisco: Jossey-Bass.

Daniel, M., & Green, L. W. (1995). Application of the Precede-Proceed planning model in diabetes prevention and control: A case illustration from a Canadian aboriginal community. *Diabetes Spectrum, 8*(2), 74-84.

Davis, K. (1987). The world's most expensive survey. *Sociological Forum, 2*, 829-835.

Davis, K., & Blake, J. (1956). Social structure and fertility: An analytic framework. *Economic Development and Cultural Change, 14*, 211-235.

Davis-Floyd, R. E. (1994). The technocratic body: American childbirth as cultural expression. *Social Science and Medicine, 38*, 1125-1140.

de Bocanegra, H. T. (1992). Cancer patients' interest in group support programs. *Cancer Nursing, 15*, 347-352.

Decosas, J., & Pedneault, V. (1992). Women and AIDS in Africa: Demographic implications for health promotion. *Health Policy and Planning, 7*, 227-233.

Desai, S., Chase-Lansdale, P. L., & Michael, R. T. (1981). Mother or market? Effects of maternal employment on the intellectual ability of 4-year-old children. *Demography, 26*, 545-561.

Dohrenwend, B. P. (1998). Some epidemiological approaches to the search for causes of psychiatric disorders. *Social Psychiatry and Psychiatric Epidemiology, 33*, 355-363.

Dohrenwend, B. P., & Dohrenwend, B. S. (1969). *Social status and psychological disorder.* New York: John Wiley.

Doyal, L. (1995). *What makes women sick: Gender and the political economy of health.* New Brunswick, NJ: Rutgers University Press.

Dressler, W. W., Balieiro, M. C., & Dos Santos, J. E. (1998). Culture, socioeconomic status, and physical and mental health in Brazil. *Medical Anthropology Quarterly, 12*, 424-446.

Dressler, W. W., Bindon, J. R., & Neggers, Y. H. (1998). Culture, socioeconomic status, and coronary health disease risk factors in an African American community. *Journal of Behavioral Medicine, 21*, 527-543.

Duffy, V. B., & Bartoshuk, L. M. (1996). Sensory factors in feeding. In E. D. Capaldi (Ed.), *Why we eat what we eat: The psychology of eating* (pp. 145-171). Washington, DC: American Psychological Association.

Dunbar, F. (1943). *Psychosomatic diagnosis.* New York: Harper & Row.

Duncan, D. F., Gold, R. J., Basch, C. E., & Markellis, V. C. (1988). *Epidemiology: Basis for disease prevention and health promotion.* New York: Macmillan.

Durkheim, E. (1951). Suicide: A study in sociology. In J. Spaulding & G. Simpson (Eds. and Trans.), *Le suicide.* (New York: Free Press. (Original work published 1897)

Dutton, D. B. (1987). Social class, health, and illness. In L. H. Aiken & D. Mechanic (Eds.), *Applications of social science to clinical medicine and health policy* (pp. 31-62). New Brunswick, NJ: Rutgers University Press.

Eaton, W. W. (1980). *The sociology of mental disorders.* New York: Praeger.

Eckenrode, J., & Gore, S. (1990). *Stress between work and family.* New York: Plenum.

Eisen, A. (1994). Survey of neighborhood-based, comprehensive community empowerment initiatives. *Health Education Quarterly, 21,* 235-252.

Eisenberg, D. M., Kessler, R. C., Foster, C., Norlock, F. E., Calkins, D. R., & Delbanc, T. L. (1993). Unconventional medicine in the United States: Prevalence, costs and patterns of use. *New England Journal of Medicine, 328,* 246-252.

El-Askari, G., Freestone, J., Irizarry, C., Krowt, K. L., Mashiyama, S. T., Morgan, M. A., & Walton, S. (1998). The Healthy Neighborhoods Project: A local health department's role in catalyzing community development. *Health Education and Behavior, 25,* 146-159.

Ell, K., & Northen, H. (1991). *Families and health care.* New York: deGruyter.

Emmons, C. A., Joseph, J., Kessler, R., & Wortman, C. (1986). Psychosocial predictors of reported behavior change in homosexual men at risk for AIDS. *Health Education Quarterly, 13,* 331-345.

Eng, E., & Parker, E. (1994). Measuring community competence in the Mississippi Delta: The interface between program evaluation and empowerment. *Health Education Quarterly, 21,* 199-220.

England, P., & Farkas, G. (1986). *Households, employment, and gender: A social, economic and demographic view.* Chicago: Aldine.

Engel, E. (1882). *Das rechnungsburch der hausfrau und seine Bedeutung im wirtshaftsleben der nation.* Berlin: L. Simmion.

Engle, P. (1989). Child care strategies of working and nonworking women in rural and urban Guatemala. In J. Leslie & M. Paolisso (Eds.), *Women, work and child welfare in the Third World* (pp. 179-200). Boulder, CO: Westview.

Etkin, N. L., & Ross, P. J. (1983). Malaria, medicine, and meals: Plant use among the Hausa and its impact on disease. In L. Romanucci-Ross, D. E. Moerman, & L. R. Tancredi (Eds.), *The anthropology of medicine: From culture to method.* New York: Praeger.

Etkin, N. L., & Ross, P. J. (1991). Malaria, medicine, and meals: Plant use among the Hausa and its impact on disease. In L. Romanucci-Ross, D. E. Moerman, & L. R. Tancredi

(Eds.), *The anthropology of medicine: From culture to method* (2nd ed., pp. 230-258). New York: Praeger.

Fabrega, H., Jr. (1997). *Evolution of sickness and healing.* Berkeley: University of California Press.

Farb, P., & Armelagos, G. (1980). *Consuming passions: The anthropology of eating.* Boston: Houghton Mifflin.

Farmer, M. M., & Ferraro, K. F. (1997). Distress and perceived health: Mechanisms of health decline. *Journal of Health and Social Behavior, 39,* 298-311.

Farmer, P. (1997). Social scientists and the new tuberculosis. *Social Science and Medicine, 43,* 347-358.

Farmer, P. (1999). *Infections and inequality.* Berkeley: University of California Press.

Fee, E., & Krieger, N. (Eds.). (1994). *Women's health, politics, and power: Essays on sex/gender, medicine and public health.* Amityville, NY: Baywood.

Figueroa, J., & Breen, N. (1995). Significance of underclass residence on the stage of breast or cervical cancer diagnosis. *American Economic Review, 85,* 112-116.

Fishbein, M., Guenther-Grey, C., Johnson, W., Wolitski, R. J., McAlister, A., Rietmeyer, C. A., & O'Reilly, K. (1997). Using theory-based community intervention to reduce AIDS risk behaviors: The CDC's AIDS community demonstration project. In M. E. Goldberg, M. Fishbein, & S. E. Middlestadt (Eds.), *Social marketing: Theoretical and practical perspectives* (pp. 123-146). Mahwah, NJ: Lawrence Erlbaum.

Fishbein, M., & Middlestadt, S. (1989). Using the theory of reasoned action as a framework for understanding and changing AIDS-related behaviors. In V. Mays & G. Albee (Eds.), *Primary prevention of AIDS: Psychological approaches* (pp. 93-110). Newbury Park, CA: Sage.

Flay, B. R., & Petraitis, J. (1994). The Theory of Triadic Influence: A new theory of health behavior and implications for preventive interventions. *Advances in Medical Sociology, 4,* 19-44.

Flegal, K. M., Carroll, M. D., Kuczmarski, R. J., & Johnson, C. L. (1998). Overweight and obesity in the United States: Prevalence and trends, 1960-1994. *International Journal of Obesity, 22,* 39-47.

Flynn, B. C., Ray, D. W., & Rider, M. S. (1994). Empowering communities: Action research through healthy cities. *Health Education Quarterly, 21,* 395-405.

Folstein, M. F., Folstein, S. E., & McHugh, P. R. (1975). Mini-mental state: A practical method for grading the cognitive state of patients for clinicians. *Journal of Psychiatric Research, 12,* 189-198.

Food for Peace Reauthorization Act: *Hearing before the committee on the Committee on International Relations, House of Representatives,* 104th Congress, 1st session (1995, November 1).

Food Marketing Institute. (1997). *Trends in the United States: Consumer attitudes and the supermarket, 1997.* Washington DC: Author.

Forthofer, M. S., Janz, N. K., Dodge, J. A., & Clark, N. M. (In press). Gender differences in the associations of self-esteem and stress with change in functional health status of older adults with heart disease. *Journal of Women and Aging.*

Forthofer, M. S., Kessler, R. C., Story, A. L., & Gotlib, I. H. (1996). The effects of psychiatric disorders on the probability and timing of first marriage. *Journal of Health and Social Behavior, 37,* 121-132.

Foster, G. M. (1976). Disease etiologies in nonwestern medical systems. *American Anthropologist, 78,* 773-782.

Foster, G., & Anderson, B. G. (1978). *Medical Anthropology.* New York: John Wiley.

Fox, J. A., & Zawitz, M. W. (1999). *Homicide trends in the United States* (Crime Data Brief). Washington, DC: Bureau of Justice Statistics.

Frankish, C. J., & Green, L. W. (1994). Organizational and community change as the social scientific basis for disease prevention and health promotion policy. *Advances in Medical Sociology, 4,* 209-233.

Frankish, C. J., Milligan, C. D., & Reid, C. (1998). A review of relationships between active living and determinants of health. *Social Science and Medicine, 47,* 287-301.

Freedman, L. P., & Maine, D. (1993). Women's mortality: A legacy of neglect. In M. Koblinsky, J. Timyan, & J. Gay (Eds.), *The health of women: A global perspective* (pp. 147-170). Boulder, CO: Westview.

Freedom of Access to Clinic Entrances Act. (1994). Retrieved July 7, 2000, from the World Wide Web: http://www.msu.edu/user/schwenkl/abtrbng/s636.htm

Freire, P. (1970). *Pedagogy of the oppressed.* New York: Seabury.

Frenk, J. (1993). The new public health. *Annual Review of Public Health, 14,* 469-490.

Fries, J. F. (1980). Aging, natural death and the compression of morbidity. *New England Journal of Medicine, 303,* 130-135.

Friis, R. H., & Sellers, T. A. (1999). *Epidemiology for public health practice* (2nd ed.). Gaithersburg, MD: Aspen.

Fugiwara, P. I., Larkin, C., & Frieden, T. R. (1997). Directly observed therapy in New York City: History, implementation, results, and challenges. *Clinics in Chest Medicine, 18,* 135-148.

Gallagher, E. B. (1979). Lines of reconstruction and extension in the Parsonian sociology of illness. In E. G. Jaco (Ed.), *Patients, physicians and illness: A sourcebook in behavioral science and health* (3rd ed., pp. 162-183). New York: Free Press.

Gillert, D. (1999). *Across America youth face greatest road risks.* Retrieved March 15, 2000, from the World Wide Web: http://www.dtic.mil/afps/news/9708076.htm

Glanz, K., Marcus, F., Lewis, B., & Rimer, K. (Eds.). (1997). *Health behavior and health education: Theory, research, and practice* (2nd ed.). San Francisco: Jossey-Bass.

Glanz, K., Resch, N., Lerman, C., & Rimer, B. (1996). Black-white differences in factors influencing mammography use among employed female health maintenance organization members. *Ethnicity and Health, 1*(3), 207-220.

Gochman, D. S. (1988). Health behavior: Plural perspectives. In D. S. Gochman, (Ed.), *Health behavior: Emerging research perspectives* (pp. 3-26). New York: Plenum.

Gochman, D. S. (1997). Health behavior research: Definitions and diversity. In D. S. Gochman (Ed.), *Handbook of health behavior research* (Vol. 1, pp. 3-20). New York: Plenum.

Goldman, D. (1999, May). Paradox of pleasure. *American Demographics,* pp. 50-57.

Goodman, R. M., Steckler, A., & Kegler, M. (1997). Mobilizing organizations for health en-
hancement: Theories of organizational change. In K. Glanz, F. Marcus, B. Lewis, &
K. Rimer (Eds.), *Health behavior and health education: Theory, research and practice* (2nd
ed., pp. 287-312). San Francisco: Jossey-Bass.

Gordon, A. J. (1988). Mixed strategies in health education and community participation:
An evaluation of dengue control in the Dominican Republic. *Health and Education Research, 3*, 399-419.

Gordon, D. F. (1995). Testicular cancer and masculinity. In D. Sabo & D. F. Gordon (Eds.),
Men's health and illness: Gender, power, and the body (pp. 246-265). Thousand Oaks, CA:
Sage.

Gotlib, I. H., & McCabe, S. B. (1990). Marriage and psychopathology. In F. Fincham &
T. Bradbury (Eds.), *The psychology of marriage: Basic issues and applications* (pp.
226-255). New York: Guilford.

Gove, W. (1972). Sex, marital status, and suicide. *Journal of Health and Social Behavior, 13*,
204-213.

Gove, W. (1984). The effects of gender differences in mental and physical illness: The effects of fixed roles and nurturant roles. *Social Science and Medicine, 19*, 77-91.

Gove, W. R., & Tudor, J. F. (1973). Adult sex roles and mental illness. *American Journal of Sociology, 78*, 812-835.

Green, J. (1999). *Cultural awareness in the human services* (3rd ed.). Boston: Allyn & Bacon.

Green, L. W., & Kreuter, M. W. (Eds.). (1991). *Health promotion planning: An educational and
environmental approach.* Mountain View, CA: Mayfield.

Greener, M. (1991). Cancer self-help groups: A vital support link. *Professional Nurse, 6*,
662-664.

Greenspan, S. (1997). *The growth of the mind and the engendered origins of intelligence.* Reading, MA: Addison-Wesley.

Greenstein, T. (1993). Maternal employment and child behavioral outcomes: A household economic analysis. *Journal of Family Issues, 14*, 323-354.

Greenstein, T. (1995). Are the "most advantaged" children truly disadvantaged by early
maternal employment: Effects on child cognitive outcomes. *Journal of Family Issues,
16*, 149-169.

Griffiths, S. (1990). A review of the factors associated with patient compliance
and the taking of prescribed medicines. *British Journal of General Practice, 40*(332),
114-116.

Griffiths, S. (1996). Men's health [editorial]. *British Medical Journal, 312* (7023), 69-70.

Groger, L. (1992). Tied to each other through ties to the land: Informal support of black elders in a Southern U.S. community. *Journal of Cross-Cultural Gerontology, 7*(3), 205-220.

Guttmacher Institute. (1999). *Teenage pregnancy: Overall trends and state-by-state information.* Retrieved September 29, 1999, from the World Wide Web: http://www.
agi-usa.org/pubs/teen_preg_stats.html

Haddon, W. (1980). Options for the prevention of motor vehicle crash injury. *Israel Journal
of Medical Science, 16*, 45-68.

Hahn, R. A. (1995). *Sickness and healing: An anthropological perspective.* New Haven, CT: Yale University Press.

Hajek, P., Belcher, M., & Stapleton, J. (1987). Breath-holding endurance as a predictor of success in smoking cessation. *Addictive Behaviors, 12,* 285-288.

Haley, W. E., Han, B., & Henderson, J. N. (1998). Aging and ethnicity: Issues for clinical practice. *Journal of Clinical Psychology in Medical Settings, 5,* 393-409.

Ham, R. J., Holtzman, J. M., Marcy, M. C., & Smith, M. R. (1983). *Primary care geriatrics.* Boston: John Wright/PSG Inc.

Hamilton, J. A. (1996). Women and health policy: On the inclusion of females in clinical trials. In C. Sargent & C. B. Brettell (Eds.), *Gender and health: An international perspective* (pp. 292-325). Upper Saddle River, NJ: Prentice Hall.

Handwerker, W. P. (1983). The first demographic transition: An analysis of subsistence choices and reproductive consequences. *American Anthropologist, 85,* 5-27.

Harkness, S., & Super, D. (1994). The developmental niche: A theoretical framework for analyzing the household production of health. *Social Science and Medicine, 38,* 217-226.

Harlow, K. S., & McDonald, J. (1991). Aging in black America: Service needs and utilization patterns. *Evaluation and Program Planning, 14,* 233-39.

Harnack, L. (1998). Guess who's cooking? The role of men in meal planning, shopping, and preparation in U.S. families. *Journal of the Dietetic Association, 98,* 995-1001.

Harris, M. (1987). Foodways: Historical overview and theoretical prolegomenon. In M. Harris & E. Ross (Eds.), *Food and evolution: Toward a theory of human food habits* (pp. 57-92). Philadelphia: Temple University Press.

Harrison, F. (1998). Contemporary issues forum: Race and racism. *American Anthropologist, 100,* 609-631.

Harrison, G. A., Weiner, J. S., Tanner, J. M., & Barnicot, N. A. (1977). *Human biology* (2nd ed.). Oxford, UK: Oxford University Press.

Hassan, F. A. (1980). The growth and regulation of human population in prehistoric times. In M. N. Cohen, R. S. Malpass, & H. G. Klein (Eds.), *Biosocial mechanisms of population regulation* (pp. 305-319). New Haven, CT: Yale University Press.

Hastings, G., MacFadyen, L., MacKintosh, A., & Lowry, R. (1998). New debate: Assessing the impact of branding and tobacco marketing communications on young people in Britain. *Social Marketing Quarterly, 4*(4), 17-26.

Haug, M. R., Musil, C. M., Warner, C. D., & Morris, D. I. (1998). Interpreting bodily changes as illness: A longitudinal study of older adults. *Social Science and Medicine, 46,* 1553-1567.

Heaney, C. A., & Israel, B. A. (1997). Social networks and social support. In K. Glanz, F. Marcus, B. Lewis, & K. Rimer (Eds.), *Health behavior and health education: Theory, research and practice* (2nd ed., pp. 179-205). San Francisco: Jossey-Bass.

Heggenhougen, K., & Clements, J. (1987). *Acceptability of childhood immunization: Social science perspectives. Evaluation and planning center for health care* (Pub. No. 14). London: London School of Hygiene and Tropical Medicine.

Helman, C. G. (1994). *Culture, health and illness* (3rd ed.). Newton, MA: Butterworth-Heinemann.

Henderson, J. N. (1993). The cultural diversity epidemic [Editorial]. *Gerontological Health, 4.*

Henderson, J. N. (1997). Dementia in cultural context: Development and decline of a caregiver support group in a Latin population. In J. Sokolovsky (Ed.), *The cultural context of aging: Worldwide perspectives* (2nd ed., pp. 425-442). Westport, CT: Bergin & Garvey.

Henderson, J. N., Gutierrez-Mayka, M., Garcia, J., & Boyd, S. (1993). A model for Alzheimer's disease support group development in African-American and Hispanic populations. *The Gerontologist, 33,* 409-414.

Herman, E., & Bentley, M. E. (1992). Manuals for ethnographic data collection: Experience and issues. *Social Science and Medicine, 35,* 1369-1378.

Hernandez, G. (1992). The family and its aged members: The Cuban experience. *Clinical Gerontologist, 1,* 35-43.

Hien, T. T., & White, N. J. (1993). Qinghaosu. *Lancet, 341,* 603-608.

Hill, J. O., & Peters, J. C. (1998). Environmental contributions to the obesity epidemic. *Science, 280,* 1371-1374.

Hoffman, L. W. (1989). Effects of maternal employment in the two-parent family. *American Psychologist, 44,* 283-292.

Hoffman, S. M., Hromas, R., Amemiya, C., & Mohrenweiser, H. W. (1996). The location of MZF-1 at the telomere of human chromosome 19q makes it vulnerable to degeneration in aging cells. *Leukemia Research, 20,* 281-283.

Holden, K. C., & Smock, P. J. (1991). The economic costs of marital dissolution: Why do women bear a disproportionate cost? *Annual Review of Sociology, 17,* 51-78.

Hollingshead, A. B., & Redlich, F. C. (1958). *Social class and mental illness.* New York: John Wiley.

Holmes, E. R., & Holmes, L. D. (1995). *Other cultures, elder years* (2nd ed.). Thousand Oaks, CA: Sage.

Holmes, T. H., & Rahe, R. H. (1967). The Social Readjustment Rating Scale. *Journal of Psychosomatic Research, 11,* 213-218.

Homedes, N., & Ugalde, A. (1994). Research on patient compliance in developing countries. *Bulletin of the Pan American Health Organization, 28*(1), 17-33.

Horowitz, I. L. (1966). *Three worlds of development.* New York: Oxford University Press.

House, J. S., Lepkowski, J. M., Kinney, A. M., Mero, R. P., & Kessler, R. C. (1994). The social stratification of aging and health. *Journal of Health and Social Behavior, 35,* 213-234.

House, J. S., Robbins, C., & Metzner, H. M. (1982). The association of social relationships and activities with mortality: Prospective evidence from the Tecumseh Community Health Study. *American Journal of Epidemiology, 116,* 123-140.

House, J. S., Umberson, D., & Landis, K. R. (1988). Structures and processes of social support. *Annual Review of Sociology, 14,* 293-318.

Huang, Y., & Manderson, L. (1992). Schistosomiasis and the social patterning of infection. *Acta Tropica, 51,* 175-194.

Huffman, S. L. (1984). Determinants of breastfeeding in developing countries: Overview and policy implications. *Studies in Family Planning, 15*(4), 170-183.

Hunt, L. M., Jordan, B., Irwin, S., & Browner, C. H. (1989). Compliance and the patient's perspective: Controlling symptoms in everyday life. *Culture, Medicine and Psychiatry, 13*, 215-234.

Hunt, L. M., Valenzuela, M. A., & Pugh, J. A. (1998). Porque me toco a mi? Mexican American diabetes patients' causal stories and their relationship to treatment. *Social Science and Medicine, 46*, 959-969.

Hursh-Cesar, G. (1988). *UNICEF KAP Studies: Report to Office of Evaluation, Office of Programme Communication, UNICEF.* Washington, DC: Intercultural Communication, Inc.

Hurtado, A. M., Hurtado, I. A. D., Sapien, R., & Hill, K. (1999). The evolutionary ecology of childhood asthma. In W. Travathan, E. Smith, & J. McKenna (Eds.), *Evolutionary medicine* (pp. 101-134). New York: Oxford University Press.

Huttenlocher, P. R. (1994). Synaptogenesis: Synapse elimination and neural plasticity in human cerebral cortex. In C. A. Nelson (Ed.), *Threats to optimal development: Integrating biological, psychological, and social risk factors* (pp. 35-54). Minneapolis: Minnesota Symposia in Child Psychology.

Illich, I. (1976). *Medical nemesis: The expropriation of health.* New York: Pantheon.

Israel, B. A., Checkoway, B., Schulz, A., & Zimmermann, M. (1994). Health education and community empowerment: Conceptualizing and measuring perceptions of individual, organizational, and community control. *Health Education Quarterly, 21*, 149-170.

Israel, B. A., Schulz, A. J., Parker, E. A., & Becker, A. B. (1998). Key principles of community-based research. *Annual Review of Public Health, 19*, 173-202.

Janzen, J. M. (1978). *The quest for therapy in Lower Zaire.* Berkeley: University of California Press.

Jelliffe, D. B. (1957). Social culture and nutrition: Cultural blocks and protein malnutrition in early childhood in rural West Bengal. *Pediatrics, 20*, 12.

Jenkins, C. D. (1988). Epidemiology of cardiovascular diseases. *Journal of Consulting and Clinical Psychology 56*(3), 324-332.

Jessor, R. (1977). *Problem behavior and psychosocial development.* San Diego, CA: Academic Press.

Johns, T. (1991, September/October). The well-grounded diet. *The Sciences,* 39-43.

Johnson, J., & Lane, C. (1993). Role of support groups in cancer care. *Supportive Care in Cancer, 1*, 52-56.

Johnson, T. P. (1991). Mental health, social relations, and social selection: A longitudinal analysis. *Journal of Health and Social Behavior, 32*, 408-423.

Jordan, B. (1990). Technology and the social distribution of knowledge: Issues for primary health care in developing countries. In J. Coreil & J. D. Mull (Eds.), *Anthropology and primary health care* (pp. 98-136). Boulder, CO: Westview.

Joseph, J., Montgomery, S., Emmons, C.-A., & Kirscht, J. (1987). Perceived risk of AIDS: Assessing the behavioral and psychosocial consequences in a cohort of gay men. *Journal of Applied Social Psychology, 17*, 231-250.

Kamerman, S., & Hayes, C. D. (1982). *Families that work: Children in a changing world.* Washington, DC: National Academy Press.

Kane, R. L., Ouslander, J. G., & Abrass, I. B. (1984). *Essentials of clinical geriatrics.* New York: McGraw-Hill.

Kanner, A. D., Coyne, J. C., Schaefer, C., & Lazarus, R. S. (1981). Comparison of two modes of stress measurement: Daily hassles and uplifts versus major life events. *Journal of Behavioral Medicine, 4,* 1-39.

Kaplan, H. B. (1991). Social psychology of the immune system: A conceptual framework and review of the literature. *Social Science and Medicine, 33,* 909-923.

Katz, S. J., Kessler, R. C., Frank, R. G., Leaf, P., & Lin, E. (1997). Mental health care use, morbidity, and socio-economic status in the United States and Ontario. *Inquiry, 34,* 38-49.

Kausler, D. H., & Kausler, B. C. (1996). *The graying of America.* Urbana: University of Illinois Press.

Kawachi, I., & Kennedy, B. P. (1997). The relationship of income inequality to mortality: Does the choice of indicator matter? *Social Science and Medicine, 45,* 1121-1127.

Kawachi, I., Kennedy, B. P., & Wilkinson, R. G. (1999). Crime: Social disorganization and relative deprivation. *Social Science and Medicine, 48,* 719-731.

Keefe, S. (1992). Ethnic identity: The domain of perceptions of and attachment to ethnic groups and cultures. *Human Organization, 51,* 35-43.

Kellam, S. G., Koretz, D., & Moscicki, E. K. (1999). Core elements of developmental epidemiologically based prevention research. *American Journal of Community Psychology, 27,* 463-482.

Kellerman, A. L., Fuqua-Whitley, D. S., Rivara, F. P., & Mercy, J. (1998). Preventing youth violence: What works. *Annual Review of Public Health, 19,* 271-292.

Kempe, H. C., Silverman, F. N., Steele, B. F., Droegemueller, W., & Silver, H. K. (1962). The battered child syndrome. *Journal of the American Medical Association, 181,* 17-24.

Kessler, R. C., & Essex, M. (1982). Marital status and depression: The importance of coping resources. *Social Forces, 61,* 484-507.

Kessler, R. C., McGonagle, K. A., Zhao, S., Nelson, C. B., Hughes, M., Eshleman, S., Wittchen, H.-U., & Kendler, K. S. (1994). Lifetime and active prevalence of *DSM-III-R* psychiatric disorders in the United States: Results from the National Comorbidity Survey. *Archives of General Psychiatry, 51,* 8-19.

Kessler, R. C., & McRae, J. A. (1984). A note on the relationships of sex and marital status to psychological distress. *Research in Community and Mental Health, 4,* 109-30.

Kessler, R. C., Walters, E. E., & Forthofer, M. S. (1998). The social consequences of psychiatric disorders: III. Probability of marital stability. *American Journal of Psychiatry, 155,* 1092-1096.

King, K. B. (1997). Psychologic and social aspects of cardiovascular disease. *Annals of Behavioral Medicine, 19,* 264-270.

Kirby, G. C. (1997). Plants as a source of antimalarial drugs. *Tropical Doctor, 27*(Suppl. 1), 7-11.

Kittler, P., & Sucher, K. (1989). *Food and culture in America.* New York: Van Nostrand Rienhold.

Klein, A. M. (1995). *Life's too short to die small.* Thousand Oaks, CA: Sage.

Klein, S. (Ed.). (1998). *National agenda for geriatric education: White papers* (Vol. I). Washington, DC: Department of Health and Human Services, Public Health Service, Health Resources and Services Administration.

Kleinman, A. (1980). *Patients and healers in the context of culture: An exploration of the borderland between anthropology, medicine, and psychiatry.* Berkeley: University of California Press.

Kleinman, A. (1988). *The illness narratives: Suffering, healing and the human condition.* New York: Basic Books.

Kodner, D. L. (1996). Foreseeing the future of long-term care: The highlights and implications of the Delphi Study. In R. H. Binstock, L. E. Cluff, & O. von Mering (Eds.), *The future of long-term care: Social and policy issues* (pp. 275-291). Baltimore: John Hopkins University Press.

Kolbe, L. J. (1988). The application of health behavior research: Health education and health promotion. In D. S. Gochman (Ed.), *Health behavior: Emerging research perspectives* (pp. 381-396). New York: Plenum.

Kolker, A. (1996). Thrown overboard: The human costs of health care rationing. In C. Ellis & A. P. Bochner (Eds.), *Composing ethnography: Alternative forms of qualitative writing* (pp. 132-159). Thousand Oaks, CA: Sage.

Koseki, L. K., & Reid, S. E. (1991). Elderly self-care education: A low technology primary health care option for developing countries. *Asia-Pacific Journal of Public Health, 5,* 322-330.

Kosorok, M. R., Omenn, G. S., Diehr, P. Koepsell, T. D., & Patrick, D. L. (1992). Conditions associated with restricted activity days among older adults. *American Journal of Public Health, 82,* 1263-1267.

Koss, M. P., Goodman, L. A., Browne, A., Fitzgerald, L. F., Keita, G. P., & Russo, N. F. (1994). *No safe haven: Male violence against women at home, at work, and in the community.* Washington DC: American Psychological Association.

Kotarba, J. A., & Seidel, J. V. (1984). Managing the problem pain patient: Compliance or social control. *Social Science and Medicine, 19,* 1393-1400.

Kotler, P., & Andreasen, A. (1991). *Strategic marketing for nonprofit organizations.* Englewood Cliffs, NJ: Prentice Hall.

Kotler, P., & Armstrong, G. (1996). *Principles of marketing* (7th ed.). Englewood Cliffs, NJ: Prentice Hall.

Kreuter, M. W. (1992). PATCH: Its origin, basic concepts, and links for contemporary public health policy. *Journal of Health Education, 23*(3), 135-139.

Krieger, N. (1994). Epidemiology and the web of causation: Has anyone seen the spider. *Social Science and Medicine, 39,* 887-903.

Krondl, M., & Coleman, P. (1986). Social and biocultural determinants of food selection. *Progress in Food and Nutrition Science, 10,* 179-203.

Kunitz, S. J., & Levy, J. E. (1981). Navajos. In A. Harwood (Ed.), *Ethnicity and medical care* (pp. 337-396). Cambridge, MA: Harvard University Press.

Lam, D. S., & Shaw, L. R. (1997). Development and application of the Family Involvement Questionnaire in brain injury rehabilitation. *Brain Injury, 11,* 219-231.

Last, J. M. (1998). *Public health and human ecology.* Stamford, CT: Appleton & Lange.

Lawrence, R. A., & Lawrence, R. M. (1999). *Breastfeeding: A guide for the medical professional* (5th ed.). St. Louis, MO: C. V. Mosby.

Leavitt, J. W. (Ed.). (1984). *Women and health in America: Historical readings.* Madison: University of Wisconsin Press.

Lee, R. B. (1968). What hunters do for a living, or how to make out on scarce resources. In R. B. Lee & I. Devore (Eds.), *Man the hunter* (pp. 30-48). Chicago: Aldine.

Lee, R. B. (1980). Lactation, ovulation, infanticide, and women's work: A study of hunter-gatherer population regulation. In M. N. Cohen, R. S. Malpass, & H. G. Klein (Eds.), *Biosocial mechanisms of population regulation* (pp. 321-348). New Haven, CT: Yale University Press.

Lefebvre, R. C., Doner, L., Johnston, C., Loughrey, K., Balch, G. I., & Sutton, S. M. (1995). Use of database marketing and consumer-based health communication in message design: An example from the Office of Cancer Communications' "5 a Day for Better Health" Program. In Maiback, E. & R. L. Parrott (Eds.), *Designing health messages: Approaches from communication theory and public health practice* (pp. 217-246). Thousand Oaks, CA: Sage.

Lefebvre, R. C., & Flora, J. (1988). Social marketing and public health intervention. *Health Education Quarterly, 15,* 299-315.

Leighton, A. H. (1959). *My name is legion.* New York: Basic Books.

Leininger, M. (1970). Some cross cultural universal and non-universal functions, beliefs, and practices of food. In J. Dupont (Ed.), *Dimensions of nutrition* (pp. 153-179). Boulder: Colorado University Press.

Lemert, E. M. (1967). *Human deviance, social problems, and social control.* Englewood Cliffs, NJ: Prentice Hall.

Leslie, J. (1989). Women's time: A factor in the use of child survival technologies? *Health Policy and Planning, 4,* 1-16.

Leslie, J., & Gupta, G. R. (1989). *Utilization of formal services for maternal nutrition and health care in the Third World.* Washington, DC: International Center for Research on Women.

Leventhal, H., Leventhal, E. A., & Contrada, R. J. (1998). Self-regulation, health, and behavior: A perceptual-cognitive approach. *Psychology and Health, 14,* 717-133.

Levine, M. (1988). An analysis of mutual assistance. *American Journal of Community Psychology, 16,* 167-188.

Levine, M., & Perkins, D. V. (1987). *Principles of community psychology: Perspectives and applications.* New York: Oxford University Press.

Lewis, F., & Daltroy, L. (1990). How causal explanations influence health behavior: Attribution theory. In K. Glanz, F. Lewis, & B. Rimer (Eds.), *Health behavior and health education: Theory, research, and practice* (pp. 92-114). San Francisco: Jossey-Bass.

Lieblich, A., Tuval-Mashiach, R. & Zilber, T. (1998). Narrative research: Reading, analysis and interpretation. *Applied Social Research Methods Series, 47.*

Ling, J. C., Franklin, B. A., Lindsteadt, J. F., & Gearon, S. A. N. (1992). Social marketing: Its place in public health. *Annual Review of Public Health, 13,* 341-362.

Link, B. G., & Phelan, J. (1995). Social conditions as fundamental causes of diseases. *Journal of Health and Social Behavior, 47,* 80-94.

Livingstone, F. (1962). On the non-existence of human races. *Current Anthropology, 3,* 279-281.

Looy, H., & Weingarten, H. P. (1992). Facial expressions and genetic sensitivity to 6-n-propylthiouracil predict hedonic response to sweet. *Physiology and Behavior, 52,* 75-82.

Lorber, J. (1997). *Gender and the social construction of illness.* Thousand Oaks, CA: Sage.

Luchina, L., Bartoshuk, L. M., Duffy, V. B., Marks, L. E., & Ferris, A. M. (1995). 6-n-propylthiouracil perception affects nutritional status of independent-living older females [Abstract]. *Chemical Senses, 20,* 735.

Luke, D. A., Roberts, L., & Rappaport, J. (1993). Individual, group context, and individual-group fit predictors of self-help group attendance. *Journal of Applied Behavioral Science, 29,* 216-238.

Lupton, D. (1995). *The imperative of health: Public health and the regulated body.* Thousand Oaks, CA: Sage.

Luthar, S. S., & Zigler, E. (1991). Vulnerability and competence: A review of research on resilience in childhood. *American Journal of Orthopsychiatry, 6,* 6-22.

Manderson, L. (1987). Hot-cold food and medical theories: Overview and introduction. *Social Science and Medicine, 25,* 329-330.

Manderson, L., & Aaby, P. (1992). An epidemic in the field? Rapid assessment procedures and health research. *Social Science and Medicine, 35,* 839-852.

Manoff, R. K. (1984). *Social marketing and nutrition education: A pilot project in Indonesia. Assignment Children, 65/68,* 95-113.

Maren, M. (1997). *The road to hell: The ravaging effects of foreign aid and international charity.* New York: Free Press.

Markides, K. S., & Coreil, J. (1986). The health of Southwestern Hispanics: An "epidemiologic paradox"? *Public Health Reports, 101,* 253-265.

Marks, J. B. (1998). Diabetes management in the future: A whiff and a long shot? *Clinical Diabetes, 16,* 140-145.

Marks, N. F. (1996). Socioeconomic status, gender, and health at midlife: Evidence from the Wisconsin Longitudinal Study. In J. J. Kronefeld (Ed.), *Research in the sociology of health care* (Vol. 13A, pp. 135-152). Greenwich, CT: JAI.

Marmot, M., Bobak, M., & Smith, G. D. (1995). *Explanations for social inequalities in health society and health.* New York: Oxford University Press.

Marmot, M., Ryff, C. D., Bumpass, L. L., Shipley, M., & Marks, N. F. (1997). Social inequalities in health: Next questions and converging evidence. *Social Science and Medicine, 44,* 901-910.

Marmot, M. G., Shipley, M. G., & Rose, G. (1984). Inequalities in death—Specific explanations or a general pattern? *Lancet, 1,* 1003-1006.

Marmot, M. G., Smith, G. D., Stansfeld, S., Patel, C., North, F., Head, J., White, I., Brunner, E. J., & Feeney, A. (1991). Heath inequalities among British civil servants: The White-hall II Study. *Lancet, 337,* 1387-1393.

Matthews, H. F., Lannin, D. R. & Mitchell, J. P. (1994). Coming to terms with advanced breast cancer: Black women's narratives from eastern North Carolina. *Social Science and Medicine, 38,* 789-800.

McCombie, S. C. (1999). Folk flu and viral syndrome: An anthropological perspective. In R. A. Hahn (Ed.), *Anthropology in public health: Bridging differences in culture and society* (pp. 27-43). New York: Oxford University Press.

McGrath, J. W., Schumann, D., Pearson-Marks, J., Rwabukwali, C. B., Mukasa, R., Namande, B., Nakayiwa, S., & Nakyobe, L. (1992). Cultural determinants of sexual risk behavior for AIDS among Baganda women. *Medical Anthropology Quarterly, 6*(2), 153-161.

McIntosh, W. A., & Shiffleet, P. A. (1984). Dietary behavior, dietary adequacy, and reli-gious social support: An exploratory study. *Review of Religious Research, 26*(2), 158-175.

McKenna, J. J., Mosko, S., & Richard, C. (1999). Breastfeeding and mother-infant cosleeping in relation to SIDS prevention. In W. R. Trevathan, E. O. Smith, & J. J. McKenna (Eds.), *Evolutionary medicine* (pp. 53-74). New York: Oxford University Press.

McNicoll, G. (1992). Changing fertility patterns and policies in the Third World. *Annual Review of Sociology, 18,* 85-108.

McWilliam, C. L., Desai, K., & Greig, B. (1997). Bridging town and gown: Building re-search partnerships between community-based professional providers and acade-mia. *Journal of Professional Nursing, 13,* 307-315.

Mead, M. (1935). *Sex and temperament in three primitive societies.* New York: William Mor-row.

Mechanic, D. (1978). *Medical sociology: A comprehensive text* (2nd ed.). New York: Free Press.

Menninger, W. C. (1935). Psychological factors in the etiology of disease. *Journal of Ner-vous and Mental Diseases, 81,* 1-13.

Merikangas, K. R. (1982). Assortative mating for psychiatric disorders and psychological traits. *Archives of General Psychiatry, 39,* 1173-1180.

Mezey, M. D. (1996). Challenges in providing care for persons with complex chronic ill-ness. In R. H. Binstock, L. E. Cluff, & O. von Mering (Eds.), *The future of long-term care: Social and policy issues* (pp. 119-142). Baltimore: Johns Hopkins University Press.

Michelson, I. (Ed.). (1985). Meta analysis and clinical psychology [Special issue]. *Clinical Psychology Review, 5*(1).

Middlestadt, S. E., Schechter, C., Peyton, J., & Tjugum, B. (1997). Community involve-ment in health planning: Lessons learned from practicing social marketing in a con-text of community control, participation and ownership. In M. E. Goldberg, M. Fishbein, & S. E. Middlestadt (Eds.), *Social marketing: Theoretical and practical perspec-tives* (pp. 291-311). Mahwah, NJ: Lawrence Erlbaum.

Miles, L. (1993). Women, AIDS, and power in heterosexual sex: A discourse analysis. *Women's Studies International Forum, 16*, 497-511.

Milliken, W. (1997). Malaria and anti-malarial plants in Roraima, Brazil. *Tropical Doctor, 27*(Suppl. 1), 20-25.

Minkler, M., & Wallerstein, N. (1997). Improving health through community organization and community building. In K. Glanz, F. M. Lewis, & B. K. Rimer (Eds.), *Health behavior and health education: Theory, research and practice* (2nd ed., pp. 241-342). San Francisco: Jossey-Bass.

Minkler, M., & Wallerstein, N. (1998). Improving health through community organization and community building: A health education perspective. In M. Minkler (Ed.), *Community organizing and community building for health* (pp. 30-52). Gaithersburg, MD: Aspen.

Moerman, D. (1982). General medical effectiveness and human biology: Placebo effects in the treatment of ulcer disease. *Medical Anthropology Quarterly, 14*(4), 13-15.

Mogelonsky, M. (1998, January). Food on demand. *American Demographics*, 57-60.

Moore, M. J. (1987). The human life span. In P. Silverman (Ed.), *The elderly as modern pioneers* (pp. 54-72). Bloomington: Indiana University Press.

Moos, R. H. (1964). Personality factors associated with rheumatoid arthritis: A review. *Journal of Chronic Diseases, 17*, 18-29.

Moos, R. H., & Schaefer, J. A. (1986). Life transitions and crises: A conceptual overview. In R. H. Moos (Ed.), *Coping with life crises: An integrated approach* (pp. 3-28). New York: Plenum.

Morgan, L. (1991). The multiple consequences of divorce: A decade review. In A. Booth (Ed.), *Contemporary families: Looking forward, looking back* (pp. 150-160). Minneapolis, MN: National Council on Family Relations.

Morgan, L., & Kunkel, S. (1998). *Aging: The social context.* Thousand Oaks, CA: Pine Forge Press.

Morisky, D. E., & Cabrera, D. M. (1997). Compliance with antituberculosis regimens and the role of behavioral interventions. In D. S. Gochman (Ed.), *Handbook of health behavior research* (pp. 269-284). New York: Plenum.

Mortimer, J. A. (1995). The Continuum Hypothesis of Alzheimer's disease and normal aging: The role of brain reserve. *Alzheimer's Research, 1*, 67-70.

Mosko, S., Richard, C., McKenna, J., & Drummond, S. (1996). Infant sleep architecture during bedsharing and possible implications for SIDS. *Sleep, 19*, 677-684.

Mosley, W. H., & Chen, L. C. (1984). An analytical framework for the study of child survival in developing countries. *Population and Development Review, 10*(Suppl.), 25-45.

Mosley, W. H., Jamison, D. T., & Henderson, D. A. (1990). The health sector in developing countries: Problems for the 1990s and beyond. *Annual Review of Public Health, 11*, 335-357.

Murdock, G. P. (1980). *Theories of illness: A world survey.* Pittsburgh, PA: University of Pittsburgh Press.

Murray, C. J. L., Yang, G., & Qiao, X. (1992). Adult mortality: Patterns and causes. In R. G. A. Feachem, T. Kjellstrom, M. Over, & M. A. Phillips (Eds.), *The health of adults in the developing world* (pp. 123-222). New York: Oxford University Press.

Mutaner, C., Eaton, W. W., Diala, C., Kessler, R. C., & Sorlie, P. D. (1998). Social class, assets, organizational control and the prevalence of common groups of psychiatric disorders. *Social Science and Medicine, 47,* 2043-2053.

Nadakavukaren, A. (1995). *Our global environment.* Prospect Heights, IL: Waveland.

Nair, N. K., & Smith, L. (1984). Reasons for not using contraceptives: An international comparison. *Studies in Family Planning, 15*(2), 84-92.

Nathanson, C. A. (1991). *Dangerous passage: The social control of sexuality in women's adolescence.* Philadelphia: Temple University Press.

National Abortion Federation. (1998). *Violence and disruption statistics.* Retrieved October 6, 1999, from the World Wide Web: http://www.naral.org/publications/facts/clinic.html

National Center for Health Statistics. (1997). *Preventing teenage pregnancy.* Retrieved January 26, 1999, from the World Wide Web: http://www.cdc.gov/nchswww/about/major/natality/teenpreg.htm

National Center for Health Statistics. (1998). *Preventing teenage pregnancy.* Retrieved February 28, 2000, from the World Wide Web: http://www.cdc.gov/nchswww/about/major/natality/teenpreg.htm

National Center for Health Statistics. (1999). *Teen birth rate down in all states.* Retrieved October 16, 1999, from the World Wide Web: http://www.cdc.gov/nchswww/releases/99news/99news/97natal.htm

National Committee for Injury Prevention and Control. (1989). *Injury prevention: Meeting the challenge.* New York: Oxford University Press.

National Institute on Aging. (1998). *Progress report on Alzheimer's disease* (NIH Pub. No. 99-3616). Washington, DC: U.S. Department of Health and Human Services, Public Health Service, National Institutes of Health.

Neese, R. M., & Williams, G. (1996). *Why we get sick: The new science of Darwinian medicine.* New York: Vintage.

Nestle, M., Wing, R., Birch, L., Disogra, L., Drwnowski, A., Middleton, S., Sigman-Grant, M., Sobal, J., Winston, M., & Economos, C. (1998). Behavioral and social influences on food choice. *Nutrition Reviews, 56*(5), S50-S74.

Nolen-Hoeksema, S. (1987). Sex differences in unipolar depression: Evidence and theory. *Psychological Bulletin, 101,* 259-282.

Notestein, F. (1983). On population growth and economic development. *Population and Development Review, 9,* 345-360.

Nuckolls, K., Cassel, J., & Kaplan, B. (1972). Psychosocial assets, life crisis and the prognosis of pregnancy. *American Journal of Epidemiology, 95,* 431-441.

Oaks, S. C., Jr., Mitchell, V. S., Pearson, G. W., & Carpenter, C. C. J. (Eds.). (1991). *Malaria: Obstacles and opportunities.* Washington, DC: National Academy Press.

Ogden, L., Shepherd, M., & Smith, W. A. (1996). *The Prevention Marketing Initiative (PMI): Applying prevention marketing.* Washington, DC: Academy for Educational Development for the Centers for Disease Control and Prevention.

Olds, D. L., Kitzman, H., Cole, R., & Robinson, J. (1997). Theoretical foundations of a program of home visitation for pregnant women and parents of young children. *Journal of Community Psychology, 25,* 9-25.

Olds, D. L., Pettitt, L. M., Robinson, J., Henderson, C., Eckenrode, J., Kitzman, H., Cole, B., & Powers, J. (1998). Reducing risks for antisocial behavior with a program of prenatal and early childhood home visitation. *Journal of Community Psychology, 26,* 65-84.

Omran, A. R. (1983). The Epidemiologic Transition Theory: A preliminary update. *Journal of Tropical Pediatrics, 29,* 305-316.

Orenstein, D., Nelson, C., Speers, M., Brownstein, J. N., & Ramsey, D. C. (1992). Synthesis of the four PATCH evaluations. *Journal of Health Education, 23*(3), 187-192.

Orenstein, W. A., Atkinson, W., Mason, D., & Bernier, R. H. (1990). Barriers to vaccinating preschool children. *Journal of Health Care for the Poor and Underserved, 1,* 315-330.

Ortega, S. T., & Rushing, W. A. (1983). Interpretation of the relationship between socioeconomic status and mental disorder: A question of the measure of mental disorder and a question of the measure of SES. *Research in Community and Mental Health, 3,* 141-161.

Ory, M., & Schulz, R. (1996). Resources for Enhancing Alzheimer's Caregiving in Health (REACH). *The Gerontologist, 36,* 100-101.

Oshansky, S. J., & Rudberg, M. A. (1997). Postponing disability: Identifying points of decline and potential intervention. In T. Hickey, M. A. Speers, & T. R. Prochaska (Eds.), *Public health and aging* (pp. 237-251). Baltimore: Johns Hopkins University Press.

Paige, D. M., Augustyn, M., Adih, W. K., Witter, F., & Chang, J. (1998). Bacterial vaginosis and preterm birth: A comprehensive review of the literature. *Journal of Nurse-Midwifery, 43*(2), 83-89.

Palinkas, L. A., Downs, M. A., Petterson, J. S., & Russel, J. (1993). Social, cultural, and psychological impacts of the Exxon Valdez oil spill. *Human Organization, 52,* 1-13.

Parcel, T. L., & Menaghan, E. G. (1994). Early parental work, family social capital, and early childhood outcomes. *American Journal of Sociology, 99,* 972-1009.

Parsons, T. (1951). *The social system.* New York: Free Press.

Patrick, D. L., & Wickizer, T. M. (1995). Community and health. In B. Amick, S. Levine, A. R. Tarlov, & D. Chapman (Eds.), *Society and health* (pp. 64-92). New York: Oxford University Press.

Paul, B. D. (1955). *Health culture and community: Case studies of public reactions to health programs.* New York: Russell Sage Foundation.

Pavlov, I. P. (1927). *Conditioned reflexes* (G. V. Anrep, Trans.). New York: Oxford University Press.

Payer, L. (1988). *Medicine and culture.* New York: Penguin.

Pearlin, L. I., & Aneshensel, C. S. (1987). Coping and social supports: Their functions and applications. In L. Aiken & D. Mechanic (Eds.), *Applications of social science to clinical medicine and health policy* (pp. 417-437). New Brunswick: Rutgers University Press.

Pelto, G. H., & Vargas, L. A. (1992). Introduction: Dietary change and nutrition. *Ecology of Food and Nutrition, 27,* 159-161.

Pelto, P. J., Bentley, M. E., & Pelto, G. H. (1990). Applied anthropological research methods: Diarrhea studies as an example. In J. Coreil & J. D. Mull (Eds.), *Anthropology and primary health care* (pp. 253-277). Boulder, CO: Westview.

Pescosolido, B. A. (1992). Beyond rational choice: The social dynamics of how people seek help. *American Journal of Sociology, 97,* 1096-1138.

Petersen, A., & Lupton, D. (1996). *The new public health: Health and self in the age of risk.* Thousand Oaks, CA: Sage.

Pfuhl, E. H., & Henry, S. (1993). *The deviance process* (3rd. ed.). Chicago: Aldine.

Phillips, D. R. (1991). Problems and potential of researching epidemiological transition: Examples from Southeast Asia. *Social Science and Medicine, 33,* 395-404.

Phillips, M., Feachem, R. G. A., Murray, C. J. L., Over, M., & Kjellstrom, T. (1993). Adult health: A legitimate concern for developing countries. *American Journal of Public Health, 83,* 1527-1530.

Pilisuk, M., McCallister, J., & Rothman, J. (1996). Coming together for action: The challenge of contemporary grassroots community organizing. *Journal of Social Issues, 52,* 15-37.

Pillai, V. K., & Shannon, L. W. (1995). Introduction: Definition and distribution of developing areas. In V. K. Pillai & L. W. Shannon (Eds.), *Developing areas: A book of readings and research* (pp. 1-13). Oxford, UK: Berg.

Pillsbury, B. (1990). *Immunization: The behavioral issues.* Washington, DC: Agency for International Development.

Pillsbury, B., & Brownlee, A. (1989). *Household and community beliefs and practices that influence maternal health and nutrition.* Washington, DC: International Center for Research on Women.

Piper, S. (1997). The limitations of well men clinics for health education. *Nursing Standard 11*(30), 47-49.

Plough, A., & Olafson, F. (1994). Implementing the Boston Healthy Start Initiative: A case study of community empowerment and public health. *Health Education Quarterly, 21,* 221-234.

Polednak, A. (1989). *Racial and ethnic differences in disease.* New York: Oxford University Press.

Polgar, S. (1964). Evolution and the ills of mankind. In S. Tax (Ed.), *Horizons of anthropology* (pp. 200-211). Chicago: Aldine.

Polgar, S., & Marshall, J. F. (1978). The search for culturally acceptable fertility regulating methods. In M. H. Logan & E. E. Hunt (Eds.), *Health and the human condition* (pp. 328-340). New York: Duxbury.

Pollak, R. A., & Watkins, S. C. (1993). Cultural and economic approaches to fertility: Proper marriage or misalliance? *Population and Development Review, 19,* 467-496.

Popkin, B. M. (1994). The nutrition transition in low-income countries: An emerging crisis. *Nutrition Reviews, 52*(9), 285-298.

Population summit of the world's scientific academies. (1994). Washington, DC: National Academy Press.

Porterfield, H. A. (1997). Perspectives on prostate cancer treatment: Awareness, attitudes and relationships. *Urology, 49*(Suppl. 3A), 102-103.

Powell, T. J. (1994). *Understanding the self-help organization: Frameworks and findings.* Thousand Oaks, CA: Sage.

President's Commission on Mental Health. (1978). *Report to the President* (Stock No. 040-000-00390-8, Vol. I). Washington, DC: Government Printing Office.

Prince, R. (1997). Diet and the prevention of osteoporotic fractures. *New England Journal of Medicine, 337,* 701.

Prochaska, J. O. (1989). With science and service we can survive and thrive. In S. Soldz & L. McCullough (Eds.), *Reconciling empirical knowledge and clinical experience: The art and science of psychotherapy* (pp. 241-252). Washington, DC: American Psychological Association.

Prochaska, J. O., & DiClemente, C. C. (1986). Toward a comprehensive model of change. In W. R. Miller & N. Heather (Eds.), *Treating addictive behaviors: Process of change. Applied clinical psychology* (pp. 3-27). New York: Plenum.

Prochaska, J. O., & DiClemente, C. C. (1992). Stages of change in the modification of problem behaviors. *Progress in Behavior Modification, 28,* 183-218.

Prochaska, J. O., Redding, C. A., & Evers, K. E. (Eds.). (1997). *The Transtheoretical Model and stages of change* (2nd ed.). San Francisco: Jossey-Bass.

Prochaska, J. O., & Velicer, T. (1997). The Transtheoretical Model of Health Behavior Change. *American Journal of Health Promotion, 12,* 38-48.

Prochaska, J., Velicer, T., Rossis, J., Goldstein, M., Marcus, B., Rakowski, W., Fiore, C., Harlow, L., Redding, C., Rosenbloom, D., & Rossi, S. (1992). Stages of change and decisional balance for 12 problem behaviors. *Health Psychology, 13,* 39-46.

Profet, M. (1991). The function of allergy: Immunological defense against toxins. *Quarterly Review of Biology, 66,* 23-62.

Prokop, C. K., Bradley, L. A., Burish, T. G., Anderson, F. O., & Fox, J. E. (1991). *Health psychology: Clinical methods and research.* New York: Macmillan.

Radley, A. (1994). *The social psychology of health and disease.* Thousand Oaks, CA: Sage.

Rangun, V. K., & Karim, S. (1991). *Teaching note: Focusing the concept of social marketing.* Cambridge, MA: Harvard Business School Press.

Raspa, R. (1984). Exotic foods among Italian-Americans in Mormon Utah: Food as nostalgic enactment of identity. In L. K. Brown & K. Mussel (Eds.), *Ethnic and regional foodways in the United States* (pp. 185-194). Knoxville: University of Tennessee Press.

Rees, C., & Jones, M. (1995). Exploring men's health in a men-only group. *Nursing Standard, 9*(43), 38-40.

Reese, F. L., & Smith, W. R. (1997). Psychosocial determinants of health care utilization in sickle cell disease patients. *Annals of Behavioral Medicine, 19,* 171-178.

Reiss, A. J., & Roth, J. A. (1993). *Understanding and preventing violence.* Washington, DC: National Academy Press.

Rentoul, L., & Appleboom, N. (1997). Understanding the psychological impact of rape and serious sexual assault of men: A literature review. *Journal of Psychiatric and Mental Health Nursing, 4,* 267-274.

Reynolds-Scanlon, S., Reynolds, S. L., Peek, M. K., Polivka, L., & Peek, C. (1999). *Profile of older Floridians.* Tampa, FL: State Department of Elder Affairs, The Florida Policy Exchange Center on Aging, University of South Florida.

Rhodes, L. A. (1996). Studying biomedicine as a cultural system. In C. F. Sargent & T. M. Johnson (Eds.), *Handbook of medical anthropology* (pp. 165-180). Westport, CT: Greenwood.

Riessman, F., & Carroll, D. (1995). *Redefining self-help: Policy and practice.* San Francisco: Jossey-Bass.

Rise, J., Astrom, A. N., & Sutton, S. (1998). Predicting intentions and use of dental floss among adolescents: An application of the theory of planned behavior. *Psychology and Health, 13,* 223-236.

Robert, S. (1998). Community-level socioeconomic status effects on adult health. *Journal of Health and Social Behavior, 19,* 18-37.

Robertson, A., & Minkler, M. (1994). New health promotion movement: A critical examination. *Health Education Quarterly, 21,* 295-312.

Robertson, S. (1995). Men's health promotion in the U.K.: A hidden problem. *British Journal of Nursing, 4,* 382-401.

Robey, B., Rutstein, S. O., Morris, L., & Blackburn, R. (1992). The reproductive revolution: New survey findings. *Population Reports,* 1-43.

Robins, L. N., & Regier, D. A. (Eds.). (1991). *Psychiatric disorders in America: The Epidemiologic Catchment Area Study.* New York: Free Press.

Rodin, J., & Ickovics, J. R. (1990). Women's health: Review and research agenda as we approach the 21st century. *American Psychologist, 45,* 1018-1034.

Rogers, E. M. (1995). *Diffusion of innovations* (4th ed.). New York: Free Press.

Romanucci-Ross, L. (1969). The hierarchy of resort in curative practices: The Admiralty Islands, Melanesia. *Journal of Health and Social Behavior, 10,* 201-209.

Rook, K. (1992). Detrimental aspects of social relationships: Taking stock of an emerging literature. In H. O. F. Veiel & U. Baumann (Eds.), *The meaning and measurement of social support* (pp. 157-169). Washington, DC: Hemisphere.

Rose, M. (1995). Effects of an AIDS education program for older adults. *Journal of Community Health Nursing, 13*(3), 141-148.

Rosen, G. (1993). *A history of public health.* Baltimore: Johns Hopkins University Press.

Rosenfeld, J. A. (1992). Maternal work outside the home and its effect on women and their families. *Journal of the American Medical Women's Association, 47*(2), 47-53.

Rosenfield, S. (1982). Sex roles and societal reactions to mental illness: The labeling of "deviant" deviance. *Journal of Health and Social Behavior, 23,* 18-24.

Rosenstock, I. M. (1974). Historical origins of the health belief model. *Health Education Monographs, 2,* 328-335.

Ross, E. (1987). An overview of trends in dietary variation from hunter-gatherer to modern capitalist societies. In M. Harris & E. Ross (Eds.), *Food and evolution: Toward a theory of human food habits* (pp. 7-56). Philadelphia: Temple University Press.

Rothman, J., & Tropman, J. E. (1987). Models of community organizing and macro practice: Their mixing and phasing. In F. M. Cox, J. L. Erlich, J. Rothman, & J. E. Tropman (Eds.), *Strategies of community organization* (4th ed., pp. 25-45). Itasca, IL: F. E. Peacock.

Rothschild, M. (1997). A historic perspective of social marketing. *Journal of Health Communication, 2,* 308-309.

Rothschild, M. (1999). Carrots, sticks and promises: A conceptual framework for the management of public health and social issue behaviors. *Journal of Marketing, 63,* 4-24.

Rowe, J., & Kahn, R. (1998). *Successful aging.* New York: Pantheon.

Royston, E., & Ferguson, J. (1985). The coverage of maternity care: A critical review of available information. *World Health Statistics Quarterly, 38,* 267-273.

Rozin, P. (1982). Human food selection: The interaction of biology, culture and individual experience. In L. M. Barker (Ed.), *The psychobiology of human food selection* (pp. 189-203). Westport, CT: AVI.

Rozin, P. (1996). Sociocultural influences on human food selection. In E. D. Capaldi (Ed.), *Why we eat what we eat: The psychology of eating* (pp. 233-265). Washington, DC: American Psychological Association.

Rubel, A. J., & Garro, L. C. (1992). Social and cultural factors in the successful control of tuberculosis. *Public Health Reports, 197,* 262-238.

Rush, D., Alvir, J. M., Kenney, D. A., Johnson, S. S., & Horvitz, D. G. (1988). Historical study of pregnancy outcomes. *American Journal of Clinical Nutrition, 48,* 412-425.

Rush, D., Leighton, J., Sloan, N. L., Alvir, J. M., Horvitz, D. G., Seaver, W. B., Garbowski, G. C., Johnson, S. S., Kulka, R. A., Holt, M., Lynch, J. T., Virag, T. G., Woodside, M. B., & Schanklin, D. S. (1988). Study of infants and children. *American Journal of Clinical Nutrition, 48,* 484-511.

Rushing, W. A. (1995). *The AIDS epidemic: Social dimensions of an infectious disease.* Boulder, CO: Westview.

Rushing, W. A., & Ortega, S. T. (1979). Socioeconomic status and mental disorder: New evidence and a sociomedical formulation. *American Journal of Sociology, 84,* 1175-1200.

Rutter, M. (1985). Resilience in the face of adversity: Protective factors and resistance to psychiatric disorders. *British Journal of Psychiatry, 147,* 598-611.

Sabo, D., & Gordon, D. F. (Eds.). (1995). *Men's health and illness: Gender, power and the body.* Thousand Oaks, CA: Sage.

Sainz, S., & Saito, M. (1997). *Hispanic involvement in motor vehicle accidents* (Transportation Research Record 1560) . Washington, DC: Transportation Research Board.

Schafe, G. E. & Bernstein, I. L. (1996). Taste aversion learning. In Capaldi, E. D. (Ed.), *Why we eat what we eat: The psychology of eating.* (pp. 31-52). Washington, DC: American Psychology Association.

Schafer, J., Caetano, R., & Clark, C. L. (1998). Rates of intimate partner violence in the United States. *American Journal of Public Health, 88,* 1702-1704.

Schlegel, A., & Barry, H. B., III. (1991). *Adolescence: An anthropological inquiry.* New York: Free Press.

Schoenfeld, D., Malmrose, L., Blazer, D., Gold, D., & Seeman, T. (1994). Self-rated health and mortality in the high functioning elderly. A closer look at healthy individuals: MacArthur field study of successful aging. *Journal of Gerontology, 49,* M109-115.

Schopper, D., Doussantousse, S., & Orav, J. (1993). Sexual behaviors relevant to HIV transmission in rural African populations: How much can a KAP survey tell us? *Social Science and Medicine, 37,* 401-412.

Schulz, A. J., Parker, E. A., Israel, B. A., Becker, A. B., Maciak, B. J., & Hollis, R. (1999). Conducting a participatory community-based prevention: Programs that work. In R. C. Brownson, E. A. Baker, & L. F. Novick (Eds.), *Community-based prevention: Programs that work* (pp. 84-105). Gaithersburg, MD: Aspen.

Schwartz, N. E., & Borra, S. T. (1997). What do consumers really think about dietary fat? *Journal of the American Dietetic Association, 97*(Suppl.), S73-S75.

Sclar, D. A. (1991). Improving medication compliance: A review of selected issues. *Clinical Therapeutics, 13,* 436-440.

Segall, A. (1997). Sick role concepts and health behavior. In D. S. Gochman (Ed.), *Handbook of health behavior research* (Vol. 1, pp. 289-301). New York: Plenum.

Segerstrom, S. C., Taylor, S. E., Kemeny, M. E., & Fahey, J. L. (1998). Optimism is associated with mood, coping, and immune change in response to stress. *Journal of Personality and Social Psychology, 74,* 1646-1655.

Sekhon, S. (1996). Insights into South Asian culture: Food and nutrition values. *Topics in Clinical Nutrition, 11*(4), 47-56.

Selye, H. (1956). *The stress of life.* New York: McGraw-Hill.

Shedler, J., & Block, J. (1990). Adolescent drug use and psychological health: A longitudinal inquiry. *American Psychologist, 45,* 612-630.

Sherris, J. D., Blackburn, R., Moore, S. H., & Mehta, S. (1986). Immunizing the world's children. *Population Reports: Issues in World Health, Series L*(5), 1-44.

Siddique, C. M., & D'Arcy, C. (1985). Marital status and psychological well-being: A cross-national comparative analysis. *International Journal of Comparative Sociology, 26,* 129-166.

Sidell, M. (1995). *Health in old age.* Philadelphia: Open University Press.

Siegel, M., & Donner, L. (1998). *Marketing public health.* Gaithersburg, MD: Aspen.

Sigman-Grant, M. (1997). Can you have your low-fat cake and eat it too? The role of fat-modified products. *Journal of the American Dietetic Association, 97*(Suppl.), S76-S81.

Skegg, D., Corwin, P., Paul, C., & Doll, R. (1982). Importance of the male factor in cancer of the cervix. *Lancet, 2,* 581-583.

Skinner, B. F. (1953). *Science and human behavior.* New York: Macmillan.

Slaninka, S. C. (1992). Support groups help cancer patients reduce stress; enhance healing. *Practical Nursing, 42*(4), 6-11.

Smedley, A. (1998). "Race" and the construction of human identity. *American Anthropologist, 100,* 690-702.

Smith, G. S., & Barss, P. (1991). Unintentional injuries in developing countries: The epidemiology of a neglected problem. *Epidemiologic Reviews, 13,* 228-266.

Smith, W. A., Helquist, M. J., Jimerson, A. B., Carovano, K., & Middlestadt, S. E. (Eds.). (1993). *A world against AIDS: Communication for behavior change.* Washington, DC: Academy for Educational Development.

Smith, W. A., & Middlestadt, S. E. (1993). The applied behavior change framework. In W. A. Smith, M. J. Helquist, A. B. Jimerson, K. Carovano, & S. E. Middlestadt (Eds.), *A world against AIDS: Communication for behavior change* (pp. 1-38). Washington, DC: Academy for Educational Development.

Smolin, L. A., & Grosvenor, M. B. (1997). *Nutrition: Science and applications* (2nd ed.). Philadelphia: Saunders.

Somers, A. (1995). W(h)ither public health? *Public Health Reports, 110,* 657-661.

Srole, L., Langner, T. S., Michael, S. T., Opler, M. K. & Rennie, T. A. L. (1962). *Mental health in the metropolis: The Midtown Manhattan Study.* New York: McGraw-Hill.

Standing, H. (1993). AIDS: Conceptual and methodological issues in researching sexual behaviour in Sub-Saharan Africa. *Social Science and Medicine, 34,* 475-483.

Staples, R. (1995). *Health among African American males.* Thousand Oaks, CA: Sage.

Stebbins, K. R. (1990). Transnational tobacco companies and health in underdeveloped countries: Recommendations for avoiding a smoking epidemic. *Social Science and Medicine, 30,* 227-235.

Stein, H. (1982). The annual cycle and the cultural nexus of health care behavior among Oklahoma wheat farming families. *Culture, Medicine, and Psychiatry, 6,* 81-99.

Stein, H. F. (1990). *American medicine as culture.* Boulder, CO: Westview.

Stewart, A. L., & Hays, R. D. (1997). Conceptual, measurement, and analytical issues in assessing health status in older populations. In T. Hickey, M. A. Speers, & T. R. Prochaska (Eds.), *Public health and aging* (pp. 174-176). Baltimore: Johns Hopkins University Press.

Stuart-Macadam, P., & Dettwyler, K. A. (Eds.). (1995). *Breastfeeding: Biocultural perspectives.* Chicago: Aldine.

Suchman, E. (1965). Stages of illness and medical care. *Journal of Health and Human Behavior, 6,* 114-128.

Sukkary-Stolba, S. (1990). *Oral rehydration therapy: The behavioral issues.* Washington, DC: U.S. Agency for International Development.

Svarstad, B. (1987). Physician-patient communication and patient conformity with medical advice. In L. H. Aiken & D. Mechanic (Eds.), *Applications of social science to clinical medicine and health policy* (pp. 438-459). New Brunswick, NJ: Rutgers University Press.

Sweet, J. A., Bumpass, L. L. & Call, V. R. A. (1988). *The design and content of the National Survey of Families and Households* (NSFH Working Paper No. 1). Madison: University of Wisconsin.

Syme, L. S. (1986). The social environment and disease prevention. *Advances in Health Education and Promotion, 1,* 237-265.

Takeuchi, D. T., & Speechley, K. N. (1989). Ethnic differences in the marital status and psychological distress relationship. *Social Psychiatry and Psychiatric Epidemiology, 24,* 288-294.

Taplin, S., & Montano, D. (1991). A test of an expanded theory of reasoned action to predict mammography participation. *Social Science and Medicine, 32,* 733-741.

Taylor, S. E., & Armor, D. A. (1996). Positive illusions and coping with adversity. *Journal of Personality, 64,* 873-898.

Templeton, A. (1998). Human races: A genetic and evolutionary perspective. *American Anthropologist, 100,* 632-650.

Than, T. T., Delay, E. R., & Maier, M. E. (1994). Sucrose threshold variation during the menstrual cycle. *Physiology and Behavior, 56,* 237-239.

Thoits, P. A. (1995). Stress, coping, and social support processes: Where are we? What next? *Journal of Health and Social Behavior, Extra Issue,* 53-79.

Timyan, J., Brechin, S. J. G., Measham, D. M., & Ogunleye, B. (1993). Access to care: More than a problem of distance. In M. Koblinsky, J. Timyan, & J. Gay (Eds.), *The health of women: A global perspective* (pp. 217-234). Boulder, CO: Westview.

Townsend, P. (1979). *Poverty in the United Kingdom.* New York: Penguin.

Trevathan, W. R., & McKenna, J. J. (1994). Evolutionary environments of human birth and infancy: Insights to apply to contemporary life. *Children's Environments, 11*(2), 88-104.

Trevathan, W. R., Smith, E., & James, J. M. (Eds.). (1999). *Evolutionary medicine.* New York: Oxford University Press.

Trostle, J. A. (1997). The history and meaning of patient compliance as an ideology. In D. S. Gochman (Ed.), *Handbook of health behavior research* (Vol. 2, pp. 109-124). New York: Plenum.

Tucker, J. S., Friedman, H. S., Wingard, D. L., & Schwartz, J. E. (1996). Marital history at midlife as a predictor of longevity: Alternative explanations to the protective effect. *Health Psychology, 15,* 94-105.

Turner, R. J., & Lloyd, D. A. (1995). Lifetime traumas and mental health: The significance of cumulative adversity. *Journal of Health and Social Behavior, 36,* 360-376.

Turner, R. J., Wheaton, B., & Lloyd, D. S. (1995). The epidemiology of social stress. *American Sociological Review, 60,* 104-125.

Turshen, M. (1989). *The politics of public health.* New Brunswick, NJ: Rutgers University Press.

U.N. Development Program. (1999). *World population trends.* Retrieved September 30, 1999, from the World Wide Web: http://www.undp.org/popin/wtrends/gubhaju/table8.htm

UNICEF. (1999). *The state of the world's children.* New York: Author.

U.S. Administration on Aging. (1994). *Old age in the 21st century: A report to the Assistant Secretary for Aging, U.S. Department of Health and Human Services, regarding his responsibilities in planning for the aging of the baby boom.* Syracuse, NY: National Academy on Aging, Maxwell School of Citizenship and Public Affairs, Syracuse University.

U.S. Bureau of Alcohol, Tobacco, and Firearms. (1999). *Abortion clinic violence 1982-1998.* Washington, DC: U.S. Department of the Treasury. Retrieved October 6, 1999, from the World Wide Web: http://www.atf.treas.gov/core/explarson/information/cibarbl.jpg

U.S. Census Bureau. (1996). *Statistical abstract of the United States.* (116th ed.). Washington, DC: Government Printing Office.

U.S. Department of Health and Human Services. (1995a). *Planned approach to community health: Guide for the local coordinator.* Atlanta, GA: U.S. Department of Health and Human Services, Centers for Disease Control and Prevention, National Center for Chronic Disease Prevention and Health Promotion.

U.S. Department of Health and Human Services. (1995b). *Report to Congress on out-of-wedlock childbearing* (DHHS Pub. No. PHS 95-1257). Hyattsville, MD: Author.

U.S. Department of Health and Human Services. (1996). *Physical activity and health: A report of the Surgeon General* Atlanta, GA: Author.

U.S. Department of Health and Human Services. (1997). *Teen birth rate down in all states: Drives U.S. birth rate to record low* [DHHS news release]. Retrieved April 29, 1999, from the World Wide Web: http://www.cdc.gov/nchswww/releases/99news/99news/97natal.htm

U.S. Department of Health and Human Services. (1999a). *Health, United States, 1999.* Washington, DC: National Center for Health Statistics.

U.S. Department of Health and Human Services. (1999b, December 3, 1999). *Healthy people 2010.* Retrieved December 15, 1999, from the World Wide Web: http://web.health.gov/healthypeople/

U.S. Department of Health and Human Services. (1999c). *The Initiative to Eliminate Racial and Ethnic Disparities in Health.* National Vital Statistics System, Linked Birth and Infant Death Set. Retrieved January 31, 2000, from the World Wide Web: http://raceasndhealth.hhs.gov/

Valente, T. W., & Rogers, E. M. (1995). The origins and development of the Diffusion of Innovations Paradigm as an example of scientific growth. *Science Communication, 16,* 238-269.

Veblen, T. (1925). *The theory of the leisure class and travel in contemporary societies.* New York: Vanguard.

Ventura, S. J., Martin, J. A., Curtin, S. C., & Mathews, T. J. (1997). *Births: Final data for 1997, National Vital Statistics Report* (Table 2). Washington, DC: U.S. Department of Health and Human Services.

Verbrugge, L. M. (1989). The twain meet: Empirical explanations of sex differences in health and mortality. *Journal of Health and Social Behavior, 30,* 282-304.

von Mering, O. (1996). American culture and long-term care. In R. H. Binstock, L. E. Cluff, & O. von Mering (Eds.), *The future of long-term care: Social and policy issues* (pp. 261-264). Baltimore: John Hopkins University Press.

Wadsworth, M. E. J. (1986). *Serious illness in childhood and its association with later-life achievement.* London: Tavistock.

Waldron, I. (1995). Contributions of changing gender differences in behavior and social roles to changing gender differences in mortality. In D. Sabo & D. F. Gordon (Eds.),

Men's health and illness: Gender, power and the body (pp. 22-45). Thousand Oaks, CA: Sage.

Waldron, I. (1997). Changing gender roles and gender differences in health behavior. In D. S. Gochman (Ed.), *Handbook of health behavior research* (Vol. 1, pp. 303-328). New York: Plenum.

Walker, C. (1995, January). Meet the new vegetarian. *American Demographics*, 9-10.

Wallace, A. F. C. (1970). *Culture and personality* (2nd ed.). New York: Random House.

Wallace, R. (1997). Variability in disease manifestations in older adults: Implications for public and community health programs. In Hickey, T., Speers, M., & Prohaska, T. (Eds.), *Public health and aging* (pp. 75-86.) Baltimore: Johns Hopkins University Press.

Walsh, J., & Warren, K. S. (1979). Selective primary health care: An interim strategy for disease control in developing countries. *New England Journal of Medicine, 301*, 967-974.

Wambach, K. (1997). Breastfeeding intentions and outcome: A test of the Theory of Planned Behavior. *Research in Nursing and Health, 20*, 51-59.

Warde, A. (1997). *Consumption, food and taste: Culinary antinomies and commodity culture.* Thousand Oaks, CA: Sage.

Wardwell, W. I. (1994). Alternative medicine in the United States. *Social Science and Medicine, 38*, 1061-1068.

Warner, L. A., Kessler, R. C., Hughes, M., Anthony, J. C., & Nelson, C. B. (1995). Prevalence and correlates of drug use and dependence in the United States: Results from the National Comorbidity Survey. *Archives of General Psychiatry, 52*, 219-229.

Warrell, D. A. (1997). Herbal remedies for malaria. *Tropical Doctor, 27*(Suppl. 1), 5-6.

Waxler, N. E. (1981). The social labeling perspective on illness and medical practice. In L. Eisenberg & A. Kleinman (Eds.), *The relevance of social science for medicine* (pp. 283-306). Dordrecht, The Netherlands: Reidel.

Weich, S., & Lewis, G. (1998). Poverty, unemployment, and common mental disorders: Population based cohort study. *British Medical Journal, 317*, 115-119.

Weidman, H. H. (1988). A transcultural perspective on health behavior. In D. S. Gochman (Ed.), *Health behavior: Emerging research perspectives* (pp. 261-280). New York: Plenum.

Weiner, B. (1980). A cognitive (attribution) emotion–action model of motivated behavior: An analysis of judgements of help-giving. *Journal of Personality and Social Psychology, 39*, 186-200.

Weiner, H. (1977). *Psychobiology and human disease.* New York: Elsevier.

Weller, S. C., Patcher, L. M., Trotter, R. T., II, & Baer, R. D. (1993). *Empacho* in four Latino groups: A study of intra- and inter-cultural variation in beliefs. *Medical Anthropology, 15*, 109-136.

Weller, S. C., Ruebush, T. R., & Klein, R. E. (1997). Predicting treatment-seeking behavior in Guatemala: A comparison of the health services research and decision-theoretic approaches. *Medical Anthropology Quarterly, 11*(2), 224-245.

Wellner, A. S. (1998, March). Eat, drink and be healed. *American Demographics*, 55-59.

Wennemo, I. (1993). Infant mortality, public policy and inequality—A comparison of 18 industrialized countries 1950-85. *Sociology of Health and Illness, 15*, 429-446.

West, P. (1991). Rethinking the health selection explanation for health inequalities. *Social Sciences and Medicine, 32*, 373-384.

West Central Florida Area Agency on Aging. (1990). *Florida: Highest proportion of elders in the nation.* Tampa, FL: Author.

Weston, J. (1997, October). Striving for balance: Health, economics, and the natural world. *Newsletter from the Sierra Madre, 35*, 1-3.

Whiteford, L. M. (1996). Political economy, gender, and the social production of health. In C. F. Sargent & C. C. Brettell (Eds.), *Gender and health: An international perspective* (pp. 244-259). Englewood Cliffs, NJ: Prentice Hall.

Wilkinson, R. G. (1992). Income distribution and life expectancy. *British Medical Journal, 304*, 165-168.

Wilkinson, R. G. (1994). The epidemiological transition: From material scarcity to social disadvantage? *Daedalus, 123*, 61-77.

Wilkinson, R. G. (1996). *Unhealthy societies. The afflictions of inequality.* Boston: Routledge & Kegan Paul.

Wilkinson, R. G. (1998). Letter to the Editor. *Social Science and Medicine, 47*, 411-412.

Williams, C. D., Baumslag, N., & Jelliffe, D. B. (1994). *Mother and child health: Delivering the services* (3rd ed.). New York: Oxford University Press.

Williams, D. R., Takeuchi, D. T., & Adair, R. K. (1992). Marital status and psychiatric disorders among blacks and whites. *Journal of Health and Social Behavior, 33*, 140-157.

Williams, F. T., & Temkin-Greener, H. (1996). Older people, dependency, and trends in supportive care. In R. H. Binstock, L. E. Cluff, & O. von Mering (Eds.), *The future of long-term care: Social and policy issues* (pp. 51-57). Baltimore: Johns Hopkins University Press.

Williamson, P. (1995). Men's health: Their own worst enemies. *Nursing Times, 91*(48), 24-26.

Wilson, L. (1990). The historical decline of tuberculosis in Europe and America: Its cause and significance. *Journal of the History of Medicine and Allied Sciences, 45*, 366-396.

Wittchen, H.-U., Zhao, S., Kessler, R. C., & Eaton, W. W. (1994). DSM-III-R Generalized Anxiety Disorder in the National Comorbidity Survey. *Archives of General Psychiatry, 51*, 355-364.

Wolinsky, F. D. (1988). *The sociology of health: Principles, practitioners and issues* (2nd ed.). Belmont, CA: Wadsworth.

World Bank. (1993). *Investing in health.* New York: Oxford University Press.

World Health Organization. (1981). *Contemporary patterns of breastfeeding: Report on the WHO collaborative study on breastfeeding.* Geneva, Switzerland: Author.

World Health Organization. (1992). *International classification of diseases and related health problems* (10th revision). Geneva: Author.

World Health Organization. (1995). *How research findings have improved diarrhea case management guidelines.* Geneva, Switzerland: Author.

World Health Organization. (1998). *Global tuberculosis control.* Geneva, Switzerland: Author.

Worthington-Roberts, B., & Williams, S. R. (1989). *Nutrition in pregnancy and lactation* (5th ed.). St. Louis, MO: C. V. Mosby.

Yach, D. (1992). The use and value of qualitative methods in health research in developing countries. *Social Science and Medicine, 35,* 603-612.

Young, J. C. (1981). *Medical choice in a Mexican village.* New Brunswick, NJ: Rutgers University Press.

Zimicki, S. (1993). Understanding the diarrhea problem in the Philippines: Research as a basis for message design. In R. E. Seidel (Ed.), *Notes from the field in communication for child survival* (pp. 7-16). Washington DC: Academy for Educational Development.

Zuckerman, M. (1989). *Biological basis of sensation seeking, impulsivity, and anxiety.* Hillsdale, NJ: Lawrence Erlbaum.

Index

incidence, 47
prevalence, 47
Distal determinants. *See* Causality continuum
Dix, D., 286
Durkheim, E., 112

Ecological models:
developing country research, 240-241
See also Social ecology paradigm; Social ecology of health model
Efficiency:
cult of, 177
Elderly, abuse of. *See* Family violence
multiple pathologies, 307
nutrition, 270
polypharmacy, 307
Emic, 167-168
Empowerment, 192
Enabling factors. *See* Precede model
Epidemiologic paradox, 65-66
Epidemiologic transition, 27
Epidemiologic polarization, 28
health problems (table), 27
Epidemiology, 47
Equilibrium. *See* Theories of disease, metamodels
Ethnic groups:
aging, 304
African Americans, 66-68
Choctaws, 311-313
crossover effect, 53
dietary practices, 272-273
Hispanics, 65-66
identity, 140
selective survival, 56
Ethnicity, 138-140
categorical model, 139
situational, 139
transactional model, 140
Ethnocentrism, 167
Etic, 167-168
Ethnomedicine, 168
Evolutionary medicine, 32-34

Darwinian medicine, 32
Explanatory model of illness, 171, 184
of dementia, 311-313
See also Illness episode
Exxon Valdez oil spill, 7-8

Faith, 172
Family planning:
developing countries, 247-248
Family resource models:
and health care utilization, 93-94
Family systems:
and health, 123-125
Family violence, 162-166
Fertility, 18
cross-national trends in adolescent fertility, 24 (table)
age-adjusted fertility rate, 18
total fertility, 18
Folk flu, 184-186
Food:
and ethnicity, 272-273
and social ties, 273-275
availability, 261-163
symbol of prestige, 271-272
Foraging groups, 30-32, 36
!Kung Bushmen, 31
Four Ps. *See* Social marketing

Gender:
and food, 264-265
and health, 104-112
anthropological perspective, 105
biological perspective, 104
culture, 109
epidemiologic perspective, 104
gap, 106
men's health, 110-112
sociological perspective, 105
General adaptation syndrome, 113
General theory of help-seeking, 91-92
Generational inversion, 165
Geophagia, 268-270
Geriatric patient, 306-308

About the Authors

Jeannine Coreil, Ph.D., is Professor in the Department of Community and Family Health at the University of South Florida (USF). She has a background in medical anthropology and sociomedical sciences. Her research interests include maternal and child health, international health, comparative health cultures, and qualitative methods. She has published an edited volume, *Anthropology and Primary Health Care,* and numerous articles and book chapters on psychosocial aspects of health. She coordinates the academic program in social and behavioral sciences in the College of Public Health at USF.

Carol Bryant, Ph.D., is Associate Professor in the Department of Community and Family Health and is Co-Director of the Florida Prevention Research Center at the University of South Florida. She has a background in nutritional anthropology and social marketing. Her research interests include community-based social marketing and the determinants of public health service utilization. She has coauthored a textbook, *The Cultural Feast: An Introduction to Food and Society,* and numerous articles about social marketing and breastfeeding promotion. Before joining the faculty at USF, she was Deputy Commissioner for Nutrition and Health Education at the Lexington-Fayette County Health Department. She is cofounder of Best Start Social Marketing in Tampa, Florida and editor of the *Social Marketing Quarterly.*

J. Neil Henderson, Ph.D., is Associate Professor of Medical Anthropology in the Department of Community and Family Health at the University of South Florida. His research interests are aging, health, and long-term care in biocultural context.

He is editor-in-chief of the *Journal of Cross-Cultural Gerontology*. Most recently, his research has been in American Indian communities on the topic of dementing diseases. He is an enrolled, voting member of the Choctaw Nation of Oklahoma.

Melinda S. Forthofer, Ph.D., is Assistant Professor in the Department of Community and Family Health in the College of Public Health at the University of South Florida and Director of the Methods and Evaluation Unit at the Florida Prevention Research Center at the University of South Florida. She has an interdisciplinary background in sociology, family studies, and health behavior/health education. Her research interests include prevention science methodology, academic and community partnerships, community-based evaluation, mental health, and social disparities in public health. She also has been a leader in the development of technology-based curricula for public health education at USF and in the application of that experience to explore the potential of technology-based systems for community collaboration in academic and community partnerships.

Gwendolyn P. Quinn, Ph.D., is Research Assistant Professor in the Department of Community and Family Health at the University of South Florida. She is an educational psychologist and is Director of the National Training Center for Social Marketing. Her research interests include maternal and child health, personality and individual differences, social marketing, and program evaluation. She serves as a qualitative research consultant to the Lawton and Rhea Chiles Center for Healthy Mothers and Babies and to the H. L. Moffitt Cancer Research Center.